DATE DUE

The   oach

Promoting Health

The Primary Health Care Approach

2nd edition

Andrea Wass

Honorary Fellow, School of Health
University of New England

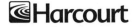

Sydney Edinburgh London New York Philadelphia St Louis Toronto

W. B. Saunders
is a Harcourt Health Sciences Company

Harcourt Australia
30–52 Smidmore Street, Marrickville, NSW 2204

Harcourt Publishers International
Harcourt Place, 32 Jamestown Road, London, NW1 7BY

Harcourt Health Sciences
1–3 Baxter's Place, Leith Walk, Edinburgh EH1 3AF

Harcourt Health Sciences, The Curtis Centre
Independence Square West
Philadelphia PA 19106–3399

Harcourt Health Sciences
11830 Westline Industrial Drive
St Louis MO 63146

This edition © 2000
by Harcourt Australia ACN 000 910 583

Reprinted 2000, 2001

First edition © 1994; reprinted 1995, 1998

National Library of Australia Cataloguing-in-Publication Data

Wass, Andrea, 1960 - .
Promoting health : the primary health care approach

   2nd ed.
   Includes bibliography.
   Includes index.
   ISBN 0 7295 3425 1.

   1. Health promotion. 2. Health promotion – Australia. 3.
   Health promotion. I. Title.

613

Publishing Services Manager: Helena Klijn
Edited and project managed by Science Desk International
Cover design by Maria Miranda
Typeset by Science Desk International
Printed in Australia by Southwood Press

CONTENTS

FOREWORD

Creating, supporting and maintaining health continues to be the most neglected area of health policy and public health practice. Despite the ever-increasing knowledge of health determinants — most of which are firmly positioned outside of the health sector — implementation strategies are more often than not focused on individual and behavioural factors. Primary Health Care and health promotion aim to address this serious imbalance. They focus instead on strategies that create the political and social environment for health improvement and allow for the full participation of the communities concerned. They consistently try to remind health professionals and policy makers of the implementation level that matters most in terms of population health. As a consequence they sit uncomfortably both in the world of practice and of research.

Health professionals committed to Primary Health Care and health promotion are often faced with the difficulty of serving two masters: their respective agencies and the community. Too frequently, evaluation expectations bypass a central public health theorem: that a small change in the health of a large population is of more public health significance than a large change in a small population. The author of this book proposes to consider Primary Health Care and health promotion as 'investment packages' with a wide-ranging long-term effect, not only on health but also on quality of life and wellbeing. She gives very practical guidance and illustrations of how to go about implementation at various levels of intervention.

There exists urgency and a need to teach Primary Health Care and health promotion strategies and the specific skills needed to implement them more systematically in schools of public health. This book is an excellent starting point to do so. At the same time it offers practitioners ample materials for self-study and continuing education. And the examples show it is being done, it can be done: it just needs to be done a lot more.

Ilona Kickbusch
Professor of International Health
Yale University School of Medicine

PREFACE

In the years since the early 1990s, when this book was first written, there has been a significant change in the political context in which health promotion workers operate, both within Australia and at the international level. Support for principles such as social justice, equity and community participation can no longer be assumed to be part of the espoused values of governments or international bodies. Economic rationalism and the 'new right' thinking from which it developed have now asserted themselves as the dominant force influencing government policy. The principles of comprehensive Primary Health Care are looking increasingly at odds with this dominant paradigm.

These changes have served to highlight how very important the principles of the Primary Health Care approach are and how vital it is that they continue to have a place in contemporary society. The role of health workers in implementing these principles is thus even more important than when this book was first written. As the year 2000 comes and goes, we each have an important role to play in renewing our commitment to the concept of 'Health For All', through comprehensive Primary Health Care and health promotion. It is hoped that this updated edition will contribute to the process of enabling and supporting health workers in their endeavours to promote the health of their communities.

The late 1980s and early 1990s was a period of significant enthusiasm and activity among community health workers, as they worked to implement the principles of Primary Health Care and health promotion in their practice. Some of this work was funded by specific Commonwealth and State grants, while the remainder was funded by the enthusiasm of health workers and their communities. As a result, there has been a significant increase in the number of published examples of good practice, in refereed journal articles, books and booklets, and in proceedings of conferences held around Australia. Therefore, rather than increasing the number of practice examples included within the book, this second edition includes an annotated bibliography of some of the key sources of these examples. This provides an opportunity to review these examples as they were reported by the health workers involved, in many cases with a level of depth which would not be possible within this book.

At the same time, many of the examples presented in the first edition have been revisited by their authors and brought up to date. This has served to highlight how, in some instances, situations change and programs move with them or cease to be required. In other instances, the examples highlight how the programs have continued for extended periods, often by responding to changing circumstances, touching on some of the issues of importance in ensuring sustainability of health promotion work.

The structure of this second edition remains basically the same as in the first edition. The major historical developments have been brought up to date and there is fuller discussion of the barriers to the Primary Health Care approach. More recent developments in Primary Health Care practice have been incorporated and the references and further reading at the end of each chapter have been updated. Discussion of the settings approach, in particular, has been strengthened.

What has steadfastly been resisted, however, is weakening the commitment to a Primary Health Care approach, despite these increasing challenges to its key principles. Commitment by health workers to these principles is the foundation for effective, balanced, appropriate and just health systems. If we do not retain unwavering commitment to the Primary Health Care approach, we will have little hope of seeing it prosper.

Andrea Wass
1999

ACKNOWLEDGEMENTS

In completing this second edition, there are a number of people whose contributions must be acknowledged. Firstly, thanks are once again owed to the students and practitioners who continue to provide feedback on the ideas presented here and who challenge me to think more clearly. Thanks also to those who have provided updated examples of their practice or other contributions to this edition.

Several people contributed importantly to the development of the first edition of the book, and their impact is still reflected in this second edition. Lyn Backhouse, with whom I co-taught the unit for which this book was first developed, challenged me to develop many of the ideas presented in this book. Pamela Griffith critically reviewed drafts of most chapters, and added much to the depth of the material presented. Rod Menere reviewed a number of chapters and ideas, Jane Dixon provided a critical review of the community development chapter and Garth Ritchie reviewed the health education chapter. Lyn Backhouse prepared a draft of the health education chapter and Fran White prepared the original section on working with people from other cultures. The friendship and support provided by Pamela Griffith, Garry Griffith, Nicola Wass, Rod Menere and Rob Edwards was also instrumental in ensuring that the first edition was completed.

Staff of the Department of Public Health, Flinders University of South Australia, and the Centre for Primary Health Care, University of Queensland, provided a supportive study leave environment in which planning and early work for this edition took place. Particular thanks are owed to Fran Baum, Bronnie Veale, Michael Crotty, John Coveney, John Palmer, Colin MacDougall, Robert Bush, Allyson Mutch and Fran Boyle. Colleagues at the School of Health, University of New England, tolerated my absent-mindedness as usual.

Thanks are also owed to Paul Butler, Helen Keleher and Marilyn Harris for their constructive feedback on the draft manuscript. My apologies for those comments that time and a dull mind prevented me from addressing.

Gina Brandwood, Helena Klijn and Rhiain Hull at Harcourt Australia provided editorial assistance for this edition. Julian McAllan acted as project manager, editor and typesetter.

My family and friends once again provided the support and encouragement that I needed to complete the project. Particular thanks are due to Nicola Wass, for commenting on a number of chapters and acting as emergency interlibrary loans officer when material was urgently required.

Finally, a special debt of gratitude is owed to Pat Nielsen and Michael Crotty, whose capacity for wisdom, integrity, love and good humour remain an inspiration. I was extraordinarily lucky to have known them both.

The authors and the publishers wish to thank the following for permission to reproduce copyright material:

- Extract, p. 39, from Health Targets and Implementation ('Health for All') Committee, *Health for All Australians*, Australian Government Publishing

Service, Canberra, 1988, p. 9. Commonwealth of Australia copyright reproduced by permission.

- Extract, p. 39, from Nutbeam, D., Wise, M., Bauman, A., Harris, E. and Leeder, S., *Goals and Targets for Australia's Health in the Year 2000 and Beyond*, Department of Public Health, University of Sydney, 1993.

- Figure 2.1, p. 68, reprinted from Brown, V., 'Towards an epidemiology of Health: a basis for planning community health programs', *Health Policy*, Vol 4, 1985, pp. 331–40, with permission from Elsevier Science.

- Extract, p. 95, from Selener, D., *Participatory Action Research and Social Change*, The Cornell Participatory Action Research Network, Cornell University, Ithaca, New York, 1997, pp. 18–21.

- Extract, p. 139, from Legge, D., Wilson, G., Butler, P., Wright, M., McBride, T. and Attewell, R. *Best Practice in Primary Health Care*, Centre for Development and Innovation in Health and Commonwealth Department of Health and Family Services, Vic, 1996, pp. 8–9.

- Extract, p. 140, from 'Australian Health and Community Services Standards: Health and Community Services Core Module' and 'Australian Health and Community Services Standards: Community and Primary Health Care Services Module'. Reproduced with permission from the Quality Improvement Council Limited.

- Extract, p. 149, from the Victorian Health Promotion Foundation, 'Quit Smoking' and 'Active at any age' billboard posters, Victorian Department of Health.

- Extract, p. 157, from "Martin St residents' unhappy anniversary", 15 January 1991, by courtesy of *The Armidale Express*.

- Extract, p. 171 from Butler, P. and Cass, S. (eds), 'Introduction' to *Case Studies of Community Development in Health*, Centre for Development and Innovation in Health, Vic, 1993, p. 10.

- Figure 6.1, p. 176, from Tones and Tilford, 1994, *Health Education: Effectiveness, efficiency and equity,* 2nd edn. Reproduced with the permission of Stanley Thornes Publishers Ltd.

- Extract, p. 177, from Werner, D., 'The Village Health Worker: Lackey or Liberator?', *World Health Forum*, 1981, 2 (1), pp. 46–68.

- Extract, pp. 187–8, from VicHealth Strategic Directions 1999–2002, Victorian Health Promotion Foundation, Victorian Department of Health.

- Extract, p. 195, from Consumer's Health Forum, *Guidelines for Consumer Representatives: Suggestions for Consumer or Community Representatives Working on Committees*, Consumers' Health Forum of Australia, ACT, 1999.

- Extract, p. 204, from WHO Regional Office for Europe, *Vienna Recommendations on Health Promoting Hospitals,* WHO Regional Office for Europe, Copenhagen, April, 1997.

- Extract, p. 205, from Fawkes, S., 'Aren't Health Services Already Promoting Health?', *Australian and New Zealand Journal of Public Health*, 1997, 21 (4), p. 392.

- Extract, p. 209, from Dommers, E., Ingoldby, M. and Heart Foundation (Victorian Branch), *The Health Promotion Handbook: Action Strategies for Healthy Schools*, Addison Wesley Longman, 1996, p. 17.

- Extract, p. 221, from Bundey, C., Cullen, J., Denshire, L., Grant, J., Norfor, J. and Nove, T. 1989, *Group Leadership, a Manual About Group Leadership and a Resource for Group Leaders*, Western Sydney Area Health Promotion Centre, 1989, p. 40.
- Extract, p. 225, from The Conflict Resolution Network, *Rules for Fighting Fair*, The Conflict Resolution Network, NSW.
- Extract, p. 231, from Ewles, L. and Simnett, I., *Promoting Health: a Practical Guide*, Baillière Tindall in association with the Royal College of Nursing, Edinburgh, 1999, p. 254.
- Extract, p. 241, from Ewles, L. and Simnett, I., *Promoting Health: a Practical Guide to Health Education*, Copyright John Wiley & Sons Limited, 1985, p. 28. Reproduced with permission.
- Extract, p. 242, from Minkler, M. and Cox, K., 'Creating Critical Consciousness in Health: Application of Freire's Philosophy and Methods to the Health Care Setting', *International Journal of Health Services*, 10 (2), Baywood Publishing Co, NY, 1980, p. 312.
- Extract, p. 249, from World Health Organisation, *Education for Health: a Manual on Health Education in Primary Health Care*, World Health Organisation, Geneva, 1988, p. 175.
- Extract, p. 253, from Minkler, M. 'Ten Commitments for Community Health Education', Health Education Research, 9 (4), reproduced by permission of Oxford University Press, 1994, pp. 527–34.
- Appendix 1, pp. 273–5, from the World Health Organisation, 'The Declaration of Alma-Ata', *World Health,* August/September 1988, pp. 16–17.
- Appendix 3, pp. 283–7, from the World Health Organisation, 'The Jakarta Declaration on Leading Health Promotion into the 21st Century', *Health Promotion International,* 12 (4), pp. 261–4.

While all reasonable attempts have been made to contact the copyright owners whose material is reproduced in this text, some have remained untraceable. The publisher would be pleased to hear from any copyright holders who have not already been acknowledged.

CONTRIBUTORS

Trish Abbott

Nurse Librarian, Manning Base Hospital, PO Box 35, Taree, New South Wales 2430

Bob Berry

Clinical Nurse Consultant (Mental Health), 12 Campbell Street, Taree, New South Wales 2430

Jennifer Brett

Manager, St Agnes Lodge and Mt Carmel House, Lochinvar Place, Port Macquarie, New South Wales 2444

Pat Brodie

Senior Research Midwife, Australian Midwifery Action Project, University of Technology, Sydney, 11 The Terraces, PO Box 123, Broadway, NSW 2007

Sandy Brooks

Clinical Nurse Specialist (Mental Health Promotion), Taree Community Health Centre, PO Box 35, Taree, New South Wales 2430

Margaret Brown

Chairperson, Health Consumers of Rural and Remote Australia Inc., PO Box 120, Lameroo, South Australia 5302

Joan Byrne

Consumer and arthritis activist, 2 Shirley Avenue, Syndal, Victoria 3150

Margaret Carroll

'Redbank', Molong, New South Wales, 2866

Judyth Collard

Director of Nursing, and Chief Executive Officer, Springwood Retirement Villages, PO Box 159, Springwood, New South Wales 2777

Pamela Griffith

Lecturer, School of Health, University of New England, Armidale, New South Wales 2351

Sue Lauder

Community Health Nurse, PO Box 1211, Geelong, Victoria 3220

Jenny MacParlane

Senior Lecturer, School of Health, University of New England, Armidale, New South Wales 2351

Liz Meadley

Immunisation Program Manager, Hunter Urban Division of General Practice, 123 King Street, Newcastle, NSW 2300

Alison Miles

Promotion Coordinator, Prometheus Information, PO Box 160, Dickson, ACT 2602

Lorna Neal

Area Coordinator (Women's Health), Mid North Coast Area Health Service (Southern Sector), PO Box 35, Taree, New South Wales 2430

Northcote Hydrotherapy and Massage Group

c/- Northcote Community Health Centre, 42 Separation Street, Northcote, Victoria 3070

Christopher Roberts

Business Manager, Prometheus Information, PO Box 160, Dickson, ACT 2602

Leonie M. Short

Senior Lecturer in Oral Health, Centre for Public Health Research, Queensland University of Technology, Victoria Park Road, Kelvin Grove, Queensland 4059

Cynthia Spurr

Manager, Health Promotion Unit, Flinders Medical Centre, Bedford Park, South Australia 5042

Anna Treloar

Registered Nurse , Kempsey District Hospital, River St, Kempsey West, New South Wales 2440

Karen Williams

Paediatric Case Manager, Brain Injury Service, 313 Darby Street, Bar Beach, New South Wales 2300

INTRODUCTION

This book examines the Primary Health Care approach to health promotion. It does so from the position that health promotion is an important component of Primary Health Care, and that health promotion is a more potent force if it is driven by the Primary Health Care philosophy.

Primary Health Care was formally endorsed as an important framework for improvement of the world's health in 1978, when the *Declaration of Alma-Ata* provided the blueprint for Primary Health Care and 'Health for All by the year 2000'. This Declaration, supported by representatives from 134 nations, emerged from international concern that health care systems had developed with a focus on costly high technology care, usually at the expense of the provision of even basic health services for the majority of the world's people.

Primary Health Care was seen as a solution to the inadequate illness management systems which had developed. By providing a balanced system of treatment and disease prevention, through affordable, accessible and appropriate services, it was hoped that Primary Health Care would address some of the major inequalities in health observed both within countries and between countries. At the same time, though, there was recognition that new health services alone were not the answer, and that a major reorientation was needed in the way in which we both think about and act on issues which impact on health.

Primary Health Care is therefore about much more than the provision of new health services. Central to Primary Health Care is the Primary Health Care philosophy or approach, which should guide all action on health issues. It is the Primary Health Care approach which tells us *how* we should do what we do. The Primary Health Care approach emphasises social justice, equity, community participation and responsiveness to the needs of local populations. It emphasises using approaches which are affordable, and therefore sustainable. It emphasises the need to work with people, in order to enable them to make decisions about which issues are most important to them and which responses are most useful, and to work with other sectors and groups to address the root causes of ill-health. This Primary Health Care approach, to be effective, needs to be applied at all levels of the health system and in every interaction between health workers and community members. Such a comprehensive approach is so much more than the delivery of primary-level services. With the use of the term 'primary health care' to refer to such services, 'Primary Health Care' is used throughout this book to reflect this comprehensive Primary Health Care approach.

Following the development of Primary Health Care, and its application to varying degrees in different countries, has come a focus on health promotion. One key reason for this is that greater emphasis on health promotion is needed if we are to develop the more balanced health system required in Primary Health Care. The *Ottawa Charter for Health Promotion,* developed in 1986, reflects the same principles seen in the *Declaration of Alma-Ata,* and very much builds on the Declaration, by providing a clear framework for action by health workers. This same approach was carried through in the *Jakarta Declaration on Leading Health Promotion into the 21st Century* (1997). This approach to health promotion recognises that action to promote health must work to change the environments that structure health chances, as well as to help individuals to change those things over which they have control. As a result, these documents present a comprehensive definition of health promotion, which is about so much more than health education.

Health workers will need a broad range of skills not traditionally regarded as central to the health system if they are to effectively implement the Primary Health Care approach to health promotion. This book focuses on those strategies which have emerged as central to health promotion practice, but which have been largely neglected in the education of health workers until the recent past. It is designed to provide both a theoretical introduction and practical strategies for action.

Health promotion is not the responsibility of any one professional group or even of the health professions as a whole. Health promotion is everyone's responsibility. Health promotion is a broad ranging activity which must be embraced by as many people as possible if it is to be effective.

Much health promotion work occurs outside the health sector, and therefore requires the active involvement of people who would not regard themselves as 'health' workers at all. Teachers, police, road safety workers, engineers, mediators, human rights investigators and many more play a central role in health promotion. Similarly, all health workers, no matter where in the health system they find themselves, have opportunities to promote health, whether it be lobbying for changes to reduce the socioenvironmental dangers to health, working to make health services more health promoting settings, educating individuals about health enhancing behaviour or engaging people meaningfully in the decision-making processes that affect their health.

Members of the community have a central role to play in using the democratic process to work for change at a societal level, and where possible making choices at an individual level to promote their health. Their role, through a process of participatory democracy, as a broad constituency for change, is a potentially very powerful one.

Within this context, though, it is worth focusing to some extent on the particular roles which health workers have to play. Firstly, they have an espoused commitment to improving the health of people, a goal which should be fundamental to all health professions. Should they choose to ignore the importance of health promotion, they will be ignoring the values which are the very foundation of their professions. In addition, they are able to advocate for a health perspective on issues outside the health sector which have an impact on health. They are also able to work with community members, encouraging and supporting them where necessary, or providing expertise and advice where that is needed.

By virtue of these issues, health workers must take up a leadership role in the promotion of health. Multidisciplinary health associations, such as the Public Health Association of Australia, have an enormously important role to play here, both in advocating for the health of the community and in modelling the effectiveness of a true multidisciplinary approach.

The professional associations of the various health disciplines have an important role to play too. Without each health discipline acknowledging its responsibility for the promotion of health, as part of a multidisciplinary approach, students of the various disciplines are unlikely to adopt health promotion as their own, seeing it instead as something which other disciplines can take up. Conversely, arguments about which health discipline should 'control' health promotion only serve to tie up precious energy and detract from the urgent tasks at hand.

Having said that, this text was originally prepared as a result of the recognised need for a text on health promotion of direct relevance to nurses, who currently make up almost 70 per cent of the paid health workforce in Australia (Australian Institute of Health and Welfare 1996: 140). By virtue of their numbers alone, they can have a powerful impact if they embrace health promotion and the philosophy of Primary Health Care.

Both the International Congress of Nurses and the Australian Nursing Federation have pledged their support for Primary Health Care and the Health for All movement. Australia's nursing workforce is therefore formally committed to Health for All. The World Health Organization (WHO) is very supportive of nurses acting as change agents in the Health for All movement. Indeed, Halfdan Mahler, Director-General of WHO from 1973 to 1986, saw nurses as 'more than ready' to take up the challenges of Primary Health Care (Mahler 1987, p. 23) and urged:

> *If the millions of nurses in a thousand different places articulate the same ideas and convictions about primary health care, and come together as one force, then they could act as a powerhouse for change.*

Of course, many health workers are still working out how they see their role in Primary Health Care and health promotion, and many others are still unaware of Primary Health Care and its implications. It remains to be seen how many health workers will take up the challenge to work as health activists, to promote health in a way which enables communities and individuals to live their lives to the full. It is vital that health workers take up this challenge if their work is to have a positive impact on the health of those they are meant to serve. If we choose to ignore the shift to Primary Health Care and continue to support a burgeoning illness management system, the costs to the health of the community will be immense. If, on the other hand, the Primary Health Care challenge is taken up by all whose work impacts on health, as well as by community members who find their health being jeopardised by the circumstances in which they live, the effect could be quite profound.

Throughout this book, the term 'health worker' is used to refer to the person working to promote health. There are two reasons for this. Firstly, while the book was written originally with nurses in mind, it may be useful for all health workers or community members learning about health promotion and so should reflect a true multidisciplinary approach. As an inclusive term, 'health worker' describes the broad range of people who may be working to promote health. Secondly, the term first came to be extensively used in the women's health movement, because it was regarded as a term which implied a more equal relationship between professionals and their patients or clients. The use of the term 'health worker', rather than professional titles, was hoped to be part of the process of breaking down the way in which professional groups related to individuals and communities, enabling the establishment of more equitable health worker–client relationships. It is in this spirit of greater equality and partnership that the term health worker is used in this book.

Health promotion draws on many areas of expertise. This means that it is difficult to make the hard choices about what to examine, and in what depth, in a text of this size. In deciding which skills and issues need to be addressed in a book such as this, consideration has been given to which topics are normally examined in undergraduate nursing and health science education. For example, it is expected that readers will already have a grounding in sociology, psychology and health and disease. Hence, a number of topics, including the structural basis of ill-health, communication skills and health and disease processes, while referred to, are not examined in any great depth. Readers who are using this book without having previously examined these issues are encouraged to supplement their reading in these areas. The references and further readings at the end of each chapter should be a useful starting point.

The book is divided into 10 chapters. Chapter 1 examines the development of Primary Health Care and the new public health movement, internationally and in Australia. It explores some of the major barriers to the implementation of Primary Health Care, while also demonstrating how the principles of the Primary Health Care approach have been consistently reiterated by the WHO, some national governments and professional organisations. The second half of this chapter examines some of the major policy development processes in Australia and examines the extent to which these have embraced Primary Health Care.

Chapter 2 examines definitions of health and health promotion, and some of the major values-based issues which arise in Primary Health Care and health promotion. These are by no means simple issues, and the chapter raises a number of questions for readers to consider.

Chapter 3 introduces the reader to research in the area of health promotion, and examines the major issues in community assessment. Chapter 4 then explores the key issues in evaluation of Primary Health Care and health promotion. These chapters are built on the premises that assessment and evaluation of health promotion are both forms of research, that they should be integrated into practice, and that the line between them is often blurred.

Chapters 5 to 9 then explore a number of strategies useful in promoting health — working with the mass media, community development, working for public policy change, group work and health education. Although these issues are examined in different chapters, the lines between these different strategies are often not clear and any number of permutations and combinations are possible should the need arise in practice. This is particularly so when health promotion takes on a settings approach, and this issue is explored in Chapter 7.

Chapter 10 then makes a number of suggestions about how to incorporate the range of material presented in this book into your own practice and into developing health promotion activities. Finally, the conclusion briefly examines where to go from here if you wish to continue developing your skills in health promotion.

Included throughout this book are a number of examples of how some of the concepts presented in the book have been put into practice. These examples will add to the growing list of case studies being presented in recent Australian publications which address health promotion and Primary Health Care. It is hoped that these examples will add to your understanding of the issues of relevance in health promotion work. It is also hoped that they will encourage budding health promoters to become involved, by demonstrating that health promotion is already a meaningful part of a great many health workers' practice.

However, these examples are not meant to be definitive; rather, they represent part of an evolving practice. Many of the more difficult areas of health promotion, including dealing with the root causes of ill-health, are not as well represented as health education designed to prevent specific diseases, because we are still coming to grips with how to address these issues. You are encouraged to read widely and examine the great many other examples currently available, and to work with your colleagues to develop your own ways of working. This book includes an annotated bibliography and list of relevant journals (Appendix 4) and a list of useful web sites (Appendix 5) to guide you to a great many other examples of Primary Health Care and health promotion practice.

The emergence of Primary Health Care and the new public health movement has provided us with a strong framework for health promotion, within which health and welfare workers, policy makers, and members of the wider community can work together. The opportunity exists for all those whose work impacts on health to take up the challenge of working in such a broad health promotion framework. I hope that this book reflects the spirit of Primary Health Care, and that it will contribute to our growing understanding of how to work to promote the health of our communities, both local and worldwide.

CHAPTER 1

Health promotion in context: Primary Health Care and the new public health movement

*T*he last century has seen quite dramatic improvements in the health and life expectancy of much of the world's population. With changes to the environments in which people live, followed later by improvements in medical practice, have come reductions in population mortality and morbidity and, in many cases, improvements in standards of living and quality of life.

However, all is not well for all of the world's population. There are major disparities in the health of people around the world, with serious differences in life expectancy between people living in various countries, as well as similarly serious differences between groups of people within countries. While some people experience better access to health and other resources than ever before, many others do not.

It was out of recognition of this fact and concern for its impact on the lives of many of the world's people that the World Health Organization began a process to work towards achieving health for all of the world's population. This process was endorsed by many of the world's governments and health professions.

This chapter will review the development of this international 'Health For All' policy process, including Primary Health Care and the new public health movement, and identify the values behind such an approach. It will examine the implications of these developments, and the barriers to their implementation. Finally, it will outline patterns of health and ill-health in Australia, then examine Australia's response to the Health For All movement.

The World Health Organization responds to international health problems

The World Health Organization (WHO) is an agency of the United Nations. It was established in 1948, as the major body to deal with international health issues. The WHO is made up of around 190 countries who, as member states, work together to promote the health of the world's people (Curtis & Taket 1996, p. 250). Included in its constitution are two important statements about health. The first is the WHO's definition of health: 'Health is a complete state of physical, mental and social well-being, and not merely the absence of disease or infirmity'. The second is about the role that the WHO sees governments playing in health promotion: 'Governments have a responsibility for the health of their peoples, which can be fulfilled only by the provision of adequate health and social measures' (WHO 1958, cited by Roemer 1986, p. 58).

Despite these statements, however, there was growing concern in the 1970s that all was not well with the world's health and health care systems. Since the end of World War II, there had been a rapid growth in the international health care industry without an increase in the health status of many people. As medical technologies and medical knowledge developed, there had been the belief that these things would solve the health problems facing people around the world. However, it became increasingly apparent that this was not the case, and that high-technology acute medical care services had a limited effect on the health of populations. There was growing evidence that it was public health in its broadest sense, rather than medical care, that was responsible for most population health improvement (McKeown 1976, 1979; Eckholm 1977). At the same time, there was a growing scepticism of the role and power of medicine itself and the value of medical treatment (Illich 1975).

Vast amounts of money were spent in industrialised countries on high-technology treatments that benefited a relative few, while some people lacked access to even basic health care services (Roemer 1986). These disparities existed and continue to do so within industrialised countries as well as between industrialised and developing countries.

Furthermore, few countries had acted to improve health by reducing poverty, improving housing and food availability and stopping political oppression, despite the wide-ranging evidence that social conditions have a greater impact on health than do health services, and that poverty is the single biggest determinant of health.

As a result of growing recognition of these concerns, the WHO and United Nations International Children's Emergency Fund (UNICEF) held a major international conference in the former USSR in 1978, attended by representatives from 134 nations. This conference is now regarded as an important milestone in the promotion of world health.

Primary Health Care

The outcome of the conference was the *Declaration of Alma-Ata* (see Appendix 1, p. 263). Contained in its 10 principles was the blueprint for Primary Health Care, which was seen as the key to achieving 'an acceptable level of health for all the people of the world by the year 2000' (WHO 1978; reproduced in WHO 1988, p. 16). This became known as 'Health for All by the year 2000'.

Several concepts stand out in the *Declaration of Alma-Ata:*
- equity;
- community participation and maximum community self-reliance;
- use of socially acceptable technology;
- health promotion and disease prevention;
- involvement of government departments other than health;
- political action;
- cooperation between countries;
- reduction of money spent on armaments in order to increase funds for Primary Health Care;
- world peace.

Pulling these important concepts together into a simple definition is a difficult task. The commonly cited definition of Primary Health Care is contained in one section of the *Declaration of Alma-Ata:*

Primary Health Care is essential health care based on practical, scientifically sound and socially acceptable methods and technology made universally accessible to individuals and families in the community through their full participation and at a cost that the community and country can afford to maintain at every stage of their development in the spirit of self-reliance and self-determination

(WHO 1978; reproduced in WHO 1988, p. 16).

This definition, however, fails to reflect the whole spectrum of Primary Health Care and the fact that it is more than just a particular type of health service. As the concepts above demonstrate, the movement for Primary Health Care is pushing for more than just changes in health services. 'It is a movement calling for new democratic actions, major health system changes and social equity' (Roemer 1986, p. 63). In order to achieve this, the WHO states that 'primary health care should be a philosophy permeating the entire health system, a strategy for organising health care, a level of care and a set of activities' (WHO, cited by Chamberlain & Beckingham 1987, p. 158). It is in its entirety that Primary Health Care has the most potential to be revolutionary in its impact on the health of the world's population.

Primary Health Care as a philosophy

The Primary Health Care philosophy is the foundation of Primary Health Care and its goal of achieving Health For All. The Primary Health Care philosophy emphasises social justice, equity, community participation, socially acceptable and affordable technology, the provision of services on the basis of the needs of the population, health education and work to improve the root causes of ill-health. It emphasises working *with* people to enable them to make decisions about their needs and how best to address them. These principles reflect the Primary Health Care philosophy — using approaches that are affordable, appropriate to local needs and, therefore, sustainable.

To be effective, this Primary Health Care approach needs to be applied throughout the health system and in every interaction between health workers and community members. All health workers and components of the health care system should be guided by the principles of Primary Health Care. No matter where in the health system consumers find themselves, these principles should be present. Indeed, given the recognition of the need for action outside the health sector to improve health and the impact of social services on health, the Primary Health Care philosophy has implications way beyond the health system.

Primary Health Care as a strategy for organising health care

When the philosophy of Primary Health Care is implemented, a particular strategy for the organisation of health care becomes apparent. A balanced system of illness treatment, rehabilitation, disease prevention and health promotion should be developed, with the entire system built to meet the goals of Primary Health Care.

Primary Health Care as a set of activities

The *Declaration of Alma-Ata* (WHO 1978) highlights a minimum set of activities that need to occur if Primary Health Care is to be implemented. These are:

- education concerning prevailing health problems and the methods of preventing and controlling them;
- promotion of food supply and proper nutrition;
- provision of an adequate supply of safe water and basic sanitation;
- provision of maternal and child health care, including family planning;
- immunisation against the major infectious diseases;
- prevention and control of locally endemic diseases;
- appropriate treatment of common diseases and injuries;
- provision of essential drugs.

Other potential priorities are also acknowledged by the WHO — for example, mental health (WHO 1990) and priorities set by local communities themselves.

Primary Health Care as a level of care

The term 'Primary Health Care' is often used to refer to primary-level health services — that is, the first point of contact with the health system for people with health problems. In a Primary Health Care system, this level of care should be the most comprehensive. In this way, problems can be dealt with where they begin. Primary-level services include community health centres, domiciliary nursing care and general medical practitioners. Non-government organisations and community groups can also be an important part of Primary Health Care services.

However, these services can only be regarded as Primary Health Care services if the Primary Health Care philosophy underpins the way in which those first-level services are provided. That is, Primary Health Care practitioners' work is guided by the principles of consumer control over decision making; collaboration with other health and welfare workers to deal effectively with health issues in their local area; equity and social justice (reflected in part, in the case of general medical practitioners, by bulk-billing or salaried medical officers attached to community health centres); and incorporation of health promotion into their work.

In recent years there appears to have been a significant increase in use of the terms 'primary health care' and 'primary care' by government, as a way of legitimising those services, without any actual reorientation of such services. However, without an orientation to the Primary Health Care philosophy, such services cannot take their place as central to the achievement of Health For All. Because of the now common use of the term primary health care to refer to community or first-level services, notably, primary medical services, 'Primary Health Care' will be used throughout this book to reflect the Primary Health Care approach or comprehensive Primary Health Care (see below).

Challenges to the Primary Health Care approach

Since the *Declaration of Alma-Ata* and the development of the Health For All by the Year 2000 program, a number of major challenges to the Primary Health Care approach have emerged. Given the enormity of the issues necessary to achieve Health For All, this is hardly surprising. However, these challenges have presented some serious threats to implementation of the Primary Health Care approach and the values of social justice, equity and community participation.

These challenges were present almost from the very day the Health For All by the Year 2000 program began. However, they were accelerated in the late 1980s

---

What Primary Health Care is not

Many people confuse Primary Health Care with a number of other concepts. Some of these are listed below.

Primary medical care (or primary care)

Primary medical care (or primary care) is medical care provided for individuals at their first point of contact with the health system. It may be provided in the out-patients section of a hospital, or by a general medical practitioner. As the first point of contact with the health system, it is an important opportunity to identify health problems early and provide timely treatment. It is not, however, by itself, Primary Health Care.

Primary nursing

Primary nursing is a system of nursing in which an individual nurse takes primary responsibility for particular patients. The focus is still on illness care rather than health promotion, and the individual, not the whole environment, is the target for change. (For a more detailed comparison of primary nursing and Primary Health Care, see Dowling, Rotem & White 1983.)

Community based health care

Community-based health care is an important component of Primary Health Care, but Primary Health Care is not only community-based care. The Primary Health Care approach has implications throughout the entire health system, and the Primary Health Care approach is about much more than the provision of health services (Tarimo & Webster 1994, p. 6).

Third World health care

Contrary to what some people believe, Primary Health Care is applicable to all countries of the world, not just developing countries. The need to address inequalities in access to health and health care, and the need for a balanced affordable health system, is equally relevant to industrialised and developing countries. Also, the Primary Health Care approach recognises the interconnections between developing and industrialised countries, and the impact that actions of the industrialised world have on the health of those living in developing countries. Changes all around the world are required to implement the Primary Health Care approach.

---

and 1990s. They resulted in the Primary Health Care approach being taken up as rhetoric by many countries, but with little fundamental change occurring or, where it did, being quickly undermined. To some extent this may be explained by a lack of understanding of the concept of Primary Health Care, due to the complexity of the definition, and a belief that it was relevant to developing countries only (WHO 1982, p. 2).

It was also to be expected that there would be resistance to the concept from those committed to the current system. Primary Health Care requires a balanced system of health promotion, prevention of ill-health, rehabilitation and accessible affordable health care. The impact of Primary Health Care represents a real threat to the Western model of health care systems because such systems would have to redistribute their resources and reorient their approach if Primary Health Care and health promotion became an important priority. This has become even more so with the increased emphasis on privatisation of health care because the provision of high-technology acute care services — not preventing illness and caring for people with a timely and low technology approach — offers the greatest potential for profit. The 'medico-industrial complex', comprised of all those companies that profit from the production and sale of medical technologies is an extremely powerful force as a national and international business lobby (George & Davis 1998, p. 179).

Primary Health Care would also require a major shift in the focus of many health workers' roles, away from the provision of acute high-technology treatments to a greater focus on the provision of low-technology community services, health promotion and advocacy for health. Not all health professionals have responded positively to this prospect.

The first major threat to implementation of the Primary Health Care approach came from efforts to narrow down the focus of Primary Health Care, to a form less threatening to the status quo.

Comprehensive versus selective Primary Health Care

Implementation of the Primary Health Care approach is clearly a massive task involving considerable political will and major changes in health systems that are significant industries in almost every country of the world. It is therefore not surprising that there was a push to identify priorities for action. Given the history of health care internationally and the urgent need for basic medical services in some parts of the world, it is also not surprising that people would wish to set priorities based on the medical model of health care. This was the beginning of the more limited form of Primary Health Care which has become known as selective Primary Health Care.

Although the need to set priorities is important, this argument was used to support a version of Primary Health Care whose philosophy is diametrically opposed to that proposed at the Alma-Ata conference. The issues surrounding this debate are by no means simple. While many people regard the *Declaration of Alma-Ata* as reflecting comprehensive Primary Health Care, some writers argue that it embraces both approaches (Taylor & Jolly 1988), while others suggest that its intent has supported selective Primary Health Care (Navarro 1984). Others suggest that the Declaration was necessarily vague in its definitions in order to gain the political support of so many countries (Van der Geest et al. 1990). Discussion of the debate on selective versus comprehensive Primary Health Care is important because the philosophical differences between the two approaches have broad implications for how we view and implement Primary Health Care and the achievement of Health For All.

Comprehensive Primary Health Care is a developmental process that emphasises social justice, equity, community control and working for social changes that impact on health and wellbeing. In comprehensive Primary Health Care, emphasis is on the conditions that generate health and ill-health. Therefore, provision of medical care is just one aspect of comprehensive Primary Health Care. As a result, comprehensive Primary Health Care has been referred to as 'medicine in its place' (Macdonald 1993).

Selective Primary Health Care, on the other hand, concentrates on providing 'medical interventions aimed at improving the health status of the most individuals at the lowest cost' (Rifkin & Walt 1986, p. 560). Thus, while comprehensive Primary Health Care focuses on the process of empowerment and increasing control over all those influences that impact on health, selective Primary Health Care operates in a way that assumes that medical care alone creates health and ensures that control over health is maintained by health professionals.

Rifkin and Walt (1986, pp. 561–2) identify four key areas in which selective Primary Health Care compares poorly with comprehensive Primary Health Care:

1. By focusing on the eradication and prevention of diseases, selective Primary Health Care assumes that health is the absence of disease rather than, as in the broader WHO definition, a state of complete physical, mental and social well-being. This then locates action for health almost solely within the realms of specialists trained to treat disease;

2. Through its emphasis on those diseases and problems most likely to respond to treatment, selective Primary Health Care ignores the need to address issues of equity and social justice, which are at the root of many health problems, but which are more difficult to treat;

3. In establishing medical interventions as the most important part of Primary Health Care, selective Primary Health Care ignores the importance of all those non-medical interventions, such as the provision of education, housing and food, which may have a greater bearing on health than health services themselves;

4. Selective Primary Health Care limits the value of community development as a strategy for improving health to being a technique for increasing community compliance with medically defined solutions, rather than as a mechanism for community empowerment. It thus identifies expertise as residing with medical workers and denies the great expertise that people have with regard to their own lives and the issues that affect them.

Selective Primary Health Care might be seen in the short term to reduce prevalence rates of specific diseases but in the longer term it does not deal with the root causes of ill-health, nor does it generate community control over health services or other factors affecting a community's health chances. Rifkin and Walt cite a measles immunisation program which, although it reduced the number of deaths from measles, did not actually reduce the number of deaths overall. Those children who might have died from measles died from some other cause because the root cause of the problem — poverty — was not addressed (Kasongo Project Team 1981, cited by Rifkin and Walt 1986, p. 563).

Indeed, a WHO study group identified five studies that demonstrated similar findings from various projects in Africa (World Bank 1993, cited in WHO Study Group on Integration of Health Care Delivery 1996, p. 12). Turshen (1989, p. 24) argues that the eradication of smallpox had the same impact in the Third World: people are simply dying of other illnesses, and overall mortality and morbidity rates remain about the same. There seems to be growing evidence that the single disease focus of selective Primary Health Care is of limited, short-term value. Conversely, it is argued that the greater benefits of comprehensive Primary Health Care are apparent in the longer term and are likely to be more sustainable.

Arguing for comprehensive over selective Primary Health Care is not to argue against the importance of addressing specific diseases. Clearly we must address those diseases that cause human suffering and death. However, by only addressing those illnesses, we risk perpetually attempting to address the end result of the problem instead of addressing the root causes of the diseases themselves or the social conditions that perpetuate disease and other suffering. Comprehensive Primary Health Care addresses these illnesses and other issues in their social context, using a process that recognises the expertise that ordinary people have and their right to exert control over their own lives.

The rise of economic rationalism

The second major threat to comprehensive Primary Health Care has been the international rise of neo-liberalism, or economic rationalism as it is more commonly known in Australia. This philosophy is built around the belief that as much of national and international life as possible should be left to the effects of the market and that governments should minimise their involvement in public life (Baum & Sanders 1995, p. 154). Central to this approach is the notion that success is best achieved by economic growth, with improvements in the standard of living for the poor expected to come from the 'trickle down' of wealth.

The rise of economic rationalism has led to a number of developments that have had a grave impact on the health of the world's population and undermined the very foundations of the Health For All movement. Inequality has increased with a marked increase in the concentration of wealth in the hands of a few. As a consequence, health inequalities between rich and poor have worsened (WHO 1998b, p. 3). This is true for both industrialised and developing countries. Many multinational corporations now have larger budgets than many countries, with the world's largest 100 companies now being larger than most United Nations member countries, and the top 500 companies now controlling more that 70% of world trade (Morehouse 1997, p. 4). As a result, the richest 358 billionaires together now own more than the poorest 45% of the world's population (UN 1996, cited by Kawachi & Kennedy 1997, p. 1037).

At least some of these consequences have resulted from the implementation of 'structural adjustment programs' in many developing countries around the world, which are contributing to the further transfer of wealth from poor to rich.

The impact of structural adjustment programs

Throughout the 1970s, Third World countries had been encouraged to borrow large amounts of money from the major banks. With changes to the international financial situation, interest rates skyrocketed in the 1980s, resulting in those countries owing huge debts which they could not pay (Werner et al. 1997, p. 81). This situation continues today, and has resulted in vast quantities of money being moved each year from poor countries to rich countries, in order to service the debt. The impact of this drain on resources is felt most heavily by the poor, especially children (UNICEF 1992, cited by Werner et al. 1997, p. 82).

Because of concern by the banks that these countries would not be able to repay their loans, the International Monetary Fund and the World Bank stepped in. They offered to refinance the loans, on the proviso that countries accepted 'structural adjustment programs', designed to ensure that countries serviced the debt owed, but with major consequences for their internal policies. Among other things, these structural adjustment programs required countries to reduce their spending on health, education and other social services, move away from food production to production of export goods, freeze local wages and open the economy up for overseas goods and investors (Werner et al. 1997, p. 83). It is not difficult to imagine the impact that these changes have had on the health of the country's poor. The WHO notes that 'the least developed countries faced difficulty even in maintaining basic minimum services in the social sector, including health' (WHO 1998b, p. 3). In addition, the reduction in land for food production and subsistence farming means that many of the poor can no longer get enough food to eat. That these policies are being implemented at the same time as the international community is paying lip service to the notion of Health For All by the Year 2000 is nothing short of tragic.

Economic rationalism in the industrialised world

Industrialised countries, in the meantime, had been undergoing their own self-imposed structural adjustment programs as a result of the acceptance of economic rationalism (Sanders 1997). In Australia, there have been significant reductions in real terms in expenditure on health, education and other social services (see, for example, Botsman 1998, p. 15). There has also been significant support for privatisation of services, with little consideration of the consequences for those aspects of health, education and social welfare that do not fit comfortably within a market model. The gap between rich and poor in Australia has increased significantly.

In addition, publicly provided services themselves have been required to implement management techniques from the private sector. This corporatisation of the public sector has had a significant impact on the focus of public services and the philosophy that drives them. This consequence of economic rationalism, known as managerialism, or new public management, is based on a set of values fundamentally at odds with the Primary Health Care approach. Baum has summarised these as a focus on customers rather than citizens, a focus on private profit rather than public service, and a focus on what is easily measurable in the short term, rather than what may be more meaningful in the long term (Baum 1996).

Pressure from managerialist values has made it extremely difficult for health workers to develop or maintain practice based on the principles of Primary Health Care, and have led many to question how committed the Australian government is to the Primary Health Care approach.

The growing impact of the World Bank on international health policy

In 1993 the World Bank in collaboration with the WHO released its annual development report, this year focusing on *Investing in health* (World Bank 1993). With the power of the World Bank, particularly in developing countries, this document is likely to be a significant indicator of future developments in health policy.

Investing in health analyses the health systems around the world and proposes a range of health policy reforms. However, it is a document full of contradictions, and this seems to have stemmed from the fact that it is attempting to address both the WHO's Health For All agenda and the agenda of the World Bank (Baum & Sanders 1995, p. 155).

Investing in health identifies a range of important issues. It identifies the importance of poverty in creating ill-health, and the need for effective health systems to have a strong focus on public health rather than excessive emphasis on expensive high-technology care. It also recognises the importance of education for health, and the need to change economic systems in order to change the health chances of people around the world (Baum & Sanders 1995, p. 154).

At the same time, however, it takes a largely uncritical stance towards the role of markets in health, and a largely negative stance towards the value of government in service provision. It suggests greater involvement of the private sector in health services in developing and former socialist countries, without acknowledging the shortcomings of market involvement in the health systems of industrialised countries (Curtis & Taket 1996, p. 273). It recommends that government take on the role of dealing with market failure in health care, rather than one of providing a comprehensive high quality service themselves.

Concern has been expressed that, through *Investing in health*, the World Bank is working to maintain underdevelopment in some nations, with considerable negative consequences for the poor, in order to address its own agenda, which is not primarily about health (Curtis & Taket 1996, p. 276). With its focus on providing clinical services, *Investing in health* reflects a focus on selective Primary Health Care, an approach likely to become even narrower because of the report's focus on private provision of health and health-related services.

Investing in health largely ignores the negative effects of structural adjustment programs, even though they are undermining some of the very recommendations that the report makes (Baum & Sanders 1995, p. 155). *Investing in health* may well result in health issues becoming a more visible part of the international agenda. However, its support for greater 'marketisation', its assumption that benefits will trickle down to the poor, and its inadequate concern with dealing directly with inequity, seem to reflect an emphasis on health as an area for business investment rather than emphasising the inherent value in investing in people.

Health beyond 2000: the renewal of the Health For All program

As the year 2000 loomed large on the horizon, the WHO faced the task of evaluating the success of the Health For All by the year 2000 program, within the context of a very different social, economic and political environment to that operating when the *Declaration of Alma-Ata* was first developed. Notable among the changes were the increased power of the World Bank and multinational corporations, which threaten to significantly undermine the influence of the WHO and even national governments. Within this context, the WHO's evaluation resulted in a process designed to renew commitment to achieving Health For All and take it forward into the 21st century.

Clearly, Health For All was not able to be achieved by the year 2000, just 22 years after the concept was formalised. How does the world health community respond to the obvious failure to achieve Health For All by the year 2000? There was always the risk that some would scoff at both the failure and the concept itself, and choose the passing of the year 2000 as reason enough to abandon the concept of Health For All.

Fortunately, the WHO did not take that approach. Instead, in parallel with the third evaluation of 'Health For All by the year 2000', the WHO developed support for the renewal of Health For All. This position was officially endorsed by the World Health Assembly in May 1998, and documented in *Health for all in the twenty-first century* (WHO 1998a).

However, with the reduced influence of the WHO and the increased power of the World Bank, it is unclear to what extent countries around the world will seriously renew their commitment to the Primary Health Care approach. For many of the world's poor countries, the choice seems almost taken out of their hands as a result of the actions of the World Bank, which seems to have locked them into a system of creating markets for Western medical technologies through replication of Western health care systems at the expense of more affordable, sustainable and equitable Primary Health Care models.

Of course, even if it had been possible to achieve Health For All by the year 2000, maintenance of such a goal requires ongoing commitment to the principles of social justice, equity, community participation and sustainability. Any reduction in vigilance is likely to see gains quickly diminished. For this reason, the WHO, sympathetic governments and non-government organisations with a concern for social justice have an important role to play in maintaining these principles on the international agenda.

The Ottawa Charter for Health Promotion and the new public health movement

In a process that began some time after the Health For All program and has developed in parallel with it, the WHO worked to further develop the notion of health promotion. Developed with the aim of increasing the relevance of the Primary Health Care approach to industrialised countries, the WHO's focus on health promotion aimed to develop an approach to health promotion built on the same values as Primary Health Care and applied to those issues that would be seen as directly relevant to the industrialised world, which had largely ignored the *Declaration of Alma-Ata*.

The first WHO International Conference on Health Promotion was held in Ottawa, Canada, in 1986. The outcome of this conference was the *Ottawa Charter for Health Promotion* (WHO 1986), which set out the action required to achieve Health for All by the year 2000 (see Appendix 2, p. 267). Like the *Declaration of Alma-Ata*, the *Ottawa Charter for Health Promotion* was and is a landmark document, laying out a clear statement of action that continues to have resonance for health workers around the world. It builds on the *Declaration of Alma-Ata*, stating, in part:

> *The fundamental conditions and resources for health are peace, shelter, education, food, income, a stable eco-system, sustainable resources, social justice and equity. Improvement in health requires a secure foundation in these basic prerequisites.*

(WHO 1986).

How are we to achieve this? The *Ottawa Charter for Health Promotion* states that health promotion action must occur on five fronts:

1. We need to promote health by *building healthy public policy*. It is not health policy alone that influences health: all public policy should be examined for its impact on health and, where policies have a negative impact on health, we must work to change them. For example, if a State or local government has a policy of allowing industrial complexes near residential areas, this would need to change if it was having a negative impact on residents' health;

2. We need to promote health by *creating environments which support healthy living*. For example, we need living, work and leisure environments organised in ways that do not create or contribute to poor health. These will come through the establishment of healthy public policy. Through creating supportive environments, it is hoped to make healthy choices easier for people;

3. We need to promote health by *strengthening community action*. Communities themselves should determine what their needs are and how they can best be met. Thus, greater power and control remains with the people themselves, rather than with the 'experts'. Community development is one means by which this can be achieved;

4. We need to promote health by *helping people develop their skills* so that they can work for more control over their own health and the environment in which they live, and so that they have the skills necessary to make healthy choices. They also need the skills to deal effectively with illness and injury when they occur;

5. We need to promote health by *reorienting the health care system* so that there is a much greater balance between health promotion and curative services, and so that the health care system works more closely with other sectors whose work impacts on health. One prerequisite for this reorientation is a major change in the way in which health care workers are educated.

To ensure effective work in those five areas, the *Ottawa Charter for Health Promotion* highlights the need for health workers to be effective in *advocacy* and *mediation* in order to *enable* people to gain greater control over their lives (WHO 1986). The need for advocacy and mediation is particularly important in reorienting the system towards Primary Health Care and health promotion, and achieving greater equity in health.

The *Ottawa Charter for Health Promotion* is regarded as the formal beginning of the 'new public health movement', a term that has widespread recognition, despite having been used several times before (Holman 1992). This new public health approach to health promotion differs from traditional public health as it has been practised in recent years in three important ways. Firstly, it recognises the broad nature of health promotion, and the need to work with other sectors of government and private institutions whose work impacts on health. This 'intersectoral collaboration' has become recognised as a central feature of effective health promotion. Secondly, it recognises the need to work in partnership with communities to increase community control over issues affecting health and to 'de-medicalise' the control of health care. Thirdly, it recognises the primacy of people's environments (both physical and socioeconomic) in determining their health, and recognises the need to work for change to the environment rather than focusing on change solely at the level of the individual (Tones, Tilford &

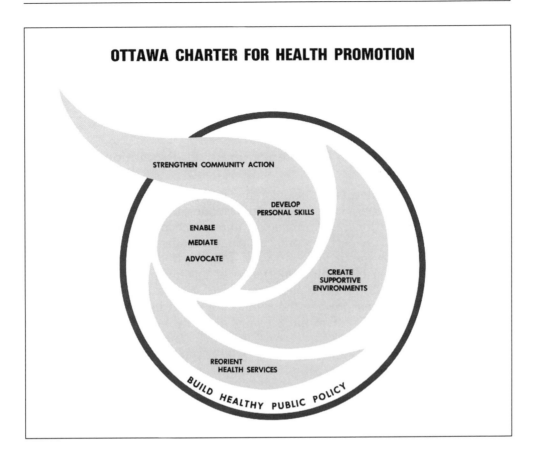

Robinson, 1990, pp. 3–4). This means that many of the changes acknowledged as vital to the new public health movement may challenge existing ways of doing things. Indeed, the WHO acknowledges the need for political action in the new public health movement to achieve the required changes.

Like the Primary Health Care approach, the new public health movement is based on a social model of health and challenges the narrow approach of the medical model. This social model of health sets very wide parameters for health promotion practice. This is exciting because it means we can actually start dealing with health problems at the point of their root cause. Indeed:

> *a social view of health implies that we must intervene to change those aspects of the environment which are promoting ill-health, rather than continue to simply deal with illness after it appears, or continue to exhort individuals to change their attitudes and lifestyles when, in fact, the environment in which they live and work gives them little choice or support for making such changes.*

(South Australian Health Commission 1988a, p. 3.)

Issues of social, political and environmental origin are largely ignored in the medical model of health, and this severely limits the ability of medical model responses to get at the root causes of ill-health. This is not to suggest that a medical model approach should be disregarded. Clearly, people will continue to get sick and require medical treatment. What is required, however, is a more balanced combination of medical model and social health approaches (Sax 1990, pp. 36–7). This is the Primary Health Care approach.

The view of health presented by the *Ottawa Charter for Health Promotion* has also been referred to as an ecological view of health because of the recognition of the importance of the environment and ecological sustainability in promoting world health. This social and ecological emphasis can be seen reflected in recommendations of the international conferences on health promotion that followed.

The Second International Conference on Health Promotion — Adelaide, Australia

The WHO's Second International Conference on Health Promotion was held in Adelaide in 1988. Its theme was healthy public policy, the key action area set out in the *Ottawa Charter for Health Promotion,* and its recommendations built very much on the spirit of the earlier work. Participants reaffirmed their commitment to the *Ottawa Charter for Health Promotion,* and urged everyone else to do so. In addition to making clear the importance of healthy public policy and the responsibility of all who produce public policy to observe and be responsive to the health impact of their policies, the conference urged industrialised countries to develop policies that reduce the growing disparity between rich and poor countries.

Furthermore, the conference identified four priority areas for action:
* support for the health of women, in recognition of their often unequal access to health and their role as health promoters within their own families;
* the elimination of hunger and malnutrition through action that takes account of agricultural, economic and environmental issues;
* the reduction of tobacco growing and alcohol production;
* the creation of more supportive environments, in particular through the alliance of the public health, peace and ecological movements (WHO/Commonwealth Department of Community Services and Health – Australia 1988).

The Third International Conference on Health Promotion — Sundsvall, Sweden

The Third International Conference on Health Promotion was held in Sundsvall, Sweden, in 1991. Its theme was supportive environments for health, and it made four recommendations for action to create such environments. These were:

* *strengthen advocacy through community action, particularly through groups organised by women;*

* *enable communities and individuals to take control of their health and environment through education and empowerment;*

* *build alliances to strengthen cooperation between health and environment campaigns;*

* *mediate between conflicting interests in society in order to ensure equitable access to a supportive environment for health.*

(WHO 1991, cited by Tassie 1992, p. 28.)

The Fourth International Conference on Health Promotion — Jakarta, Indonesia

In 1997, the WHO sponsored the Fourth International Conference on Health Promotion, held in Jakarta, with the theme of 'New Players for a New Era: Health Promotion into the 21st Century'. The purposes of this conference were to review and celebrate the achievements of the previous 10 years since the *Ottawa Charter for Health Promotion* was developed, and to make a renewed commitment to health promotion in the light of changes to the social and political environment since the *Ottawa Charter for Health Promotion* was developed. It was the first WHO health promotion conference to be held in a developing country and it actively involved the private sector in developing health promotion strategies.

There was some concern expressed at the conference about the difficulties of involving the private sector in health promotion policy development, with questions raised about the extent to which the private sector can be meaningfully involved without fundamental conflicts of interest (Hancock 1998). This is a complex issue that will remain on the agenda for some time and reflects the growing influence of neo-liberalism, as described above.

Despite these concerns, the conference produced a declaration that builds on the principles laid down in previous conferences. The *Jakarta Declaration on Leading Health Promotion into the 21st Century* reiterated the key principles of the new public health movement and identified a number of important strategies for continuing an emphasis on dealing with health problems in their social, political and economic context (see Appendix 3, p. 273).

The *Jakarta Declaration on Leading Health Promotion into the 21st Century* identifies the importance of health promotion as an investment and reiterates the need to address the significant social determinants of health. Building on the *Ottawa Charter for Health Promotion*, it identifies the following prerequisites for health:

> *peace, shelter, education, social security, social relations, food, income, empowerment of women, a stable ecosystem, sustainable resource use, social justice, respect for human rights and equity. Above all, poverty is the greatest threat to health.*

It emphasises the importance of the five strategies for action laid down in the *Ottawa Charter for Health Promotion,* noting in particular the need for comprehensive approaches that work on several levels of the Ottawa Charter, and the value of implementing broad health promotion strategies within various settings, such as cities, communities, schools, workplaces and health services. It also emphasises the importance of meaningful participation and of effective partnerships between all levels of government, non government organisations and private and public sectors. It then goes on to set five priorities for health promotion in the 21st Century:

1. *Promote social responsibility for health.* Decision makers in both the public and private sectors should demonstrate social responsibility by preventing harm to individuals and the environment, by restricting trade in harmful products and integrating concern for equity into all policy development;

2. *Increase investments for health development.* There should be an increased investment in health and areas that impact on health, including housing and education, with particular attention paid to groups that have poor health or are most vulnerable, including women, children, older people, and indigenous, poor and marginalised populations;

3. *Consolidate and expand partnerships for health.* Effective health and social development requires collaboration between all levels of government and society to make the changes necessary to improve health chances for all. These partnerships must be ethical and based on mutual respect;

4. *Increase community capacity and empower the individual.* As effective health promotion is a participatory process, communities and individuals need to be provided with the necessary skills and access to decision-making power to enable then to influence the determinants of health;

5. *Secure an infrastructure for health promotion.* Funding to establish and maintain infrastructures for health promotion locally, nationally and globally is required. Efforts need to be made to motivate government and non-government organisations to mobilise resources for health promotion. Health promoting settings are an important framework for this infrastructure. Intersectoral collaboration and international collaboration are important too. Developing local-level expertise through education and dissemination of health promotion experience is necessary, as is ensuring that all countries have the necessary 'political, legal, educational, social and economic environments to support health promotion' (WHO 1997, p. 263).

Finally, the Declaration calls for an international health promotion alliance, to raise awareness of the determinants of health and take the processes outlined in the Declaration forward into action.

As discussion of the development of Primary Health Care and health promotion demonstrates, there are many challenges to be faced in attempting to implement these processes. Nonetheless, they remain vital to the future health and wellbeing of most of the world's population, through their concern with social justice, equity, democratic processes and sustainability of the world's ecosystems. While the barriers to the implementation of the Primary Health Care approach may appear increasingly daunting, such barriers may be seen as markers of the potential for real change, rather than as a reason to back away from the important principles laid down by the international health community.

We are much more aware now of the barriers to the Primary Health Care approach but we need not lose the commitment to these principles. It is to be hoped that we can go forward, in a spirit of determined optimism, with the knowledge that, no matter what the barriers, social justice and the right of all people to live healthy, peaceful and harmonious lives is a goal worth striving for.

Australia's response to the Health for All movement

As a signatory to the *Declaration of Alma-Ata,* Australia formally committed itself to Health for All by the year 2000 in 1981. As in many other countries, this national commitment did not occur in a vacuum. The 1970s had seen the establishment of the first community health centres and the first Aboriginal Medical Service, based on the very philosophy formalised in the *Declaration of Alma-Ata.*

These foundations meant that there was a multidisciplinary cadre of health workers already developing experience and committed to a community-centred approach (Baum 1998, p. 32). This resulted in a ground swell of local level activity, as health workers throughout Australia grappled with the necessary issues, even while the government policy-making process was being established.

This local-level enthusiasm for the principles of Primary Health Care, while by no means uniform across all Australian communities, is extremely important to Australia's successes in working toward Health For All and yet can often be relatively invisible. It should not be forgotten when considering Australian responses to Health For All.

It was in the mid-1980s that Australian government policy activity started becoming apparent. Even so, most of the action to date has been in the formulation of policies. This policy development has been extremely important, although the impetus of Australia's early commitment to health and social justice seems to have dissipated in more recent policies, as more conservative government moved away from the values of social justice and equity. Nonetheless, Australia has been identified as one of the countries that has taken the new public health movement seriously. It is worth examining some of the major Australian policy developments since 1986 for their continuing influence and their potential for more comprehensive action. To consider this in context, though, a brief review of Australia's health profile and health expenditure is in order.

A snapshot of Australia's health

The pattern of health and ill-health in Australia generally reflects that which exists throughout the industrialised world. Australia has benefited from the general improvements in health that have occurred in the 20th century. Overall, the health of Australians is very good, with average life expectancies some of the best in the world. The health and quality of life of most Australians compares well with most of the world's population. This is important to celebrate and to bear in mind so that we might consider how we can contribute to improving the health of those countries less fortunate than Australia.

However, Australians are not immune to the effects of inequality on health, and some of these have become worse as income inequality in Australia has increased. While the health of Australians is on average good, there are some significant differences in the health chances of a number of population sub-groups in Australian society.

Poor socioeconomic status is the single biggest determinant of ill-health and death in Australia (National Health Strategy 1992, p. 10). People of all ages in the lower socioeconomic groups have higher rates of death and reported illness than their more affluent counterparts, with unemployed people faring worst of all. These inequalities have been noted in the statistics for sudden infant death syndrome, accidental drowning, motor vehicle accidents, other accidents, suicide, cardiovascular disease, respiratory disease and cancers, for example (National Health Strategy 1992, p. 11; Mathers 1994).

Gender is also a significant determinant of health chances in Australia. Mortality rates for males are higher than those for females for all major causes of death (Australian Institute of Health and Welfare 1998, pp. 7–9). Men are also less inclined to seek medical assistance when they experience symptoms of poor health. At the same time, however, reported morbidity rates for women are worse than those of men (Australian Institute of Health and Welfare 1998, p. 16), and women's experience of the health system is often negative. In 1996, life expectancy for men was 75.4, while for women it was 81.1 (Australian Institute of Health and Welfare 1998, p. 11).

There are also marked differences in health status according to ethnicity. While many migrants have better health on arrival than the average Australian because of the requirements of the immigration process, this advantage disappears the longer they have been in Australia, as a result of the impact of limited job opportunities, the adoption of the health habits of the country to which they have migrated and the lack of social support far from extended family and friends (Australian Institute of Health and Welfare 1998, p. 46; Bates & Linder-Pelz 1990, pp. 36–8; Minas 1990). However, this pattern of good health on arrival may be less likely to be the case for those migrants who come to Australia as refugees on the basis of humanitarian grounds. This group of migrants is likely to be suffering both physical and psychological trauma as a result of the often brutal experiences they have endured.

However, it is Australia's Aboriginal and Torres Strait Islander people who have the most serious health inequalities, with infant mortality rates two to four times higher than the national average and life expectancy 14 to 20 years less than for other Australians (Australian Institute of Health and Welfare 1998, pp. 28–32). As a result, Aboriginal and Torres Strait Islander hospitalisation rates are more than 50% higher than for other Australians (Australian Institute of Health and Welfare 1998, p. 32). As poor as these statistics are, they may actually underestimate the severity of Aboriginal and Torres Strait Islander people's poor health, as information in this area is incomplete and Aboriginal and Torres Strait Islander people are not always identified in health statistics.

This unequal access to health may sometimes be ignored if only generic national figures are used, and pockets of disadvantage may be hidden behind 'average' figures. Most of the issues that cause these health differences result from structural issues outside the traditional health care system and require health promotion action from both within the health system and outside it, in collaboration between various levels and sectors of government and non-government bodies.

However, like most Western industrialised health systems, the focus of the Australian health care system has been largely on the provision of individual treatment for individual problems. This means that attention and resources are focused on treating the end result rather than the cause of health problems, and the scope for increasing activity to prevent health problems is great.

This is reflected in how Australia spends its health budget. As Figure 1.2 demonstrates, by far the majority of Australia's health spending is allocated to the provision of illness treatment services, either in institutions such as hospitals and nursing homes or in private medical, dental and pharmaceutical services. Only a small proportion of the health budget (5.2% in the year 1993–94, the latest year for which figures are available) is allocated to community and public health. Health promotion and illness prevention account for only a proportion of this. In 1989-90 this proportion was 32% (Grant and Lapsley 1993 p 113), which would be just 1.6% of total health expenditure (though the actual figure for 1993-4 has not been made available).

This figure represents a small increase on previous years, with health promotion accounting for 1.2% of health spending in 1988–89 (Grant & Lapsley 1992, p. 106), 1.1% in 1987–88 (Grant & Lapsley 1991, p. 108), 1.0% in 1986–87 (Grant & Lapsley 1990, p. 94) and 0.9% in 1985–86 (Grant & Lapsley 1989, p. 92).

It is therefore quite apparent that health promotion has so far played a relatively minor role in the health care system in this country. Indeed, Australia's expenditure on health promotion compares poorly with other industrialised countries such as the UK, which spends 5–6% and the Netherlands, which spends 5% of its health budget on health promotion (Oldenburg et al. 1994, p. 16).

However, this does not adequately describe the money spent by the Australian government on programs that have positive health benefits, as a significant amount of money used to promote the health of the community is spent from budgets other than health. For example, money spent on safe roads, public transport systems and basic services such as water supply has a positive impact on health yet is not counted as part of health promotion expenditure (Australian Institute of Health and Welfare 1996, p. 121). At the same time, though, considerable expenditure in other areas actively promotes ill-health. Subsidies to cigarette and alcohol companies provide two examples of this unhealthy expenditure (Sax 1990, p. 37).

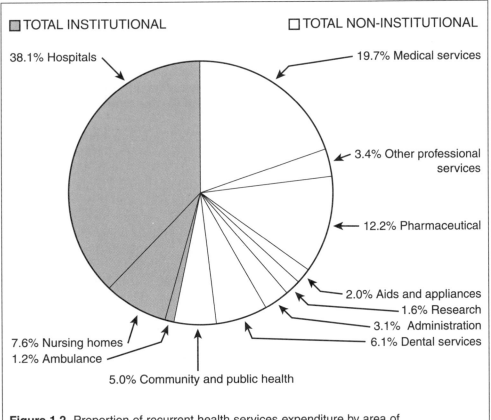

Figure 1.2 Proportion of recurrent health services expenditure by area of expenditure, 1996–97 (Australian Institute of Health and Welfare 1999, p. 161).

Clearly, there is scope for Australia to focus more of its health expenditure on the promotion and protection of health. At the same time, a comprehensive whole of government approach is needed if we are to fully protect and maximise the health of the community. Such a whole of government approach would need to consider the health consequences of public policy in all areas, including the health portfolio itself.

Setting goals and targets for Australia's health: The *Health for all Australians* report and beyond

In response to Australia's commitment to Health For All by the year 2000, the Better Health Commission was established by the federal government in 1986. It identified national health goals for Australia in its report *Looking forward to better health* (Better Health Commission 1986). These were then examined in greater detail by the Health Targets and Implementation ('Health For All') Committee, which released the *Health for all Australians* report in 1988. This was essentially Australia's plan of action to achieve Health for All by the year 2000. Some Australian States went on to produce their own health goals and targets based on the *Health for all Australians* report, and a number of health regions applied it at a more local level.

In its report, the Health Targets and Implementation Committee set five national priorities for action in the areas of control of high blood pressure, improved nutrition, injury prevention, the health of older people and the prevention of cancer (notably lung, skin, breast and cervical cancers). It also set national goals and targets in a range of areas, under the three general categories of population groups, major causes of illness and death, and risk factors (see below). In addition, it noted a number of barriers to better health and recognised the need for structural change in the health system if we are to promote the health of all Australians.

The *Health for all Australians* report represented quite an important shift in Australian health policy development. It was the first time that the federal government had formally recognised the role played by social inequalities in causing ill-health. It was also the first time that a national health strategy document setting goals and targets for the health of Australians had been drawn up (Health Targets and Implementation Committee 1988, p. 8) — quite a remarkable fact given the large amounts of money that the health system consumes each year. Furthermore, in defining the quest for better health for Australians, the report acknowledged the existence of barriers to that quest, both those outside the health system, such as economic and social factors, and those within the system, which it acknowledged is geared to illness rather than health (Health Targets and Implementation Committee 1988, p. 8).

However, the *Health for all Australians* report has been criticised on a number of grounds. For example, although it acknowledges that health inequalities exist between different groups in Australian society, it is built primarily on a biomedical rather than a social model of health. Although setting goals for population groups, major causes of illness and death, and risk factors, the report focuses largely on medical problems in the priorities for action that it sets. In addition, targets are set for disease categories, yet none are set for population groups or for conditions that severely limit people's health but which have not been categorised as a disease — for example, chronic back pain and the health consequences of sexual assault (Brown 1988, p. 33). Therefore, the solutions that the report suggests are somewhat limited. One of the main reasons for this is that the Health Targets and Implementation Committee (1988, p. 6) chose to identify changes that could be made within the health system, rather than also looking at what could be done in a comprehensive intersectoral approach to health. This was quite an unfortunate choice, as the document was meant to implement Primary Health Care, and could have been an important first step in the formal establishment of intersectoral action for health in Australia.

Furthermore, the committee chose as its priorities those problems for which action was likely to be effective (Health Targets and Implementation 1988, p. 11). Other issues may have been ignored because they were difficult to address, although they may have been urgent. It has also been suggested that the committee chose as priorities areas in which well defined goals and targets were already available, rather than areas that were most important (Consumers' Health Forum 1988, cited by McPherson 1992, p. 128). Such an approach has been criticised elsewhere for ignoring the most serious health problems that people face and thus achieving less for people's health in the longer term (Rifkin & Walt 1986). Therefore, although the *Health for all Australians* report represents an important beginning for Australia's health, it does not embrace the principles of Primary Health Care to the extent that it could have.

The *Health For All Australians* report represents the beginning of Australia's commitment to health goals and targets, carried through in several subsequent documents, including *Health Goals and Targets for Australian Children and Youth* (Child, Adolescent and Family Health Service, 1992), *Goals and Targets for Australia's Health in the Year 2000 and Beyond* (Nutbeam et al. 1993) and *Better Health Outcomes for Australians* (Commonwealth Department of Human Services and Health 1994). In addition, a draft set of Aboriginal health goals and targets was produced. The commitment to a goals and targets approach represents something of a two-edged sword for advocates of the Primary Health Care approach. On the one hand, these documents finally set goals to direct the issues that the entire health system should be addressing, and so provide an opportunity for the health system to make a bigger difference to health status in Australia. On the other hand, however, they are prescriptive and amount to some quite narrow goals being imposed from above. As described above in relation to *Health For All Australians*, goals and targets tend to be set in areas in which results are most measurable or most likely to be achievable, rather than in areas that are most important (Baum 1995a, p. 223). This can then lead to those more important areas being even further ignored. Also, because goals and targets are established at national level and drive the policy and planning process, communities are largely unable to set their own goals relevant to their own needs. This places the goals and targets approach in some contrast to a Primary Health Care approach, where community control and responsiveness to local issues is a priority.

Following on from the *Health for all Australians* report, the National Better Health Program was established to implement the report's recommendations. It provided funding for health promotion activities, particularly those that addressed the five priority areas outlined in the *Health for all Australians* report (Australian Institute of Health 1990, p. 81). The program was funded until June 1992, when it was evaluated. The evaluation report, *Towards Health For All and Health Promotion* (Commonwealth Department of Health, Housing and Community Services 1993), included recommendations for the establishment of a national Health For All Strategy, supported by legislation, and for the continuation of a strong national health promotion program as part of this strategy.

Goals and targets for Australia's health in the year 2000 and beyond

The goals and targets set in the *Health for all Australians* report were for the 5-year period following the report's release. The second set of goals and targets was developed in 1992 and released in February 1993 in a report, *Goals and Targets for Australia's Health in the Year 2000 and Beyond* (Nutbeam et al. 1993). These built on the lessons learned from the first experience with goals and targets. *Goals and Targets For Australia's Health in the Year 2000 and Beyond* revised and refined the targets set in the *Health for all Australians* report in the areas of preventable morbidity and mortality and healthy lifestyles and risk factors (Nutbeam et al. 1993). It also recognised the importance of moving beyond a mainly medical model focus by establishing additional targets in the areas of health literacy, health skills and healthy environments (see opposite). It recognised the need for the whole health system to be involved in achieving health goals and targets and, to help achieve this, identified the need to establish specific goals and targets for the health system (Nutbeam et al. 1993, pp. 13–14). Further, it urged a stronger intersectoral approach to health issues. As a result, this second set of goals and targets was broader, less medically defined and therefore much more in line with the *Ottawa Charter for Health Promotion's* broad framework.

National Health Priority Areas

The federal government responded to *Goals and Targets for Australia's Health in the Year 2000 and Beyond* by choosing four priority areas and developing more detailed goals and targets for these areas. Needless to say, this meant laying aside the many other important areas identified in *Goals and Targets for Australia's Health in the Year 2000 and Beyond*. The four priority areas chosen were cardiovascular health, cancer control, injury prevention and control, and mental health. Strategies to address these areas were presented in *Better Health Outcomes for Australians* (Commonwealth Department of Human Services and Health 1994).

In 1996, the Commonwealth government shifted its focus somewhat by moving away from specific targets. The National Health Priority Areas, which were endorsed by the Australian health ministers representing the Commonwealth and all States and Territories, were a refined version of *Better Health Outcomes for Australians* and focused attention on the four priority areas of cardiovascular health, cancer control, injury prevention and control, mental health, and added diabetes mellitus. However, the approach taken was to set indicators for monitoring progress in improvement, rather than goals and targets (Mathers and Douglas 1998, p. 139). The *First Report on National Health Priority Areas 1996* was released in 1997 (Australian Institute of Health and Welfare, and Commonwealth Department of Health and Family Services 1997). Reports on progress in each of the priority areas will be produced every two years.

The consequence of all this activity in the area of national health goals and targets was 17 years of activity but with no set of goals and targets reported on

A decade of Australian health goals and targets

Health For All Australians — 1988

Priorities

Nutrition, injury, health of older people, cancer, heart disease.

Other goals and targets
Population groups

The socioeconomically disadvantaged, Aborigines, migrants, women, men, older people, children, adolescents.

Major causes of illness and death

Heart disease and stroke, cancers (including lung, breast, cervical and skin cancers), injury, communicable disease, musculoskeletal diseases, diabetes, disability, dental disease, mental illness, asthma.

Risk factors

Drugs (including tobacco smoking, alcohol misuse, pharmaceutical misuse or abuse, illicit drugs and substance abuse), nutrition, physical inactivity, high blood pressure, high blood cholesterol, occupational health hazards, unprotected sexual activity, environmental health hazards.

Goals and Targets for Australia's Health in the Year 2000 and Beyond — 1993

Preventable mortality and morbidity

Cardiovascular disease, preventable cancer, injury, communicable diseases, HIV/AIDS, sexually transmitted diseases, maternal and infant (including perinatal) health, asthma, diabetes mellitus, mental health problems and disorders, physical impairment and disability, developmental disability and oral health.

Healthy lifestyles and risk factors

Diet and nutrition, overweight and obesity, physical activity, high blood cholesterol, high blood pressure, smoking, alcohol misuse, illicit drug use, quality use of medicines, healthy sexuality, reproductive health, sun protection, oral hygiene, safety behaviours, immunisation and mental health.

Health literacy and health skills

Health literacy, life skills and coping, safety skills and first aid, self help and self care and social support.

Healthy environments

The physical environment, transport, housing, home and community infrastructure, work and the workplace, schools and health care settings.

Better Health Outcomes for Australians — 1994

Cardiovascular health, cancer control, injury prevention and control, mental health.

National Health Priority Areas — 1997

Cardiovascular health, cancer control, injury prevention and control, mental health, diabetes mellitus.

more than once (Mathers & Douglas 1998, p. 139). Without this continuity, we can make very little comment about progress.

Examining the role of health promotion and Primary Health Care in the Australian health system

During the 1990s there have been several other processes reviewing aspects of health promotion and Primary Health Care. These reviews have been valuable in documenting the current state of play in Australia, highlighting examples of good practice and recommending several strategies for improving support for Primary Health Care and health promotion. These documents represent a valuable framework for action in Australia. Unfortunately, very little of the recommended action has been taken. However, they remain valuable guides should a federal government decide to take them seriously.

Improving Australia's health: The role of Primary Health Care

In 1991, the National Centre for Epidemiology and Population Health was commissioned by the National Better Health Program to examine the role of Primary Health Care in health promotion in Australia. In October 1992, after a year-long consultation process, the final report — *Improving Australia's health: the role of Primary Health Care* — was released (National Centre for Epidemiology and Population Health 1992). A range of issues was studied, including the state of Primary Health Care in Australia, how Primary Health Care in Australia might address the issue of more efficient, effective and equitable health promotion and how it could be strengthened. The report recommended the establishment of Primary Health Care reference centres in each State and Territory, greater education for and funding of innovative Primary Health Care activity, greater support for 'Healthy Cities' (see p. 186) and the development of a national Primary Health Care Policy and Implementation Plan. Furthermore, it acknowledged two alternative attitudes towards health promotion in Primary Health Care: health promotion as a developmental process in partnership with community members, and health promotion as a planning process imposed by a central health promotion agency. These often opposing approaches have been of concern to a number of health workers for some time and their acknowledgement in the report is valuable. However, the report did not deal with the many barriers to the implementation of Primary Health Care in Australia, a vital issue if Primary Health Care is to move beyond being token.

Despite the fact that a national Primary Health Care policy has not been developed, several Australian States have established their own Primary Health Care policies. South Australia produced *A Social Health Strategy* (South Australian Health Commission 1988a), *Primary Health Care in South Australia: a discussion paper* (South Australian Health Commission 1988b) and an implementation plan, *Strategic Directions for Primary Health Care* (South Australian Health Commission 1993). A significant commitment to these policies over a number of years saw considerable progress made in the implementation of Primary Health Care principles (Baum 1995a). Similarly, Queensland released *A Primary Health Care Policy* (Queensland Health 1992b) and a *Primary Health Care Implementation Plan* (Queensland Health 1992a) and has gone some way to implementing these policies. With a move to more conservative government throughout the early 1990s, however, the commitment to Primary Health Care appears to be fading.

The National Health Strategy

In 1991, the Australian health ministers commissioned the National Health Strategy — a two-year examination of the structure and funding of the Australian health system. Development of the National Health Strategy provided an excellent opportunity to reorient the system to a Primary Health Care approach. Unfortunately, the strategy focused on making the current system more efficient without making the major changes required of a reorientation to Primary Health Care. Indeed, the National Health Strategy only considered health promotion and Primary Health Care towards the end of its life and after issues of funding and restructuring had been considered, so this opportunity for major change was lost. This seems to reflect a continued belief that health promotion and Primary Health Care are marginal to the Australian health system.

However, the National Health Strategy paper that considered health promotion, *Pathways to Better Health* (National Health Strategy 1993), drew on previous Australian health promotion and Primary Health Care work [including *Towards Health For All and Health Promotion* (Commonwealth Department of Health, Housing and Community Services 1993b) and *Improving Australia's Health: the Role of Primary Health Care* (National Centre for Epidemiology and Population Health 1992)]. Quite a comprehensive document, it made a number of recommendations about continuing support for health promotion within the health system, including the establishment of a National Health Promotion Authority, further development of education for health promotion, the development of a stronger intersectoral approach to health promotion and the further strengthening of health promotion action by community health centres, schools, general medical practitioners, hospitals and workplaces.

Promoting the health of Australians: A review of infrastructure support for national health advancement

In 1995, the Commonwealth Department of Human Services and Health commissioned the Health Advancement Standing Committee of the National Health and Medical Research Council to conduct a review of health promotion activity and the infrastructure needed to support health promotion in Australia. Following a period of consultation and response to a discussion paper, the final report, *Promoting the health of Australians: A review of infrastructure support for national health advancement* was released by the NHMRC in December 1996. Two complementary reports, *Promoting the health of indigenous Australians: a review of infrastructure support for Aboriginal and Torres Strait Islander health advancement* (1996) and *Building Australia's capacity to promote mental health: review of infrastructure for promoting health in Australia* (1997), were also released by the NHMRC and AHMAC Mental Health Working Group, respectively.

The review was based on the *Ottawa Charter for Health Promotion's* definition of health promotion and acknowledgement of the central role of cultural and socio-economic factors in determining health, including the importance of equity, and the need for an emphasis on intersectoral action and healthy public policy. However, the emphasis in the review is on the action required within and by the health system.

The report makes a wide range of recommendations for the development of leadership and direction and for the establishment of a strong infrastructure for health promotion, beginning with the establishment of a National Public Health Partnership between State and Commonwealth governments (this has already begun). Its recommendations are comprehensive and wide ranging, although the lack of inclusion of local government in the National Public Health Partnership is of some concern given the central role of local government in public health.

Questions have been raised as to whether Australia has the necessary infrastructure in place to champion and implement the wide range of policy recommendations made in these reports (Nutbeam 1998, p. 301). At the time of publication, it remained to be seen the extent to which these documents will be effectively implemented. Like many documents before them, they hold considerable promise.

Integrating Health For All into other Australian health policy development

Several other more specific recent national policy and strategy documents have implications for Australia's health. These are *A National Aboriginal Health Strategy*; the *National Women's Health Policy: Advancing Women's Health in Australia*; the *National Non-English Speaking Background Women's Health Strategy*; *The Health of Young Australians*: *a National Health Policy for Children and Young People*; the *National Mental Health Strategy* and the *National Rural Health Strategy*. It is worthwhile briefly examining these and the approaches they take. In addition, it is worth noting some of the work that has been done towards the development of a national men's health policy.

The National Aboriginal Health Strategy

In 1989, following an extensive consultation process involving Aboriginal and non-Aboriginal communities, groups and individuals, the National Aboriginal Health Strategy Working Party produced *A National Aboriginal Health Strategy*. This policy document is extremely important, for at least three reasons. Firstly, it had been developed with the active involvement of Aboriginal people themselves over a lengthy period of consultation. Secondly, it was a consensus document achieved with representation from Commonwealth, State and Territory governments, which identified both key issues and potential solutions to some of the major Aboriginal health issues (Anderson 1997, p. 119). And thirdly, it went some considerable distance in reflecting a social health approach, more than any other Australian health strategy produced to date.

The *National Aboriginal Health Strategy* is grounded in the recognition of the importance of the structural basis of Aboriginal health, describing the inextricable link between Aboriginal health, land rights and domination of Aboriginal people by non-Aboriginal culture. Within this framework, it considers the roles of government in dealing with Aboriginal health, the necessary changes to the structure of the health system, the role of intersectoral collaboration in promoting Aboriginal health, a wide range of specific health issues, and Aboriginal health research and evaluation.

In particular, the Strategy argues for Aboriginal community control of health services and research into issues related to Aboriginal people and their health. It also argues for Aboriginal women's control of specific women's issues — that is, matters related to child bearing, family planning and gynaecological health. This is vital because Western medical control of child bearing and related issues ignores the fact that they are regarded by Aboriginal people as 'women's business' and also ignores the spiritual importance of many of these issues. In addition, it examines abuse of alcohol and other substances, and the health impact of such things as housing, food supply and education.

In suggesting strategies to deal with the specific ill-health problems facing Aboriginal people, the strategy acknowledges cardiovascular disease, diabetes, chronic lung disease, pneumonia, asthma, kidney diseases and renal failure, ear disease, diarrhoeal diseases, trauma and injury, contagious diseases of childhood, hepatitis B, sexually transmissible diseases, ocular diseases, dental health, mental health, domestic violence and child abuse as serious problems.

A National Aboriginal Health Strategy was greeted with great enthusiasm when it was released. It represented the first comprehensive response to Aboriginal health issues in their social context. Certainly, there is scope for further strengthening of the approach it takes (see Anderson 1997), but it remains an extremely good basis for action. However, despite the value of *A National Aboriginal Health Strategy* and the seriousness and urgency of the issues it raises, the Strategy still was not followed by action. In 1994 an evaluation of *A National Aboriginal Health Strategy* was conducted. This evaluation, five years after its release, found in part that *A National Aboriginal Health Strategy* was never effectively implemented, that it had been grossly underfunded, that there was inadequate accountability for the inaction, that ATSIC was used as a scapegoat for the inaction, and that there was inadequate political support for the implementation of the Strategy (National Aboriginal Health Strategy 1994, as presented in Anderson 1997, p. 121).

Commonwealth, State and Territory response to *A National Aboriginal Health Strategy* is extremely disappointing. Anderson has suggested that this inaction can be explained by lack of political will and shortcomings in the Australian health care system and other agencies that structure the relationship between Aboriginal people and the State (Anderson 1997, p. 122). Failure to address these issues and properly implement the policies of *A National Aboriginal Health Strategy* raises many questions about whether government commitment to Aboriginal health is likely to be more than lip-service. Nonetheless, *A National Aboriginal Health Strategy* remains a valuable resource for health workers committed to understanding and working to improve Aboriginal health.

National Women's Health Policy: Advancing Women's Health in Australia

The *National Women's Health Policy* was launched in 1989. It was developed after a 20-year process of lobbying by women's groups to make the health system more responsive to the needs of women. The *National Women's Health Policy* resulted from a process of extensive consultation with women's groups throughout Australia and was built on a recognition of the social model of health and the impact that the social environment has on health and health choices. It highlights seven priority health issues for women, which are not limited to standard medical classification of illness, but reflect the social health basis of the policy. These issues are reproductive health and sexuality, the health of ageing women, women's emotional and mental health, violence against women, occupational health and safety, the health needs of women as carers and the health effects of sex role stereotyping on women.

The policy also recognises that issues of concern to women and their health are not limited just to specific health issues, and so it highlights five issues related to the structure of the health system that require action. These are the need for improvements in health services for women, the need to provide relevant health information for women, the need for more research into women's health issues, the need to increase women's participation in health decision making and the need to train health workers to deal more appropriately with women and their health concerns.

A National Women's Health Program was established to implement the Policy, funded jointly by Commonwealth and State and Territory governments. After four years of implementation, the National Women's Health Program was evaluated in 1993. It identified the continuing relevance of the *National Women's Health Policy* and National Women's Health Program. It identified the need for more work to address 'the links between health status and broader cultural and socio-economic factors' and the need to continue to support innovative projects in women's health (Commonwealth Department of Health, Housing, Local Government and Community Services 1993, pp. xxiii–xxiv). The ongoing commitment of the National Women's Health Program to a social health and Primary Health Care approach remains one of its strengths.

In 1991, the *National Non-English Speaking Background Women's Health Strategy* was released. It complements the *National Women's Health Policy* by focusing on the particular needs of women from non-English speaking backgrounds. It focuses on occupational health and safety as it relates to women from non-English speaking backgrounds, the needs of carers from non-English speaking backgrounds, the need for better language services, the need for better access and choice for a range of health services for women from non-English speaking backgrounds, and the need to improve the quality of a number of health services required by women from non-English speaking backgrounds (Alcorso & Schofield 1991). Like the *National Women's Health Policy*, the *National Non-English Speaking Background Women's Health Strategy* recognises the impact of the environment on health. Many of the issues it raises will require action in a number of sectors in order to be addressed.

The National Mental Health Strategy

The National Mental Health Strategy was established in 1992, when the *National Mental Health Policy* (Australian Health Ministers 1992a) and the first *National Mental Health Plan* (Australian Health Ministers 1992b) were both released. The *National Mental Health Policy* recognised the importance of promoting the mental health of the Australian community. However, overall its focus was on better quality services for individuals with mental health problems and for their carers. It emphasised the importance of a 'community-oriented approach to the provision of mental health services' (Australian Health Ministers 1992, p. 2), although, as previous deinstitutionalisation policies have demonstrated, community-based care without sufficient funding can have disastrous consequences. Furthermore, the policy recognises the need for better access to such services as transport, accommodation and community services, and the need for better education for the community as a whole about mental health problems. It identifies the need for greater support for the carers of people with mental health problems, including greater financial support and involvement in decision making (Australian Health Ministers 1992, p. 4).

Despite their aim of improving the mental health of the community as a whole, the *National Mental Health Policy* and first *National Mental Health Plan* focused on provision of services for people with mental health disorders, in particular, those with serious mental health problems, and placed little emphasis on mental health promotion. This may have been largely a consequence of the urgent need to improve the quality of service provision for those with serious mental illness but it had some consequences that required amending. Of particular concern was the need to increase the focus on mental health promotion.

This issue was taken up in the *Second National Mental Health Plan* (Australian Health Ministers 1998). This second plan identified three priority areas: promotion and prevention, the development of partnerships in service reform, and the quality and effectiveness of service delivery. While still a significant focus on improving service provision for those with serious mental illness, the inclusion of mental health promotion and mental illness prevention was extremely important. This importance was reflected in the development of an action plan specifically designed to address these areas. The *Mental Health Promotion and Prevention National Action Plan*, released in January 1999, lays out a framework for action to promote mental health and prevent mental illness, complementing the *National Youth Suicide Prevention Strategy* and the *Depression Action Plan* already in operation (National Mental Health Promotion and Prevention Working Party 1999, p. 7).

The *National Mental Health Promotion and Prevention Action Plan* identifies a broad range of strategies to promote mental health, drawing on a range of research and other literature to support its proposals. Taking a life-span approach, it begins with proposals for action for babies and infants and progresses through to those required to promote mental health among older people. It then addresses the action needed for population groups at particular risk of developing mental health problems, notably:

• individuals, families and communities experiencing adverse life events;
• rural and remote communities;
• Aboriginal and Torres Strait Islander communities;
• people from diverse linguistic and cultural backgrounds;
• mental health service consumers, carers and community organisations.

Finally, it sets out action required for the whole of the community, the mass media and health professionals.

The *Mental Health Promotion and Prevention National Action Plan* represents a comprehensive strategy for the promotion of mental health. It identifies the difference between mental health promotion and mental illness prevention, and attempts to address both. Its approach to mental health promotion is broad and in line with the *Ottawa Charter for Health Promotion* and the Primary Health Care approach. It also identifies a series of research questions for areas where we need to improve what we know in order to act more effectively. It offers promise for a comprehensive approach to the promotion of mental health. The challenge remains for this plan to be implemented and for a comprehensive intersectoral approach to be taken to mental health promotion, by addressing the many underlying social and economic circumstances that put people at greatest risk.

The National Rural Health Strategy

Following government recognition that the health needs of people living in rural areas of Australia are different to those of their urban counterparts, the federal Department of Community Services and Health hosted the first National Rural Health Conference in February 1991. The aim of this conference was to develop a national rural health strategy.

The *National Rural Health Strategy*, released later that year, recommended the establishment of a national body to direct and coordinate:

* rural health policy and practice;
* the funding of research into the particular needs of rural dwellers and approaches to address those needs;
* the development of support and education for rural health workers;
* improvement of current equity and access problems for rural dwellers;
* the promotion of health for rural dwellers;
* effective planning to address the particular health needs of vulnerable groups (including Aboriginal and Torres Strait Islanders, older people, people with chronic illness or disabilities, women, children, adolescents and people with HIV/AIDS or at risk of contracting the virus (National Rural Health Strategy 1991, pp. 1–2).

Following on from the strategy, the National Rural Health Alliance and a National Rural Health Unit were established and funds became available through the Rural Health Support Education and Training Program.

A revised *National Rural Health Strategy* was released by the Australian Health Ministers Conference in 1994 and updated in 1996. In addition, the first national conference on rural public health, co-sponsored by the Commonwealth Department of Health and Family Services and the Department of Primary Industries and Energy, was held in 1997.

In 1997/98 a review of the National Rural Health Strategy was again conducted. *Healthy Horizons: a Health Strategy for Regional, Rural and Remote Australians* was released in March 1999 and is designed to cover the period 1999–2003. It sets seven key goals for this period:

* *improve health for areas of highest priority;*
* *improve the health of Aboriginal and Torres Strait Islander people living in regional and remote Australia;*
* *better information about the health of regional, rural and remote Australians;*
* *coordinated services developed and maintained by collaboration;*
* *a skilled and responsive health workforce;*
* *flexible funding for regional, rural and remote communities to be based on need;*
* *recognise regional, rural and remote health as an important part of Australia's health system.*

(National Rural Health Policy Forum 1999, p. 9.)

The National Rural Health Strategy and its implementation in the years before 1999 focused on issues of recruitment and retention of health workers, management models for rural health services and development of mainstream health programs for the needs of rural people. While there has been some formal acknowledgement of the Primary Health Care approach to addressing health issues, the National Rural Health Strategy has been criticised for not going far enough to promote the health of rural Australians.

The Health of Young Australians: a National Health Policy for Children and Young People

In 1995, the Australian Health Ministers endorsed *The Health of Young Australians: a National Health Policy for Children and Young People*. It was followed in 1996 by the *National Health Plan for young Australians: an action plan to protect and promote the health of children and young people*.

The Health of Young Australians: a National Health Policy for Children and Young People recognises the importance of treating children and young people's health as an investment in the future, the fact that much illness and injury in children and young people is preventable, and the role that the health sector should play in influencing the work of other sectors whose work impacts on the broader determinants of health. It identifies the importance of equity in achieving health for children and young people, noting the particular needs of Aboriginal and Torres Strait Islander children and young people, recent migrants, those with disabilities or chronic illness, those living in poverty and those who are homeless.

The Health of Young Australians: a National Health Policy for Children and Young People identifies the importance of the social environments in which children live in structuring their health chances and acknowledges the role of families, schools and the broader society, including the impact that socioeconomic status and geographical location have on health and health services. It identifies the need for action in seven key areas:

- *healthy, supportive environments for children and young people;*
- *customer-focused and participative health services;*
- *a balanced approach;*
- *addressing inequities;*
- *coordination and collaboration;*
- *research, information and monitoring;*
- *workforce and training.*

(Commonwealth Department of Human Services and Health 1995, p. 29.)

The National Health Plan for Young Australians is designed as a 5-year plan to implement the policy of the *The Health of Young Australians: a National Health Policy for Children and Young People*, and against which the progress can be evaluated in 2001. At that point it is to be expected that a revised plan will be developed. It remains to be seen to what extent the rhetoric of these documents will make a difference to the health of Australia's children and young people.

Towards a National Men's Health Policy?

In 1996, the Commonwealth Department of Health and Community Services released a *Draft National Men's Health Policy* for discussion and comment. The process of raising the profile of men's health had formally begun with the first National Men's Health Conference organised by the Commonwealth in 1995, following a concerted period of lobbying by several individuals and groups concerned about the health and wellbeing of Australian men and boys.

The draft document began by examining the major issues impacting on men's health, with a major focus on the impact of socialisation, socioeconomic status and workplace health and safety, and identified the particular needs of a number of different groups of men, including boys and young men, working-aged men, older men, Aboriginal and Torres Strait Islander men, gay men, rural men, men from non-English speaking backgrounds and men with disabilities. The draft policy itself then identified the importance of a men's health policy being based on a social model of health and a Primary Health Care approach.

The *Draft National Men's Health Policy* was designed to provide a framework for a year-long consultation process, leading to the endorsement of a men's health policy, but, with a change in government at the national level in March 1996, the new government decided against proceeding with the development of a national men's health policy. However, significant interest and concern had been generated in men's health over the previous five years, so it is unlikely that action will be curtailed. A number of Australian States are proceeding with the development of men's health policy and action.

Conclusion

The last 20 years have seen the development of numerous international and national policies and programs designed to reorient health systems towards Primary Health Care and health promotion. These developments occurred as a result of recognition of inequities in health and social development throughout the world. Within Australia, we have seen some important action based on these calls for a reorientation of our approach to health issues.

At the same time, however, commitment to the principles of social justice, equity and a responsive health system based on population need has been wavering. The impact of economic rationalism around the world and in Australia is being seen in a narrower commitment to Primary Health Care and health promotion.

Despite significant policy activity since the mid 1980s and some promising beginnings, there has not been a corresponding reorientation of action. Indeed, much of the policy activity that has occurred has been more in line with selective Primary Health Care than comprehensive Primary Health Care. This, combined with the impact of economic rationalism and its focus on economic policy at the expense of social policy, has resulted in a situation where Australia has not seriously reoriented its approach and is giving indications of an increased medicalisation of primary health care services.

This has made the need for a commitment to the Primary Health Care approach by health workers, as individuals and members of professional associations, even more important. Within the context of the national policies described in this chapter, and sometimes despite them, many community health workers around

Australia have been working to implement the principles of Primary Health Care and health promotion in their practice. The result has been some inspiring examples of what can be achieved by working in this way.

In order to do this, health workers have been drawing on a range of skills and strategies. These have been developed and discussed in the professional literature and have been integrated into the education of many health workers. This process has been taken up around the world by many in the health professions and has paralleled the activities of national governments, who cannot alone implement the changes required in a Primary Health Care approach.

The challenge for health workers is to put into practice the principles of Primary Health Care and health promotion using a social health perspective. Many of the key strategies and skills required to do this effectively are discussed in the remainder of this book. Health workers are encouraged to take up the challenge of the Primary Health Care approach by incorporating the principles of Primary Health Care into their daily practice and developing and implementing their skills in health promotion.

References and further reading

AHMAC Mental Health Working Group 1997, *Building Australia's Capacity to Promote Mental Health: Review of Infrastructure for Promoting Mental Health in Australia.* National Mental Health Strategy, Canberra.

Alcorso, C. and Schofield, T. 1991, *The National Non-English Speaking Background Women's Health Strategy,* Australian Government Publishing Service, Canberra.

Anderson, I. 1997, 'The National Aboriginal Health Strategy', in Gardner, H. (ed.), *Health Policy in Australia,* Oxford University Press, Melbourne.

Anderson, I. 1988, *Koorie Health in Koorie Hands: an Orientation Manual in Aboriginal Health for Health Care Providers,* Koorie Health Department, Health Department Victoria, Melbourne.

Australian Health Ministers Conference National Public Health Partnership Group 1998, *National Public Health Partnership Strategic Directions 1998–2000,* National Public Health Partnership, Melbourne.

Australian Health Ministers Conference 1994, *National Rural Health Strategy,* Australian Government Publishing Service, Canberra.

Australian Health Ministers 1998, *Second National Mental Health Plan,* Mental Health Branch, Commonwealth Department of Health and Family Services, Canberra.

Australian Health Ministers 1992a, *National Mental Health Policy,* Australian Government Publishing Service, Canberra.

Australian Health Ministers 1992b, *National Mental Health Plan,* Australian Government Publishing Service, Canberra.

Australian Institute of Health and Welfare, and Commonwealth Department of Health and Family Services 1997, *First Report on National Health Priority Areas 1996,* Australian Institute of Health and Welfare, and Commonwealth Department of Health and Family Services, Canberra.

Australian Institute of Health and Welfare 1999, *Health Expenditure Bulletin No. 15: Australia's Health Services Expenditure to 1997–98,* Australian Institute of Health and Welfare, Canberra.

Australian Institute of Health and Welfare 1998, *Australia's Health 1998: the Sixth Biennial Report of the Australian Institute of Health and Welfare,* Australian Institute of Health and Welfare, Canberra.

Australian Institute of Health and Welfare 1996, *Australia's Health 1996: the Fifth Biennial Report of the Australian Institute of Health and Welfare,* Australian Government Publishing Service, Canberra.

Australian Institute of Health and Welfare 1994, *Australia's Health 1994: the Fourth Biennial Report of the Australian Institute of Health and Welfare,* Australian Government Publishing Service, Canberra.

Australian Institute of Health and Welfare 1992, *Australia's Health 1992: the Third Biennial Report of the Australian Institute of Health and Welfare,* Australian Government Publishing Service, Canberra.

Australian Institute of Health 1990, *Australia's Health 1990: the Second Biennial Report of the Australian Institute of Health,* Australian Government Publishing Service, Canberra.

Australian Institute of Health 1989, *Australia's Health: the First Biennial Report of the Australian Institute of Health 1988,* Australian Government Publishing Service, Canberra.

Australian Nursing Federation 1990, *Primary Health Care in Australia: Strategies For Nursing Action,* Australian Nursing Federation, Melbourne.

Bates, E. and Linder-Pelz, S. 1990, *Health Care Issues,* Allen and Unwin, Sydney.

Baum, F. (ed.) 1995, *Health For All: the South Australian Experience,* South Australian Community Health Research Unit in association with Wakefield Press, Kent Town, South Australia.

Baum, F. 1995a, 'Goals and Targets for Health: their Limitations as an Approach to Promoting Health', *Australian Journal of Primary Health − Interchange,* 1 (1), 19−28.

Baum, F. 1996, 'Community Health Services and Managerialism', *Australian Journal of Primary Health − Interchange,* 2 (4), 31−41.

Baum, F. 1998, *The New Public Health: an Australian Perspective,* Oxford University Press, Melbourne.

Baum, F. and Sanders, D. 1995, 'Can Health Promotion and Primary Health Care Achieve Health For All Without a Return to their More Radical Agenda?', *Health Promotion International,* 10 (2), 149−60.

Bechhofer, F. 1989, 'Individuals, Politics and Society: a Dilemma for Public Health Research?', in Martin, C. J. and McQueen, D. V. (eds), *Readings for a New Public Health,* Edinburgh University Press, Edinburgh.

Better Health Commission 1986, *Looking Forward to Better Health,* Australian Government Publishing Service, Canberra.

Botsman, P. 1998, *Two Tier or New Frontier? The Challenge of Future Health Care Reform,* South West Health Care Papers No. 1, Division of Public Health/Centre for Health Outcomes and Innovations Research, University of Western Sydney, Macarthur.

Brown, S. 1988, 'Health for All Australians', *Health Issues,* 14 (June), 33−4.

Chamberlain, M. C. and Beckingham, A. C. 1987, 'Primary Health Care in Canada: in Praise of the Nurse?', *International Nursing Review,* 34 (6), 158−60.

Child, Adolescent and Family Health Service 1992, *Health Goals and Targets for Australian Children and Youth,* Child Adolescent and Family Health Service and Department of Community Services and Health, Canberra.

Commonwealth Department of Community Services and Health 1989, *National Women's Health Policy: Advancing Women's Health in Australia,* Australian Government Publishing Service, Canberra.

Commonwealth Department of Health and Family Services 1996, *The National Health Plan for Young Australians: an Action Plan to Protect and Promote the Health of Children and Young People,* Australian Government Publishing Service, Canberra.

Commonwealth Department of Health, Housing, Local Government and Community Services 1993, *National Women's Health Program: Evaluation and Future Directions,* Australian Government Publishing Service, Canberra.

Commonwealth Department of Health, Housing and Community Services 1993, *Towards Health for All and Health Promotion: the Evaluation of the National Better Health Program,* Australian Government Publishing Service, Canberra.

Commonwealth Department of Human Services and Health 1994, *Better Health Outcomes for Australians: National Goals, Targets and Strategies for Better Health Outcomes in the Next Century,* Australian Government Publishing Service, Canberra.

Commonwealth Department of Human Services and Health 1995, *The Health of Young Australians: a National Health Policy for Children and Young People,* Australian Government Publishing Service, Canberra.

Curtis, S. and Taket, A. 1996, *Health and Societies: Changing Perspectives,* Edward Arnold, London.

Dowling, M., Rotem, A. and White, R. 1983, *Nursing in New South Wales and Primary Health Care: a Survey of Perceptions,* University of New South Wales Centre for Medical Education, Research and Development, Sydney.

Eckholm, E. P. 1977, *The Picture of Health: Environmental Sources of Disease,* W. W. Norton and Co, New York.

George, J. and Davis, A. 1998, *States of Health: Health and Illness in Australia,* Longman, Melbourne.

Grant, C. and Lapsley, H. M. 1989, *The Australian Health Care System 1988,* Australian Studies in Health Service Administration No. 64, School of Health Services Management, University of New South Wales, Kensington.

Grant, C. and Lapsley, H. M. 1990, *The Australian Health Care System 1989,* Australian Studies in Health Service Administration No. 69, School of Health Services Management, University of New South Wales, Kensington.

Grant, C. and Lapsley, H. M. 1991, *The Australian Health Care System 1990,* Australian Studies in Health Service Administration No. 71, School of Health Services Management, University of New South Wales, Kensington.

Grant, C. and Lapsley, H. M. 1992, *The Australian Health Care System 1991,* Australian Studies in Health Service Administration No. 74, School of Health Services Management, University of New South Wales, Kensington.

Grant, C. and Lapsley, H. M. 1993, *The Australian Health Care System 1992,* Australian Studies in Health Service Administration No. 75, School of Health Services Management, University of New South Wales, Kensington.

Hall, J., Birch, S. and Haas, M. 1996, 'Creating Health Gains or Widening Gaps: the Role of Health Outcomes', *Health Promotion Journal of Australia,* 6 (1), 4–6.

Hancock, T. 1998, 'Caveat Partner: Reflections on Partnership with the Private Sector', *Health Promotion International,* 13, (3), 193–5.

Health Issues Centre. 1988, *Where the Health Dollar Goes,* Health Issues Centre, Melbourne.

Health Targets and Implementation ('Health For All') Committee 1988, *Health for all Australians,* Australian Government Publishing Service, Canberra.

Holman, C. D. J. 1992, 'Something Old, Something New: Perspectives on Five "New" Public Health Movements', *Health Promotion Journal of Australia,* 2 (3), 4–11.

Hill, S. 1989, '"Health For All": Bureaucracy Unravelled', *Health Issues,* 19, 14–15.

Illich, I. 1975, *Limits to Medicine,* Penguin, Harmondsworth, UK.

Kawachi, I. and Kennedy, B. P. 1997, 'Health and Social Cohesion: Why Care About Income Inequality?', *British Medical Journal,* 314, 5, 1037–40.

Keleher, H. 1999, *Rural Public Health Matters,* Australian and New Zealand Journal of Public Health, 23 (4), 342.

Labonté, R. 1998, Healthy public policy and the World Trade Organization: a proposal for an international health presence in future world trade/investment talks, *Health Promotion International,* 13 (3), 245–56.

LaFond, A. 1995, *Sustaining Primary Health Care,* Earthscan, London.

Macdonald, J. J. 1993, *Primary Health Care: Medicine in its Place,* Earthscan, London.

Mahler, H. 1987, 'A Powerhouse for Change', *Senior Nurse,* 6 (3), 23.

Mathers, C. 1994, *Health Differentials Among Adult Australians Aged 25–64 Years,* Australian Institute of Health and Welfare, Health Monitoring Series Number 1, Australian Government Publishing Service, Canberra.

Mathers, C. and Douglas, B. 1998, 'Measuring Progress in Population Health and Wellbeing', in Eckersley, R. (ed.), *Measuring Progress: is Life Getting Better?* CSIRO Publishing, Collingwood, Victoria.

McKeown, T. 1976, *The Modern Rise of Population,* Edward Arnold, London.

McKeown, T. 1979, *The Role of Medicine: Dream, Mirage or Nemesis?,* Basil Blackwell, Oxford.

McPherson, P. 1992, 'Health For All Australians', in Gardner, H. (ed.), *Health Policy: Development, Implementation and Evaluation in Australia,* Churchill Livingstone, Melbourne.

Minas, I. H. 1990, 'Mental Health in a Culturally Diverse Society', in Reid, J. and Trompf, P. (eds), *The Health of Immigrant Australia: a Social Perspective,* Harcourt Brace Jovanovich, Sydney.

Morehouse, W. (ed.) 1997, *Building Sustainable Communities: Tools and Concepts for Self-Reliant Economic Change,* The Bootstrap Press, New York, and Jon Carpenter Publishing, Charlbury, UK.

National Aboriginal Health Strategy Working Party 1989, *A National Aboriginal Health Strategy,* Department of Aboriginal Affairs, Canberra.

National Centre for Epidemiology and Population Health 1991, *The Role of Primary Health Care in Health Promotion in Australia: Interim Report,* National Centre for Epidemiology and Population Health, Australian National University, Canberra.

National Centre for Epidemiology and Population Health 1992, *Improving Australia's Health: the Role of Primary Health Care: Final Report of the Review of the Role of Primary Health Care in Health Promotion in Australia,* National Centre for Epidemiology and Population Health, Australian National University, Canberra.

National Health and Medical Research Council 1996a. *Promoting the Health of Australians: a Review of Infrastructure Support for National Health Advancement.* Australian Government Publishing Service, Canberra.

National Health and Medical Research Council 1996b. *Promoting the Health of Indigenous Australians: a Review of Infrastructure Support for Aboriginal and Torres Strait Islander Health Advancement.* Australian Government Publishing Service, Canberra.

National Health Strategy 1992, *Enough to Make You Sick: How Income and Environment Affect Health,* Research Paper No. 1, September, National Health Strategy, Canberra.

National Health Strategy 1993, *Pathways to Better Health: National Health Strategy,* Issues Paper No. 7, National Health Strategy, Canberra.

National Mental Health Promotion and Prevention Working Party 1999, *Mental Health Promotion and Prevention National Action Plan,* Mental Health Branch, Department of Health and Aged Care, Canberra.

National Rural Health Policy Forum 1999, *Healthy Horizons: a Framework for Improving the Health of Rural, Regional and Remote Australians,* National Rural Health Policy Forum and National Rural Health Alliance, for the Australian Health Ministers' Conference, Canberra.

Navarro, V. 1986, *Crisis, Health and Medicine: a Social Critique,* Tavistock, New York.

Navarro, V. 1984, 'A Critique of the Ideological and Political Position of the Brandt Report and the Alma-Ata Declaration', *International Journal of Health Services,* 14 (2), 159–72.

Nutbeam, D., Wise, M., Bauman, A., Harris, E. and Leeder, S. 1993, *Goals and Targets for Australia's Health in the Year 2000 and Beyond,* Department of Public Health, University of Sydney, Sydney.

Nutbeam, D. 1998, 'Promoting the Health of Australians: How Strong is Our Infrastructure Support?' *Australian and New Zealand Journal of Public Health,* 22 (3 Suppl.), 301–2.

Oldenburg, B., Wise, M., Nutbeam, D., Leeder, S. and Watson, C. 1994, 'Pathways to Enhancing Australia's Health', *Health Promotion Journal of Australia,* 4 (2), 15–20.

Primary Health Care Group, Commonwealth Department of Human Services and Health 1996, *Draft National Men's Health Policy,* Commonwealth Department of Human Services and Health, Canberra.

Public Health Division, Commonwealth Department of Health and Family Services 1996, 'The National Public Health Partnership — Commonwealth and State and Territory Cooperation', *Health Promotion Journal of Australia,* 6 (3), 60–63.

Queensland Health. 1992a. *A Primary Health Care Implementation Plan,* Queensland Department of Health, Brisbane.

Queensland Health. 1992b. *A Primary Health Care Policy,* Queensland Department of Health, Brisbane.

Rifkin, S. and Walt, G. 1986, 'Why health improves: defining the issues concerning "comprehensive primary health care" and "selective primary health care"', *Social Science and Medicine,* 23 (6), 559–66.

Research Unit in Health and Behavioural Change 1989, *Changing the Public Health,* John Wiley and Sons, Chichester, UK.

Roemer, M. I. 1986, 'Priority for Primary Health Care: its Development and Problems', *Health Policy and Planning,* 1 (1), 58–66.

Russell, C. and Schofield, T. 1986, *Where it Hurts: an Introduction to Sociology for Health Workers,* Allen and Unwin, Sydney.

Saggers, S. and Gray, D. 1991, *Aboriginal Health and Society: the Traditional and Contemporary Aboriginal Struggle for Better Health,* Allen and Unwin, Sydney.

Sax, S. 1990, *Health Care Choices and the Public Purse,* Allen and Unwin, Sydney.

South Australian Health Commission 1988a, *A Social Health Strategy for South Australia,* South Australian Health Commission, Adelaide.

South Australian Health Commission 1988b, *Primary Health Care in South Australia: a Discussion Paper,* South Australian Health Commission, Adelaide.

South Australian Health Commission 1993, *Strategic Directions of Primary Health Care,* South Australian Health Commission, Adelaide.

Tarimo, E. and Webster, E. G. 1994, *Primary Health Care Concepts and Challenges in a Changing World: Alma Ata Revisited,* Division of Strengthening of Health Services, World Health Organization, Geneva.

Tassie, J. 1992, *Protecting the Environment and Health: Working Together for Clean Air on the Le Fevre Peninsula,* Le Fevre Peninsula Health Management Plan Steering Committee, Port Adelaide.

Taylor, C. and Jolly, R. 1988, 'The Straw Men of Primary Health Care', *Social Science and Medicine,* 26 (9), 971–7.

Thomson, N. 1991, 'A Review of Aboriginal Health Status', in Reid, J. and Trompf, P. (eds), *The Health of Aboriginal Australia,* Harcourt Brace Jovanovich, Sydney.

Tones, K., Tilford, S. and Robinson, Y. 1990, *Health Education: Effectiveness and Efficiency,* Chapman and Hall, London.

Turshen, M. 1989, *The Politics of Public Health,* Rutgers University Press, New Brunswick, New Jersey.

Van der Geest, J., Speckmann, J. and Streefland, P. 1990, 'Primary Health Care in a Multi-Level Perspective: Towards a Research Agenda', *Social Science and Medicine,* 30 (9), 1025–34.

Warren, K. S. 1988, 'The Evolution of Selective Primary Health Care', *Social Science and Medicine,* 26 (9), 891–8.

Werner, D., Sanders, D., Weston, J., Babb, S. and Rodriguez, B. 1997, *Questioning the Solution: The Politics of Primary Health Care and Child Survival,* Healthwrights, Palo Alto, CA.

Wise, M. and Nutbeam, D. 1994, 'National Health Goals and Targets — An Historical Perspective', *Health Promotion Journal of Australia,* 4 (3), 9–13.

World Bank 1993, *World Development Report 1993: Investing in Health,* Oxford University Press, Oxford.

World Health Organization 1978, 'Declaration of Alma-Ata', reproduced in *World Health,* August/September 1988, 16–17.

World Health Organization 1982, *Primary Health Care from Theory to Action,* World Health Organization, Copenhagen.

World Health Organization 1986, *The Ottawa Charter for Health Promotion,* World Health Organization, Geneva.

World Health Organization 1990, *The Introduction of a Mental Health Component into Primary Health Care,* World Health Organization, Geneva.

World Health Organization 1997, 'The Jakarta Declaration on Leading Health Promotion into the 21st Century', *Health Promotion International,* 12 (4), 261–4.

World Health Organization 1998a, *Health For All in the 21st Century,* World Health Organization, Geneva.

World Health Organization 1998b, *The World Health Report 1998: Life in the 21st century. A vision for all.* World Health Organization, Geneva.

World Health Organization/Commonwealth Department Of Community Services And Health — Australia 1988, 'Healthy Public Policy — Strategies for Action', in Australian Nursing Federation 1990, *Primary Health Care in Australia: Strategies for Nursing Action,* Australian Nursing Federation, Melbourne.

World Health Organization Study Group on Integration of Health Care Delivery 1996, *Integration of Health Care Delivery: Report of a WHO Study Group, WHO Technical Report 861,* World Health Organization, Geneva.

CHAPTER 2

Concepts and values in health promotion

*C*hapter 1 identified a number of important principles in Primary Health Care and the new public health movement and raised some key issues in the national and international response to the WHO's Health For All movement. The centrality of poverty in creating ill-health, social justice and equity, the promotion of health through directly addressing causes of health problems, community participation and sustainability were all identified as important issues. Definitions of health and health promotion were examined in the context of their historical development.

Given the importance of these issues, and some of the challenges they have presented over the last 20 years, this chapter will explore these issues in greater depth, and present some other key concepts and values, raising a number of important questions that health workers will face as they grapple with the complexities of health promotion. Many of these serve to reiterate the particular value base of the Primary Health Care approach to health promotion.

Defining health

No examination of health promotion is possible without first considering what health is. In our predominantly Western culture, we tend to think automatically of health as an individual phenomenon and an individual responsibility. However, the health of individuals is strongly influenced by the social, cultural, political and economic conditions of the society in which they live, and it can never be fully considered outside that context.

Indeed, in many respects the whole discourse on health is politically constructed. In Western capitalist society, with its emphasis on consumption and profit making, attempts are made to define health as a consumable product. Emphasis is then placed on individual choices about which health 'products' to buy, rather than on people's unequal access to health.

Furthermore, because of the relationships between politics and industry, particularly in capitalist countries such as Australia, decisions about health are often the result of political agendas and are sometimes determined more by these than by need. In turn, decisions about health issues have the potential to have a substantial impact on political agendas both locally and internationally, as the discussion of the potential of Primary Health Care in Chapter 1 demonstrates. This relationship between health and politics is so strong because access to health is inextricably linked to access to power (Benn 1981, pp. 266–7), the basis of politics. As long as health is defined only in individual terms, these issues of power and control, and the unequal access to life chances because of socioeconomic status, ethnicity and gender, are invisible and easily ignored. One stark Australian example of these links is provided by the interconnection between the health of Aboriginal people and the struggle for Aboriginal self-determination.

In defining health, then, it is not sufficient to consider only the health of the individual. People live and work in groups, communities and societies, which have lives of their own and impact on each other quite profoundly. Any examination of health must consider the health of individuals, families, communities, societies and even the world. Two notable efforts to keep the health of individuals firmly in context have come from the Aboriginal health movement and the environmental movement, where concern for spiritual and cultural connectedness and environmental sustainability, respectively, have moved health definitions beyond the individual. And so, for example, Aboriginal health has been defined as:

> *Not just the physical well-being of the individual but the social, emotional, and cultural well-being of the whole community. This is a whole-of-life view and it also includes the cyclical concept of life-death-life.*

> (National Aboriginal Health Strategy Working Party 1989, p. x.)

Similarly, Honari (1993, p. 23), attempting a similar approach, provides an environmental definition of health by defining health as 'a sustainable state of well-being, within sustainable ecosystems, within a sustainable biosphere'.

The WHO's definition of health, with its recognition of social wellbeing, touches on this interrelationship by recognising the links between individuals and their social world. However, these broader approaches to defining health have been largely ignored in the past, with focus remaining on the health of individuals. Given that there are particular issues that arise in considering broader approaches to health and that health has been particularly individualised within Western culture, it is worthwhile examining some of the various dimensions of health at the levels of individual, family, community and world health. Remember, as you examine health on each of these levels, that the interrelationships between them are very strong and that none of them can be considered in isolation from the others.

Individual health

Health has been defined in different ways by many different people. Probably the main distinction between definitions of individual health is between those that define health as the absence of disease and those that define it more broadly as a sense of wellness.

Consider the following examples. Whom would you regard as healthy?
- a person who is free from disease but experiencing long-term grief;
- a person who has a serious chronic illness but is happy and lives an active life;
- a person who is free from disease but engages in risky behaviours;
- a person who is free from disease but culturally isolated and depressed;
- a person who is living in poverty.

As the above examples show, defining health is not an easy task. Indeed, it has kept some people busy for years! How health is defined is very important, however, because it determines what will be regarded as health problems and therefore what will be regarded as the work of health promotion. We touched on this issue briefly in Chapter 1. If we define health as merely the absence of disease, we see health promotion as disease prevention, and ignore many issues that may make people's lives uncomfortable but which are not medically classified as diseases or risk factors for disease. There are some major problems with this approach.

Ignoring those problems that do not necessarily create disease — chronic back pain and domestic violence, for example — may leave people suffering from conditions that limit their abilities or reduce their quality of life. Indeed, medical knowledge of what causes disease is still in its infancy in many respects. It is quite possible that, if we address only medically defined problems, we could be ignoring today issues that do not seem to be related to diseases only to discover in a few years that they do, in fact, play an important role in disease causation. For example, cigarette smoking was a socially acceptable habit until recently and it is not all that long ago that sunbathing was regarded as a normal healthy activity. Further-more, many environmental health issues are ignored on the grounds that there is no 'evidence' of a problem, when epidemiological evidence may take 20 years to surface and people may have already suffered greatly during this time.

The WHO's definition of health as 'a complete state of physical, mental and social wellbeing, and not merely the absence of disease or infirmity' is probably the most often cited definition of health. It has been important for the role it has played in highlighting that health is about much more than the absence of disease, and that it is much more than a physical state. This point has been reiterated recently by the WHO, with the *Ottawa Charter for Health Promotion* stating that health is 'a resource for everyday life, not the objective of living' (WHO 1986). The extent to which people value their health depends on a wide range of factors in addition to the state of their bodies. This has been described as asking the question 'health for what?' (Marsick 1988, p. 112).

However, the WHO definition has been criticised on a number of grounds (see, for example, Sax 1990, p. 1). Firstly, it has been argued that it is unrealistic and unachievable, because it describes a state of such total wellbeing that it is unlikely that anyone could achieve it for more than a very brief period in their lives. With its focus on perfection, too, it excludes those with disabilities or long-term medical conditions.

Secondly, it has been criticised for being unmeasurable, describing, as it does, a general state of wellbeing. Indeed, it has been pointed out that, despite health having been defined this way since 1946, health statistics still only enable us to measure death and disease and we remain without effective measures of health broadly defined (Mathers & Douglas 1998, p. 125).

On the other hand, some have criticised the WHO definition for not being broad enough. For example, a number of authors have noted its lack of inclusion of spiritual wellbeing, which is increasingly being recognised as important (Teshuva et al. 1997; Raeburn & Rootman 1998). And, as noted above, those in the indig-enous and environmental movements have criticised its definition of individual health out of a cultural and environmental context.

Despite these difficulties with the WHO definition of health, it remains an important concept, and is an important starting point because it has pointed the way to consideration of a broad definition of health at a time when health was under threat of being increasingly ed. Indeed, it seems that people themselves may define health along the same lines as the WHO definition of health (Blaxter 1990, p. 3). That is, many people identify themselves as healthy more by a sense of wellbeing within the context of their whole lives than by the presence or absence of disease. Indeed, it is probably because the WHO definition of health makes intrinsic sense to many people that it has endured as a useful definition of health, despite the difficulties experienced by scientists and social scientists in trying to measure it. Carlyon (1984) recognises this when he points out that health promotion is as much the realm of social philosophers as health workers because of the centrality of how people make meaning of their lives in their feelings of health or ill-health.

De Vries reminds us that a sense of wellbeing equates with a sense of wholeness, which is what the term health originally meant (de Vries 1993, p. 129). As de Vries points out (1993, p. 129), 'wholeness … is not the same as being happy or living without pain, frustration or handicaps; wholeness may be achieved in the presence of disease or infirmity'. This sense of wholeness, or integrity, seems to be an important dimension in health. It is interesting to note that this approach contradicts the WHO definition of health to some extent, as it suggests that this sense of wholeness may be present even if disease or disability are present.

It is out of recognition of these issues that the notion of quality of life has gained increased attention in health research. There is growing recognition of the importance of quality of life in people's experience of health, and the notion of health-related quality of life is gaining recognition (e.g. Bowling 1997, p. 36; Mathers & Douglas 1998, p. 147). Johnstone (1994, pp. 391–7) describes the range of attempts to define quality of life, which she points out is an extremely complex, perhaps indefinable, concept. She concludes that quality of life judgments can properly be made only by the individual because quality of life may be defined quite differently by different people and because only the individual is in a position to judge his or her own quality of life. This is significant because it alerts us to the importance of enabling people to make the decisions about their own health and quality of life, rather than imposing judgments on them.

Rijke (1993, p. 80), drawing on the work of several others, proposed a list of characteristics of health, which clearly relate to the notions of wholeness, quality of life, social wellbeing and spiritual wellbeing. Rijke's characteristics of health are:

> *autonomy, will to live, experience of meaning and purpose in life, high quality of relationships, creative expression of meaning, body awareness, consciousness of inner development, individuality: the experience of being a unique part of a greater whole, and vitality, energy.*

It is clear that this is quite a different approach to that when we consider health as absence of physical disease. How do we reconcile two such different approaches to health? The issues that arise here are so different that Mathers and Douglas (1998, p. 147) suggest that we may need to focus on two sets of information — one related to illness and another related to wellbeing or quality of life. Others suggest that they can be combined to calculate 'happy life expectancy', a combination of measures of life satisfaction and life expectancy (Ruut Veenhoven 1996, cited by Wearing & Headey 1998, p. 176).

The link between these two approaches appears to be becoming clearer. There is a growing sense that this sense of wellness or quality of life may in many instances have a direct bearing on physical health. Knowledge about the inextricable relationship between physical and mental health is growing all the time, but we still have a great deal to learn in this area (see, for example, Evans et al. 1994; Lafaille & Fulder 1993; Kennedy, Kiecolt-Glaser & Glaser 1988).

Family health

There are several issues worth noting when considering the concept of family health. Most people live their lives as members of a family, and it is within the context of family life and dynamics that they learn much about how people respond to life experiences and relate to each other. Families can influence the life of an individual quite profoundly. And, as the 1997 report into the forced removal of Aboriginal children from their families demonstrated, removal from families can have a profoundly traumatic effect (Human Rights and Equal Opportunity Commission 1997).

There are several ways in which families have been found to influence the health and wellbeing of their members. Firstly, families influence the physical health of their members through the provision of resources necessary for survival. The level of resources able to be provided within a family, by virtue of their socioeconomic status, has a significant impact on the likely access of family members to basic requirements for health and health care (Sanders 1995, p. 11). One-parent families are at particular risk of living in poverty.

Secondly, it is through the family that individuals may be exposed to, or protected from, aspects of the social, economic and physical environment. For example, it is within the context of the family that many occupational hazards are transmitted between individuals (for example, family members exposed to asbestos particles brought home on a worker's clothes) (Jackson 1985, p. 4), and individuals absorb the human cost of occupational injury.

Thirdly, people are socialised within families. It is within family life that people learn acceptable values, roles and behaviours. These significantly affect people's relationships with others and a wide variety of behaviours and values that have a direct bearing on physical and mental health, such as approaches to stress and coping, lifestyle behaviours, attitudes to health and illness and sex role stereotyping (Sanders 1995, p. 11). Families may be the source of domestic violence, for example.

Fourthly, most human caring occurs within the context of family life. This has both positive and negative consequences. There is now growing recognition of the health impact of caring for a dependent person on the carer, who is usually a woman. This is another example of the impact of sex role stereotyping within family life.

Finally, the extent of caring and support in a family can either protect family members against mental illness or increase the psychological distress of members, increasing the risk of many mental health problems (Sanders 1995, p. 12).

The notion of family is a value-laden concept, and definitions of it vary across cultures; consequently, there are different definitions of what a healthy family might be. The popular notion of family presented in the Australian press — two parents with two children — represents just one form of family currently existing in Australia and should not be assumed to represent the optimally healthy family. Within Australia, as of 1997, 83.5% of family households were couple families (two parent families or couple only), with 14.7% being one-parent families and 1.8% other forms of family, usually two related adults (for example, siblings or a parent and adult child) living together (ABS 1997, p. 7). It is worth noting that these official statistics all relate to family households, as do many definitions of family. However, this is a somewhat limited definition of family because most people regard their family as comprising a wider range of relatives than those who live under the same roof, and extended families are of particular significance for many people (Sanders 1995, p. 16).

In addition to these family households, around 25% of Australian households are not families. While some of these are people living alone, many households consist of non-family groups, such as groups of unrelated adults, sharing a house. These groups function in some respects as families, even though they do not impact on the lives of members as deeply as families may do. The dynamics of these groups can impact on the health of the people living in them in similar ways to a more traditional family. To a certain extent, then, family health may be reflected in the degree to which the family operates as an effective group (Douglas 1983). The principles that help make a group effective will be discussed in Chapter 8.

Sokalski, as coordinator of International Year of the Family (1994), suggested eight aspects of family life to aim for in encouraging a more egalitarian family life than many people experience now. These concepts may also be central to a definition of family health. These key elements are 'shared responsibility; mutual respect; trust and support; non-threatening behaviour; honesty and accountability; negotiation and fairness; economic partnership; and responsible parenting' (Sokalski 1992, cited by Edgar 1992, p. 3).

Community health

Defining community

Health at the level of the community is also vital to any consideration of health. However, in order to examine the notion of community health, we need first to clarify what is meant by the term 'community', and this is by no means a simple task. 'Community' has been defined in a variety of ways, ranging from very specific definitions to others that are broad and more general (Goeppinger & Baglioni 1985, p. 518). Indeed, some suggest that it is used in so many different ways as to be meaningless (Dalton & Dalton 1975, p. 1). However, the whole notion of community, in all its guises, has such a central role in considerations of community health and social wellbeing that it is too important to be rejected. A number of points are worthy of discussion.

Many of the broader definitions of community refer simply to 'community as "lots and lots of people" or community as population' (Hawe 1994, p. 200). In these definitions, communities are little more than large numbers of individuals. This approach may be seen in geographical definitions of community, in which communities are defined as groups of people sharing a particular geographical location, and when the term community is used to refer to society as a group of people or population.

Other definitions of community, however, are more dynamic, defining a community, for example, as 'a "living" organism with interactive webs of ties among organizations, neighbourhoods, families, and friends' (Eng et al. 1992, p. 1). These dynamic definitions of communities emphasise that they are social systems (Hawe 1994, p. 201), bound together by either shared values or shared interests. In these definitions, participation in the life of the community and identification as members of the community are important and result in a sense of belonging. This sense of belonging may also be described as a 'sense of community'.

There has also been much recognition that limiting the concept of community to shared geographical location may ignore many communities of interest. A community of interest has been defined as a group of people who share beliefs, values or interests on a particular issue (Clark 1973, p. 411). Communities of interest include such people as residents of a housing estate, groups of single parents or unemployed people, members of particular ethnic groups, and global communities, such as religious groups that span nations or social movements such as the women's movement or the environmental movement.

In addition to freeing communities from geographical boundaries by defining a community of interest around a shared perspective on a particular issue, this definition recognises heterogeneity among people and the fact that those who share an interest in one issue may have few other common interests or beliefs, and may even be sharply divided on other issues.

However, the term community is often romanticised, described in a way that assumes that communities are made up of close-knit groups of people who care for one another and experience little conflict (Labonté 1989a). Such an impression is far from the truth. Communities are very rarely, if ever, characterised by harmony and shared values on all issues and are more likely to reflect elements of conflict and competing interests. Communities may be strongly divided by opposing values, and may even be built on attitudes that reflect racism, sexism, ageism or homophobia, for example, rather than mutual care and concern (Minkler 1994, p. 529).

In addition, the term community may often be deliberately used to take advantage of its romantic connotations, such as when governments use terms like community care or community programs (Bryson & Mowbray 1981). Such programs may be seen positively because they are described in this way yet such programs are often underfunded or reliant on volunteer labour that, in the case of community care, is usually provided by women, with negative impacts on their own health and wellbeing.

Having considered some of the key issues that arise in attempting to define community, we can now turn to the question of how we might define a healthy community.

Defining community health

Building on the issues identified above, one element of what makes a community healthy is that it is more than merely a group of individuals. That is, healthy communities may be those in which there are strong local networks between individuals, groups and organisations that make up the community, and therefore that a sense of community exists.

These issues of the interactive ties that bind members of an effective community and a sense of community have much in common with the notion of social capital, a concept that is of increasing interest to social science researchers for its potential to make aspects of community and social health more visible in a world increasingly focusing on financial aspects of society at the expense of social aspects. Social capital has been defined as 'the processes between people which establish networks, norms and social trust and facilitate co-ordination and co-operation for mutual benefit' (Cox 1996, p. 15). This is clearly central to people's capacity to work effectively together.

Another concept likely to be important in a healthy community is the degree of equity, or sharing of the available resources. There is a growing range of evidence demonstrating that a socially just society is much more likely to be a healthy society. Several important studies have indicated that the level of equity in a society is associated with a number of positive social indicators, including low crime rates, high education levels and better health statistics (Wilkinson 1996). While there is scope to explore the exact nature of the relationship further, it is apparent that equity is an important indicator of community health.

Another important element of a healthy community is community capacity or community competence. A competent community has been defined as:

one in which the various component parts of the community: (1) are able to collaborate effectively in identifying the problems and needs of the community; (2) can achieve a working consensus on goals and priorities; (3) can agree on ways and means to implement the agreed upon goals; and (4) can collaborate effectively in the required actions.

(Cottrell 1976, cited by Goeppinger & Baglioni 1985, p. 508.)

Building on the notion of community competence, community capacity has been defined as the strengths, resources and problem-solving abilities of a community (Robertson & Minkler 1994, p. 303). This clearly relates to the importance of networks and interactive ties, and therefore social capital, because it is these elements that enable a community to develop the capacity to achieve something.

A healthy community, too, is likely to be one in which there is an acceptance of diversity, not one in which shared bonds are based solely on homogeneity. As Labonté (1989a, p. 87) points out, Nazi Germany was a strong community, but it was not a healthy one.

Consideration of what makes a healthy community and how this can be measured raises more questions than it answers. Moreover, Hayes and Willms (1990, p. 165) point out that definitions of a healthy community may vary between communities, depending on the cultural and political values of each community, and it may be appropriate for communities to develop their own vision of community health. However, if these values create harm for others, or in some other way cut across the principles of social justice and equity, we would have to question to what extent it is truly a marker of community health.

While the question of community health may need to be explored for some time yet, one important issue is worth reiterating: that health, at the level of the community as well as at that of the individual, relates to much more than the absence of disease, and any attempts to measure community health that focus solely or primarily on epidemiology and illness indices will not reflect the whole range of issues likely to impact on community health.

World health

The *Declaration of Alma-Ata* highlights the importance of world health in referring to the need for world peace and cooperation between countries if we are to

---

A developing country pays the price of improved standards of living in the West

In December 1984, an accident at the Union Carbide factory at Bhopal in India left at least 2850 people dead and some 200 000 injured, many of them permanently disabled. The deaths and injuries occurred as a result of a toxic cloud of methyl isocyanate, caused by a water leak in the factory, which spread over a populated area around Bhopal (Turshen 1989, p. 260–1). Many large companies from industrialised countries site dangerous industries in Third World countries because of the cheaper labour costs and lower worker and environmental safety requirements. The result is that these poor countries and their people are the ones who bear the brunt of the risks and human costs of injury in industries that often benefit industrialised nations more than developing countries.

---

achieve Health for All. It makes it quite clear that people cannot experience health if they are living in a war-torn country and are subjected to deprivation, suffering and fear as a result of war or political oppression.

The concept of world health is also extremely important because without it some communities or societies may achieve health at the expense of others, through the exploitation of resources or lack of consideration for the global environment. Indeed, Werner et al. (1997, pp. 78–86) identify how the international economy has developed as a result of some countries being able to take advantage of others. This process began as a major international force with the development of colonialism in the 17th Century and continues today with the use of developing countries as a cheap source of labour and non-renewable resources, and new markets in which to sell the products of multinational companies.

They argue that inequities between countries are not simply a result of the pace of development in some developing countries. On the contrary, they are the direct result of the international development process, which results in the advancement of some industrialised countries as a direct result of the exploitation of other, deliberately underdeveloped, countries (Werner et al. 1997, pp. 78–86; Green 1994, p. 51).

Therefore, much of the poverty and ill-health in developing countries is actually there because of the actions of industrialised countries. For example, the siting of dangerous industries and the dumping of wastes in developing countries, the use of land in developing countries to produce cash crops rather than provide food for local people and the destruction of the habitats of people in developing countries to provide raw materials for industrialised countries all have a potent impact on developing countries for the benefit of industrialised countries. Moreover, many developing countries are locked into repayment of loans from industrialised countries, which requires them to sell off their own natural resources, often just to keep up with the interest payments.

Furthermore, as Western countries introduce laws to protect their environments and residents from the dangers of illness-producing substances, many of the industries and products concerned are being transferred to the Third World. For example, tobacco products are now being aggressively marketed in the Third

Working for change globally

As members of a relatively affluent country, untroubled by civil war or other major conflict, Australian citizens have a responsibility to work for change in the international community. This can be achieved as members of professional associations, such as the Public Health Association of Australia, as members of non-government organisations with a social justice focus, and as individual citizens.

With the increasing globalisation of political and economic systems, decisions made by individuals in their everyday lives may have a marked impact both on the environment and on the living and working conditions of people throughout the world. Health workers are encouraged to be mindful of the consequences of purchasing choices they make and to take an active citizenship role and work for positive change.

Two organisations that work internationally using the principles of social justice and equity central to the Primary Health Care approach, and in which those with a concern for these principles can become actively involved are Community Aid Abroad and Amnesty International.

Community Aid Abroad

Community Aid Abroad is a voluntary organisation that works with disadvantaged communities, both within Australia (Aboriginal and Torres Strait Islander people) and overseas.

Community Aid Abroad aims to support communities in dealing with their immediate problems, while also addressing the underlying causes of inequality and powerlessness. It therefore aims to eliminate poverty and achieve social justice and environmental sustainability.

Community Aid Abroad is affiliated with Oxfam International

Amnesty International

Amnesty International is a worldwide movement of people who work through international action to prevent some of the most serious human rights violations by governments and other political groups.

Amnesty International campaigns:
- to free all 'prisoners of conscience' - people imprisoned for their beliefs or because of their colour, sex, ethnic origin, language or religion — provided they have neither used nor advocated violence;
- to ensure prompt trials for political prisoners;
- to end torture, 'disappearances', political killings and executions;
- to promote the protection of human rights generally.

World, as public opinion and public policy make them less acceptable in industrialised countries (Chapman & Wong 1990).

Australians cannot afford to concentrate on improving the health of Australians out of context of the experiences of other countries of the world. Unfortunately, most industrialised nations are focusing on health within their borders without considering the consequences of their actions in other countries of the world. Baum and Sanders (1995) have criticised this 'health in one nation' approach for undermining the very foundations of the Health for All movement.

In addition, industrialised countries consume significantly more than their fair share of the world's resources. The consequences are being felt not just in the health of people living in developing countries, but also in the health of the planet. The health of human individuals and groups cannot be considered in isolation from the physical environments in which they live, and the increasing damage to the environment is putting human health, and that of other species, at considerable risk (McMichael 1993). The definition of health as 'a sustainable state of wellbeing, within sustainable ecosystems, within a sustainable biosphere' (Honari 1993, p. 23) discussed above attempts to deal with the interrelationship between people and the physical environment but, of course, much more than definitions are required. The 1992 Earth Summit held in Rio de Janeiro was an attempt to commit the world community to environmental responsibility, but commitment is low and change will remain slow as long as sustainability requires more responsible consumption, and therefore reduction in profits.

While attempts to provide an actual definition of world health may raise many questions, it is clear that the concept of world or planetary health must be based on some recognition of the importance of respect and equity between countries and the importance of sustainable development for planetary survival.

What creates health?

As a result of the dominance of the biomedical model, there is a widespread assumption that ill-health is largely the result of individual lifestyle choices, microorganisms and other biological processes. However, individual biology is but one influence on health. If we are to deal effectively with health problems, we have to base action on a more comprehensive understanding of the factors that result in ill-health and the processes that create health. This requires us to focus attention on the social and environmental factors that promote health. Of central importance here is the role of social justice.

A case for social justice

Internationally, it has long been recognised that poverty is the single biggest determinant of ill-health. For millions of people around the world, in developing and industrialised countries alike, lack of access to sufficient basic resources is a direct cause of illness, poor quality of life, and death.

What is also becoming clear is that relative poverty is a significant determinant of ill-health. That is, inequity, or lack of access to a fair share of the available resources, is increasingly being recognised as a major cause of ill-health. Several major studies from around the world have demonstrated that, even in countries of relative wealth, people with lower socioeconomic status have significantly higher death and illness rates than those further up the socioeconomic spectrum (Wilkinson 1996).

Equally important is that the strength of this link between socioeconomic status and health varies according to the degree of differences in income between people of differing socioeconomic status. Several important studies have identified recently that countries with higher levels of equality in income distribution have higher life expectancy (Wilkinson 1996). This seems to be the case both in countries that are relatively poor and in those that are well off. Kaplan et al. (1996) have identified that US States with greater inequality in income distribution have higher mortality rates, lower birth weight rates, higher crime rates, higher levels of expenditure on medical care and higher smoking and lower exercise rates than States with more equal income distribution. They identified that this association between poor health and income equality was also associated with poor unemployment, imprisonment, social services and education levels. This work highlights the significant impact that inequality and the conditions that encourage it have on health, even in conditions of relative affluence.

Similarly, there are some significant examples from relatively poor countries of how good health has been achieved in situations in which comparatively few resources are available. In all such situations, it is the equality in distribution of resources and the related commitment to the welfare of all members of society that explains the health of the people (Beaglehole & Bonita 1997).

It is important to note that this effect of inequality in income distribution on health is not explained by effects on health caused by individual lifestyle factors such as smoking. Rather, the death rate pattern across groups with differing income levels seems far stronger than the effect of any individual risk factors for most diseases (Wilkinson 1996, pp. 26–7). Even for diseases regarded as strongly amenable to behavioural change, such as coronary heart disease, the impact of income inequality is strong.

The increasing disregard for social inequities and their impact on the lives of ordinary people seems to be a direct result of the growth of economic rationalism and the primacy of the economy. It is ironic, then, that Glyn and Miliband (1994) have identified that inequality affects more than the health of the population – it also affects the economic health of a society. Drawing together a wide range of research, they argue that social justice is actually good for a country's economy, and that inequalities in a society have detrimental effects on a country's economic growth. This flies in the face of much rhetoric arguing that countries need to accept inequality if they wish to succeed economically and have everyone benefit by a 'trickle down' process – it seems that the converse is the case. A review of several developing countries indicates that economic growth will not by itself improve health status in the developing world either (Beaglehole & Bonita 1997, p. 208).

This growing evidence of the impact of inequality on both individual health and the health and wellbeing of societies serves to highlight the importance of social justice to both the experience of individuals living in a society and the health and success of society as a whole. At a time when issues of equity and social justice seem to be increasingly out of favour with national governments and international agencies, this confirmation of the importance of social justice is extremely important. And, among other things, it serves to highlight and reconfirm the importance of the Primary Health Care approach.

What is health promotion?

Having briefly reviewed the issues of concern in any discussion of health, we are in a better position to consider what health promotion is. It is already clear that health promotion must relate not just to the health of individuals, but also to the health of groups and communities and the world, and that it must relate to more than the absence of medically defined problems. One popular definition that fits comfortably with the preceding discussion is that health promotion is:

*health education **and** related organisational, political and economic interventions that are designed to facilitate behavioural and environmental changes to improve health.*

(Green 1979, cited by Fisher et al. 1986, p. 96.)

This definition recognises the importance of health education in promoting health, but also acknowledges that health promotion is so much more than health education — it also requires structural changes on a number of levels to produce environments supportive of health. This is clearly a huge task and a political process.

The *Ottawa Charter for Health Promotion* recognises this approach to health promotion, as the discussion in the previous chapter demonstrates. It notes the central importance of increasing people's control over their health and issues that impact on it, and also notes the structural changes and community building required for that to be achieved.

The *Ottawa Charter for Health Promotion* defines health promotion as 'the process of enabling people to increase control over, and to improve, their health'. However, in essence the Ottawa Charter is itself a definition of health promotion much broader than that captured in the above definition, as the description of the five levels of action in the Ottawa Charter identified (see pp. 18–19 and Appendix 2, p. 267). In addition, health promotion has been identified as including three types of processes: 'a process of personal development towards health; a process of organisational development towards health; and a process of political development towards health' (Kickbusch 1997, p. 5)

In considering health promotion action, Labonte (1989c, p. 236) urges us to ask the question 'exactly what is a health problem, and who gets to define it?'. He argues that issues defined by communities as health problems should be regarded as such, and should therefore be the work of health promotion.

A question often raised is whether there is any difference between health promotion and disease prevention. Certainly many people seem to assume that they are the same thing. People may talk about health promotion, but all their activities may be in the area of disease prevention. Some people even talk solely of 'prevention', while others talk mistakenly of 'health prevention'. This distinction between health promotion and disease prevention is worth examining.

Disease prevention has been described as occurring on three levels. Primary disease prevention refers to activities designed to eradicate health risks, such as immunisation programs. Secondary disease prevention refers to activities that lead to early diagnosis of disease, such as bowel cancer screening. Tertiary disease prevention refers to rehabilitation work that helps people to recover from illness. While primary, secondary and tertiary disease prevention make an important contribution to health care overall, clearly they do not encapsulate health promotion as it has been developed through the *Ottawa Charter for Health Promotion*. Rather, disease prevention tends to focus on activities that prevent particular diseases, and is therefore very specific to illness and disease. More often than not, disease prevention focuses on alleviating symptoms, reducing risk factors and changing individual behaviours.

Health promotion incorporates disease prevention but extends beyond it to address broader issues impacting on health. Brown (1985, p. 332) suggests the development of a health promotion framework to complement that of disease prevention. This is extremely important because it helps to make visible the broad aspects of health promotion ignored by disease prevention. In this schema, primary health promotion refers to activities that eradicate health risks; secondary health promotion refers to activities that improve people's quality of life; and tertiary health promotion refers to activities that result in social changes conducive to health. The relationship between disease prevention and health promotion is demonstrated in Figure 2.1.

There is a real danger, however, that discussions of health promotion and disease prevention may excessively simplify any differences between the two. Perhaps more important than whether an activity is aimed at preventing disease or promoting health is whether the approach which is taken is reductionist or holistic. Both specific disease prevention or more general health promotion can be carried out in a way that is either simplistic and focuses on superficial change, or holistic and addresses the problem on a number of levels. For example, recent work in the area of smoking prevention has highlighted the political dimension of Australian and Third World tobacco sales and attempted to address these issues. On another level, attempts have been made to break the social acceptability of smoking by severing the ties between smoking and culture, sport and success (see 'The Victorian Health Promotion Foundation', p. 139, and 'Tobacco sponsorship

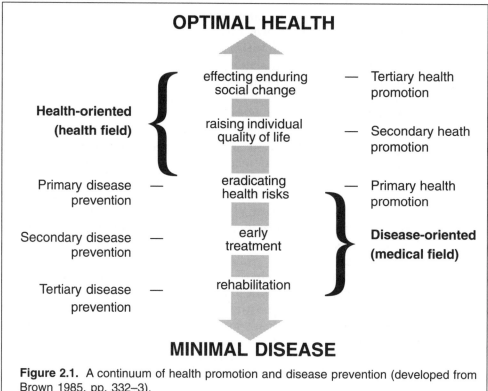

Figure 2.1. A continuum of health promotion and disease prevention (developed from Brown 1985, pp. 332–3).

replacement at the local level — a success story', pp. 186–8). Such activity challenges the profit base of tobacco companies and their role in Australian society.

Similarly, some work has been done to raise awareness of the control of the international agriculture and food industries by a small number of multinational companies. Steps have also been taken to address issues of improving nutrition by working to increase the availability of healthy food and challenge the advertising of manufactured, largely unhealthy food, rather than focusing solely on educating individuals about how to choose a healthy diet. These, then, represent broad approaches to what can be regarded as 'disease prevention' issues and demonstrate that defining an activity as disease prevention or health promotion will not by itself identify whether that activity is comprehensive or narrowly focused.

The aim of health education: compliance or empowerment?

As the definition of health promotion presented above demonstrates, health education is an integral part of health promotion. Indeed, education plays a central role in health promotion because it is not only a part of work for individual behaviour change or values clarification, but it also plays a vital role in any public policy or environmental changes, since as often as possible these should be made with the informed consent of the community, rather than imposed on it (Green & Kreuter 1991, p. 14). Having recognised the central role of health education in health promotion, we need also to examine what the aim of any health education should be. Are we aiming to have people comply with the wishes of professionals, or are we aiming to empower people to make their own informed decisions?

Compliance with the wishes of professionals appears to be the reason for a great deal of early health education, and many people continue with this aim in mind. But health education designed with this in mind does little to empower people and much to disempower them: it keeps control with the health workers rather than the people themselves. While there may be times when this is unavoidable, on the whole workers need to ensure that it does not happen unnecessarily, and that, through education, people are able to have greater control over the things that influence their lives. If people are to keep or gain control over their lives, education needs to be an enabling or liberating force. This idea has been developed by Paulo Freire (1973), who first developed the concept of empowerment education.

The line between education as compliance and education as empowerment is not always clear-cut. If we are educating people in order to empower them, are we not expecting them to comply with our wishes and empower themselves? And can we ever be sure that in presenting all sides of an issue our own biases are not reflected in how we present the argument and the emphasis we place on different points? Determining the extent to which we are working for compliance rather than empowerment is something that all health educators must do in order to evaluate the way in which they practise and to further develop their approach so that they are working for and with people rather than on them.

Attitudes of health workers towards community members

The approach health workers take towards the people they are employed to work for can have quite a marked impact on the way in which health promotion is achieved and how community members feel about the experience. A health worker's approach will influence how controlling or supportive they are of community members. It can therefore stifle or encourage the development of skills that will allow people to work more effectively for what they need in the future.

The authoritarian approach

People with an authoritarian approach believe that the experts and power holders know best, and are right in imposing their decisions on their 'target', whether this is an individual, a group or a community. They believe that, because of their expertise and status in the community, they do not need to involve community members in the decision-making process.

The paternalistic approach

The paternalistic approach is very similar to the authoritarian approach except that decision makers believe it is important to consult with the community. However, there is a strong sense of the decision makers being wiser than the community, and if people's wishes do not match professional opinion, it is assumed that they do not understand, and so efforts are made to explain the decision makers' views before they are imposed.

The partnership approach

In the partnership approach, it is assumed that members of the community have a great deal of expertise regarding their own lives and the issues of concern to them. Workers therefore involve community members actively in the decision-making and implementation process, so that instead of merely being consulted, community members become joint decision makers. Generally, people who use this approach believe that the process of involving community members in the decision making is just as important as the actual decision made. They also believe that the decision made is likely to be more valuable because of the involvement of the people themselves in the process. Workers are regarded as having expertise in their particular field, rather than expertise in all aspects of their clients' lives.

Participation

The importance of community participation in all stages of planning, implementing and evaluating policies and services that impact on health is recognised in the *Declaration of Alma-Ata,* the *Ottawa Charter for Health Promotion,* and the *Jakarta Decalaration on Leading Health Promotion into the 21st Century.* Indeed, community participation has been described as 'the heart of primary health care' (Ahmed 1980, cited in Rifkin 1986, p. 240). Since the development of the Health for All movement, community participation has been increasingly reflected in the rhetoric of health policy documents. Health workers are being urged to incorporate participation strategies into their practice.

The importance of community participation has been recognised both for the process of participation and the outcome of that participation. Through the process of meaningful participation, people can gain a sense of confidence in their ability to work for change in the world around them. At the same time, this participation enables people to develop a wide range of skills in such areas as working effectively with groups, organisation, negotiation, submission writing and working with the mass media. The confidence and improved skills developed through this process then also increase these people's ability to work effectively for change on future issues.

However, the notion of participation is not simple or value-free. Rather, community participation is often regarded in a rather romantic manner. 'The idea of citizen participation is a little like eating spinach: no one is against it in principle because it is good for you' (Arnstein 1971, p. 71). However, in many instances community participation may be used more to control people than to encourage empowerment. Decisions about what types of participation are relevant in a particular situation are not necessarily straightforward, but are important. If there are no opportunities for people to participate in the decisions which affect them, they are likely to feel disenfranchised and powerless. If, however, too much participation is expected or people are required to participate in order to obtain access to health care or other services, they are equally likely to feel powerless and the participation may feel like manipulation. It may also give the impression that the 'cost' of health related services is compulsory participation in the development of those services. Such an approach can be tantamount to victim- or community-blaming for disadvantaged communities (see pp. 62–3).

Health workers therefore have a fine line to walk in providing opportunities for participation by community members, to make those opportunities meaningful and appropriate, and to get on and do the job themselves when that is what is required. Some discussion of the different approaches to participation is therefore valuable.

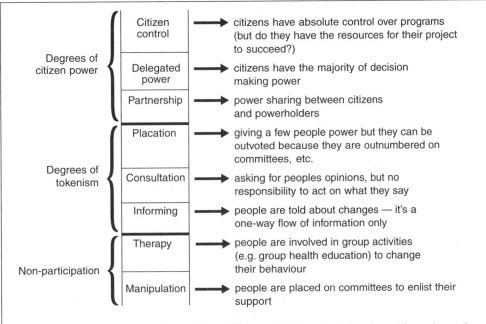

Figure 2.2. Eight rungs on the ladder of Citizen Participation (developed from Arnstein 1971, p. 70).

Sherry Arnstein (1971) has suggested that there are at least eight types of participation, ranging from forms of manipulation and co-option through to shared decision-making power. It is worthwhile examining her 'Ladder of Citizen Participation' (Figure 2.2) because it provides quite a useful framework for the forms of participation that can operate. Although other models of participation exist, Arnstein's provides the most useful one for the purposes of this discussion, and will be used throughout this book.

Arnstein describes two froms of community participation as 'non-participation', because they involve either placing people on committees in order to gain their support ('manipulation') or because they are seen as opportunities to change people's behaviour rather than give them any involvement in decision making ('therapy'). 'Informing', 'consultation' and 'placation' are described as forms of tokenism because, while people may be heard, there is no guarantee that their ideas will be acted upon, because they have no power. It is only at the levels of 'partnership' and above that people have decision-making power. There is 'delegated power' when citizens have most of the decision-making power, while with 'citizen control' citizens have total control (Arnstein 1971, p. 73). Using Arnstein's ladder as an analytical tool, it is possible to see that a great many instances of participation are actually non-participation or tokenism and few cases of participation actually result in shared power or power being handed over to community members. However, it is this power sharing that we are aiming for in a Primary Health Care approach. In many instances, power sharing will result only from the decentralisation of decision making.

However, Baum (1998, pp. 322–5) urges us not to assume that shared decision-making power is the only form of participation that is worthwhile. There may be times, for example, when consultation with a community is a valuable exercise that increases the relevance of the activity being developed. Clearly, community members cannot be partners on every health-related decision, and providing opportunities to hear their views may still be valuable. What is important is not to 'dress up' lower levels of participation as shared decision making, and to work for real shared decision making wherever possible.

Rifkin (1986, p. 246) suggests three questions that we can ask about participation to determine the extent to which it is likely to strengthen or deny people's access to power in any one instance. They are 'Why participation?', 'Who participates?' and 'How do they participate?'.

Why participation?

There are several reasons why participation by members of the community may be encouraged by health workers, although not all of these may actually benefit those being encouraged to participate. Before we start working to increase people's participation, we need to clarify just why we want them to participate. What approach do we take to participation, and are we intending to empower people through their participation or have them support our own ideas for health improvement?

Not all reasons for encouraging participation are driven by a recognition of the value of community members' contribution. People may be made to feel that they are playing an important role even when their ideas are not being given serious consideration, in the hope that the feeling of involvement will 'make them feel better'. People may be encouraged to participate because of the likely health benefits of the participation itself, rather than a belief in the value of what they may contribute. For example, members of a local support group may be permitted to have a representative on a committee looking at mental health services in the region, but this may be because it is considered to be 'good for' the members of the support group, and no real heed is taken of their opinions and ideas. This, then, is a fairly manipulative use of participation.

Participation may also be used to 'buy' people's acceptance of a preplanned change. There is evidence that people are less likely to resist a change if they have contributed to its development. Thus, in some instances, people may be encouraged to participate, not because their ideas are highly regarded and will be implemented, but because it is hoped that their involvement will prevent them from complaining about the final result. These reasons for encouraging participation are clearly in parallel with the lower levels of Arnstein's ladder of citizen participation.

However, in the Primary Health Care approach, participation is encouraged out of recognition that community members bring their own perspective and their own expertise to issues, and these may contribute a great deal more to the quality of decisions than if decisions are made by health workers alone. There is also growing evidence that this participation may itself be directly beneficial to health when it results in empowerment of community members (Wallerstein 1992).

Who participates?

In the Primary Health Care approach to health promotion, the short answer to this question is 'as many people as possible'. However, it is of particular importance to make sure that everyone has the opportunity to participate, not just the most articulate. This may mean that it is particularly important to ensure that people for whom services are supposedly planned have real opportunities for participation in decision making. Examination of participation processes to see exactly who is involved provides an opportunity to consider which avenues for participation currently exist and whether they are enabling people to participate fully.

How do they participate?

In 1989, Dwyer (1989, pp. 60–1) outlined five forms of participation in common use in Australia. They were client feedback and evaluation, voluntarism, consultation and public discussion, representative structures, and advocacy and public debate. These remain the main models of participation, although many health workers have been working at the local level to adapt them to suit particular situations, providing opportunities for community members or consumers to participate more fully in issues of concern to them. In recent years, some of the more active forms of participation have become less popular with government, challenging health workers to come up with more innovative ways of ensuring that community members have meaningful opportunities to participate.

Client feedback and evaluation

The most basic form of participation is client feedback and evaluation, which occurs when clients are asked for their opinions on how effective a service or policy is. On the basis of their responses, changes may or may not be made. The extent to which the feedback received is useful will depend in part on what feedback is sought and how it is sought.

Voluntarism

Voluntarism means that community members are actively involved in the running of a service, but as volunteers. The extent to which this includes input into how things are done varies greatly between agencies. The value of volunteerism is a matter of contention. On the one hand it can be used as a form of free labour, while on the other hand it is an opportunity for volunteers to develop skills and contribute their own expertise. It is also often used as a mechanism to change the system so that it better meets the needs of its users. Self-help groups provide some examples of how this may be done. Voluntarism has been used successfully in a number of areas, for example, the women's health movement. However, health workers working with volunteers should be mindful of the potential for exploitation and should reflect critically on their own relationships with volunteers.

Consultation and public discussion

It is argued that all members of Australian society have the right to respond to calls for public discussion on issues of relevance to them. Government departments advertise in the major Australian newspapers when they call for public comment on draft policy documents and the opportunity to respond and therefore participate in the policy-making process is open to everyone. However, not everyone has the confidence or the skills to respond to such opportunities, and the fact that calls for public response are often published only once, and only in the more prestigious newspapers in each State, means that this avenue for public participation is not as available to all community members as it might at first appear. Further development of this approach, so that it becomes more universally accessible, is needed.

Representative structures

Involving people in the management of a particular service can be very valuable because the quality of the resulting service may better meet the needs of its consumers if potential consumers are among those on the management committee. Management committees responsible for the day-to-day running of centres such as refuges, Aboriginal medical services, community health centres and women's health centres are said to enable their members to contribute quite closely to the way in which services are delivered.

In reality, however, because of the way many of these organisations are funded, committee members may find that they become caught up in the responsibilities of administrative work and have little opportunity to seriously affect the direction the organisation is taking or make an impact on public policy relevant to their areas of concern. People on management committees may have responsibility without the corresponding authority to influence the direction the service or its guiding policies take, and may find little scope to implement any innovative ideas they have. That said, community-controlled services, such as community-controlled Aboriginal health services, are often very responsive to the needs of the community they are serving and provide an excellent model that could be better incorporated into the health system.

Because of these shortcomings of the management committee approach, people may be unwilling to commit themselves to a management committee, be unable to attend enough committee meetings to affect the direction that the organisation takes, or be 'burnt out' by the work required of management committee members before they have been able to implement their ideas for improving the service. For these reasons, establishing an advisory committee may be very worthwhile. Such a committee can act in the same way as a management committee, except that it does not have responsibility for administrative management of the service. It may focus on establishing and implementing policy for the service, strategic planning and development of any new ideas, and response to public feedback. In this way, members are able to focus their energies on the elements of the service with which they want to be involved. This approach is likely to work best if the advisory committee has the authority to decide on the matters it discusses, rather than simply advising another committee which may or may not take its advice.

One way in which this idea has been implemented in recent years has been through the establishment of community advisory bodies that take up this role at district or regional level. District Health Councils in Victoria, Health and Social Welfare Councils in South Australia and District Health Forums in Tasmania provided structures through which community members are able to influence the direction of local health care and encourage an emphasis on equity and a broad approach to health (National Health Strategy 1993a, pp. 59–62). They provide a useful model for community control of health care direction, although to be effective they need to be representative of the community and, as mentioned above, they do need some power to have their decisions acted upon if they are to make an impact.

Unfortunately, Australian governments have moved away from this model in recent years. With the influence of economic rationalism, and extension of managerialism throughout the health and social service sectors, both the District Health Councils and the Health and Social Welfare Councils were dismantled, despite positive evaluation (Sanderson & Baum 1995). Despite rhetoric of consumer centredness, managerialism has seen a significant shift away from community participation. Some commentators argue that this is because corporatism, in which business interests rule unfettered, is actually anti-democratic (Saul 1997). This would help explain why participatory structures are being dismantled without reason, at the same time that participatory rhetoric is being used.

Advocacy and public debate

Relatively powerful representatives of groups can lobby for changes on their behalf, usually involving them in the process. The Office for the Status of Women is one example of this approach. Similarly, a number of smaller groups can join together to form an umbrella group under which they lobby together, pressuring the system to change. The Consumers' Health Forum of Australia is one such group. It is a national health consumer organisation that any consumer group with an interest in health issues can join. Its aim is to increase the voice of consumers and community members in the health-policy-making process. The Australian Council of Social Services (ACOSS) is another such group. In addition, many individual organisations, such as the Public Health Association of Australia, take up opportunities to advocate for issues and encourage public debate.

Encouraging effective participation

If health workers are to enable effective community participation, there are at least three complementary approaches worth taking. Firstly, we need to develop a culture of community participation in organisations, which supports and encourages meaningful community participation. Secondly, we need to establish participatory structures, which institutionalise effective participation in decision-making processes. Thirdly, we need to develop and implement a range of participation strategies so that people may participate in a way that suits them (Wass 1995). Auer et al. (1993) have developed a set of 11 keys to effective community participation that capture these three approaches (see below).

Dwyer (1989, p. 62) suggests three prerequisites for effective community participation. These are skills and resources, power sharing and appropriate agendas.

Skills and resources

In many respects, community members are not adequately prepared to participate effectively. Although Australia is regarded as a democratic society, we do not learn that we should actively participate or how we should do it. Therefore, if people are to be encouraged to participate, they need to be provided with an opportunity to develop the skills and resources they will need. One program, which was developed for use in Victoria, South Australia and Tasmania and is

---

Keys to effective participation

- Organisational policy which makes clear commitment to community participation, providing guidelines for both staff and community members on exactly what kind of participation and power sharing is supported;
- Organisational structures which include continuing community input and facilitate autonomous decision making at the local level;
- Management, staff and community commitment to processes which respect and encourage community input;
- Recognition that the agenda of consumer and community groups may not always be the same as that of the agency;
- Commitment of resources (financial, human and material) to encourage and support community participation;
- Long time lines during consultation processes, so that participation for community members can be meaningful;
- Use of clear, everyday language that does not exclude ordinary people;
- True support from staff and recognition of the positive outcomes of handing over power to community members;
- Training, which includes exploration of values and development of shared goals, for managers, staff and community members;
- 'A critical mass of enthusiastic people' to enable community participation to be an ongoing process;
- Appropriate means of evaluating the effectiveness of community participation

(Auer et al 1993, pp. 98–102).

now a national program, attempts to prepare people to participate more effectively in the health system. Known as 'Talking Better Health', it outlines a process through which health workers can enable participants to reflect critically on their experiences with the health system and identify how they can work to improve these (Commonwealth Department of Human Services and Health 1994).

Power sharing

Unless people feel that they are likely to have an impact, they may decide that it is not worth the effort of trying to participate. Organisations that decide they want to encourage participation must therefore decide to prevent manipulative tactics that exclude community members from effective decision making and to instigate affirmative action techniques in meetings and decision making so that all participants have a fair say. Otherwise, only those people who are most comfortable with meeting procedure, and are therefore the most dominant within the group, may have their voices heard and their ideas acted upon. As Sherry Arnstein (1971, p. 72) has said, 'participation without redistribution of power is an empty and frustrating process for the powerless'.

Appropriate agendas

If people are going to participate, then obviously the agendas of the organisations concerned must be relevant to them. This has an added advantage: if organisations adjust their agendas so that they are more relevant to the community and people are therefore more willing to participate, it is likely that their activities will more effectively meet the needs of their community. Consequently, organisations are made increasingly accountable to the public, which goes hand in hand with the power sharing discussed above.

It is quite apparent that the five forms of participation described above may be put into effect more often than they currently are, as do the three prerequisites for community participation. We also need to establish more effective participation and decision-making processes if we are to enable people to participate meaningfully in the decisions that affect their lives. Health workers are currently endeavouring to develop more innovative participation strategies, and you may be able to develop some yourselves.

Responsibility for health and the problem of victim blaming

The key impetus for the recent encouragement of community participation in Primary Health Care and health promotion has been the *Declaration of Alma-Ata's* call for action 'in the spirit of self-reliance'. Encouraging people to take responsibility for their own health, both individually and at the levels of the community and the country, is part of the Primary Health Care approach.

Encouraging people to take responsibility for their own health on an individual level has been gaining momentum as part of health promotion strategies since the 1970s. As the relationships between individual behaviours and illness were identified, calls for change in individual behaviour became more and more popular as an increasing number of diseases were labelled as lifestyle diseases. This recognition of the impact that individual behaviours have on health, and the role individuals have in influencing their health, is important.

Being a community representative

In the South Australian Mallee community where I live, there has always been a need for volunteers, especially in the health and welfare fields. I have always had an interest in health and welfare and started off years ago on the local hospital auxiliary and board. I also gained valuable insights into the needs in, and workings of, the mental health field through confrontation with the system about the welfare of my own son. A number of opportunities and challenges have arisen over the last few years and I am now representing consumers at regional, State and national levels.

Consumers have a right to participate in decision-making processes that may ultimately affect their health and wellbeing. They are the people who really count, but their voice is too often not heard, and their comments are quite often not taken seriously or accepted other than at the level of a token gesture.

I feel that consumer representatives have a really important role to play. They have the opportunity to put forward the 'grass roots' issues and concerns, but they must have a mandate to ensure that documents, vision statements, workshop reports and implementation plans reflect lay needs, and in terminology that can be understood by consumers.

Their voice acts as a balance to the views of government and professionals. To enable this to happen, information and sufficient time must be made available to allow consumers to participate in whatever arena they are placed. There must be continuing opportunities for consumer input and there must be structures and support systems in place to enable community members to continue in these roles, including assistance with research and with dissemination of information to other consumers and community groups. In addition, consumer representatives cannot be expected to give, and have to pay to give, hence they also need to be given allowances, for travel and child care, for example, especially in rural areas.

Consumer participation has the potential to bring consumer issues to the forefront and improve quality of life for community members. If it is to achieve this, though, this participation must result in change, not just keep consumer representatives busy.

What being a consumer representative has meant to me

Being a consumer representative means making a big commitment. In my case it has meant spending many hours on the road travelling to various towns and centres and therefore time and energy have to be accounted for as well. One needs to have an understanding and supportive family, otherwise problems could occur.

There have been times when I have felt very alone, particularly when the support mechanisms are not there. I have had to acknowledge that in the area of community representation one is often left to 'fight it alone', and I have had to work to make sure that it doesn't floor me.

I have also gained a lot from being a consumer representative, and I would like to share some of the gains, hopefully to assist and encourage other people to participate. The positives of being a consumer representative have included:

- The building up of one's self-esteem (especially if one hasn't worked for quite a while) allows one to feel confident enough to step out into the public forum.
- Acceptance of the consumer voice by Australia-wide professionals and service providers, through chances for input at policy, planning and implementation levels, is a definite plus.
- Being given the opportunity to represent rural and remote consumers on State and National committees and organisations.
- Continuing to network with other consumers and service providers is important in the learning process about the 'who and where' of seeking

assistance and action. The recognition that true partnerships between
health professionals and consumers are needed is encouraging.
- The opportunities to present the views, issues and needs of rural and
  remote consumers has increased in recent years and this is just wonderful.
  I am very proud to be a volunteer representative. All those hours of
  travelling, and communicating via phone and fax are starting to bring
  about change and acceptance of the consumer voice.
- Meeting some very genuine and warm people in my travels.

Yes, I enjoy what I do!

Margaret Brown
Chairperson, Health Consumers of Rural and Remote Australia Inc.

However, individuals live their lives in a social context and there are many
barriers that may constrain the choices they are able to make. As the previous
discussion points out, a great many of the determinants of health are the result of
the social, economic and political structures in which people live their lives. There
are some real dangers, therefore, in focusing only on the role of individual
behaviours in disease. People may be blamed for ill-health, and for some of the
determinants of ill-health, when they do not have control over the factors affecting
their health or the freedom to make healthy choices. This has become known as
blaming the victim.

Blaming the victim occurs when the structural causes of ill-health are ignored
and attention is focused on the individual or individuals affected by the problem,
with the aim of changing their behaviour (Crawford 1977). Victim blaming is a
subtle process. Ryan (1976, p. 8) has described it as 'cloaked in kindness and
concern'. It occurs not only when people fail to see the structural causes of
deprivation and ill-health, but also when they see them but still seek to solve the
problem by working to change the individual (Ryan 1976, pp. 8–9).

One of the real strengths of the *Ottawa Charter for Health Promotion's* five-
pronged approach to health promotion action is that it minimises the chance of
victim blaming occurring: if health promotion action occurs at the level of working
for healthier public policy as well as at the level of further developing the skills of
the individual, the structural barriers to ill-health are likely to be addressed. It is
vital, therefore, that the broad approach to health promotion action described in the
Ottawa Charter for Health Promotion is not watered down to the point where structural action disappears and is replaced by more action at the level of the individual.

Victim blaming does not happen only at the level of the individual. With a
focus on community development and community-based action, when many
problems stem from national or international issues, there is a danger that
disadvantaged communities may be blamed if they are unable to pick themselves
up by their bootstraps (Labonté 1989a, p. 88).

The issues surrounding individual responsibility for health versus social
responsibility for health are complex and interrelated. It is not a case of choosing
one over the other, but of what balance there is between the two. Unfortunately,
because they have come to represent opposing philosophical viewpoints, many
discussions present them as opposite to each other, which does not help individual

workers clarify how they will address health issues and assist individuals in making changes in their lives. Health workers may need to clarify for themselves how to work with the tension between these two aspects of health promotion, to be aware of their biases, and to keep clear in their minds how both aspects of a problem need to be addressed in whatever balance is appropriate for the issue in question.

The influence of labelling

The concept of labelling is very much related to the notion of victim blaming. Our response to issues and problems that arise may well be influenced by our beliefs and expectations about particular groups of people, stages of life or illness experiences. The stereotyping or labelling of people, often because of their ethnicity, gender, age or socioeconomic status, can have a powerful impact on the way in which they are treated. For example, an older person who suffers pain when walking may be told that it is just part of getting old and is to be tolerated, while a younger person may not be treated in the same way. Similarly, stories of the development of labels such as 'Mediterranean back' demonstrate that health workers do not always respond to a migrant working in a factory who develops back pain in the same way as they respond to non-migrants with a similar problem, and stereotypical responses to women suffering with depression has resulted in over-prescription of addictive, so-called 'minor' tranquillisers. Many such stories demonstrate the assumptions people may make about the behaviour of others and their underlying motives. The consequences of this labelling may be very disempowering.

Similarly, there have been recent examples in Australia of disadvantaged communities complaining of the way in which they are regularly victimised, particularly through the mass media. Such communities want to be recognised for their strengths as well as their needs. Constantly being depicted in a negative light results in these communities experiencing the negative consequences of labelling, while the positive qualities and resources of these communities are denied. The resultant disempowerment itself becomes a major health problem for the community.

Working with people from other cultures

It is not surprising that health workers may spend much of their time working with people from cultures different from their own, given the diversity of backgrounds from which Australians come. Indeed, work to improve the health of people from non-Anglo cultures is a high priority for many health workers because of the poor health of many Aboriginal people and Australian immigrants and the fact that these groups tend to be over-represented among those living in poverty, and so are at risk of experiencing health problems. We therefore need to consider some of the general principles guiding work with people from different cultures, given the important role that culture plays in determining values and meanings. You are encouraged to read further on this topic if you have not already examined it in some depth (see, e.g. Eckermann et al. 1992; Pauwels 1995; Reid & Trompf 1990, 1991).

As discussed previously, the notion of working in partnership with people is central to the Primary Health Care approach. This partnership approach really comes to the fore when working with people from cultures different from your own because the expertise they bring in relation to the norms and values of their own culture is vital to the communication process and the promotion of health. However, this awareness of the norms and values of the culture with which we identify does not come automatically to health workers or community members. Culture develops within a social, political and historical context and expresses a group's preferred ways of thinking about the world. These world views permeate all social structures, and are reflected in the policies and procedures that govern the system itself. 'Culture presents a way of perceiving, behaving and evaluating one's world. It provides the blueprint or guide for determining one's values, beliefs and practices' (Boyle & Andrew 1989, pp. 11–12). It defines relationships and roles within society, by describing rights and obligations. In some instances, culture constrains individual behaviour, while in others it results in shared meanings and understandings, leaving room for the beliefs and interpretations of individuals. As a result, the culture of a society, community or group is integrated into the daily lives of individuals and groups, and is largely hidden from our awareness.

The interrelationship between culture and history is reflected in the fact that the shared meanings that make up a culture have often developed from the history of that cultural group. While some of that history may be in the distant past, other history may be relatively recent and very alive for the people concerned. The history of European treatment of Aboriginal people in Australia is a stark example of this point, and this history may be very present in determining attitudes, including wariness of mainstream health systems and wariness or stereotypical behaviour in Aboriginal–non-Aboriginal communication (Eckermann et al. 1992, p. 156).

Because culturally driven beliefs and practices are so unconscious, we are often unable, unless we make a conscious effort, to recognise the culturally influenced values and behaviours we portray to others. Furthermore, because our own culture is so familiar to us, we tend to believe that the way we think, act and judge our world is shared by all others, and tend to judge unfavourably others who do not portray similar values, assuming that ours is the 'right' way. Our upbringing, our education and our own 'enculturation' make it difficult for us to reflect on and challenge notions that are considered common sense or traditional in our culture. If we are going to work effectively with others, we need to ensure that we reflect on those beliefs and values that we take for granted, so that we can respond effectively in the face of differing values.

Language plays a key role in transmitting and reproducing the dominant culture, and can be a major barrier to effective communication. This can be the case even when you are communicating in English with people from another culture, as meanings and nuances can be culture specific even when the same language is apparently being spoken. In addition, non-verbal communication is just as much culturally driven as verbal communication and so greater awareness of your own non-verbal communication and that of others is vital. Be mindful of the fact that other people's non-verbal communication may not mean what it appears to, and that your own non-verbal communication may be misinterpreted.

When people find they need to work with someone from another culture, their initial reaction is often to begin to find out about the other culture, and people usually attempt to do this by reading. Certainly, reading can be an important beginning, but it is by no means the only way to learn. Books and articles are a limited way of finding out about another culture. Firstly, they tend to portray a static picture of a culture, when in fact culture is dynamic and constantly changing. Secondly, because they provide little or no room to individualise cultural beliefs and interpretation, books present an image of a culture as uniformly shared by all its members. Just as members of your own culture vary widely in the acceptance of its values, so too do members of other cultures vary in their acceptance of the values of their particular culture. Thirdly, books often represent a very limited view of the cultures they discuss. For example, many anthropological accounts of cultures ignore women's roles, and present a one-sided picture of cultural life. Therefore, reading about other cultures may be useful, but your understanding will be strengthened by listening to the people themselves and coming to conclusions tentatively.

While the particular issues of relevance to communities may vary across communities and according to the issue at hand, issues that commonly vary across cultures and of which you may need to have an understanding are time orientation, personal space, the interrelationship between culture and religion, family practices (such as avoidance relationships), status rules according to gender and age, philosophies and beliefs about health and illness, and forms of non-verbal communication.

Perhaps the most useful skill for a health worker working with people from other cultural backgrounds is sensitivity, including, but certainly not limited to, intercultural sensitivity. Intercultural sensitivity is built on a recognition of the value base of our own and others' cultures. It is reflected by preparedness to listen and to learn from those with whom you are working. Being culturally sensitive includes not attributing all difference to 'culture' as such, but recognising that there is scope within culture for individual difference. Indeed, there is as much variety and conflict within communities from other cultures as there is within communities generally. Being culturally sensitive therefore includes recognising the need to canvass the opinions of as many people as possible, rather than assuming that the opinions of one small group of people reflects the opinions of the community overall. This sensitivity to the people with whom you are working provides a basis on which trust can develop and effective communication can occur.

Miller identifies two important points for working with people from other cultures:

- *treat all facts you have ever heard or read about cultural values as hypotheses, to be tested anew with each [person]*

- *remember that people can be bicultural, or engaged in the process of integrating two value systems that are often in conflict.*

(1992, cited by Hopkins 1996, p. 5.)

Working with people from other cultures presents a challenge for a variety of reasons. The health problems they face are often quite urgent, and the challenges of intercultural communication quite strong. The challenges to their own values can also often present a personal challenge for health workers. Nonetheless, the principles of effective intercultural work provide important guidance for health workers, both for working with individuals and groups from other cultures and for working with individuals and groups from subcultures different from their own.

Vic Health struggles with political opposition

The promulgation of the Tobacco Act 1987 and the establishment of the Victorian Health Promotion Foundation was an excellent example of what can be done at a social level to work creatively for health promotion (see pp. 186–88). It also gave rise to several examples of the sort of opposition and political pressure that can surface when practices that are profit-making, but which have a negative impact on health, are challenged. In this case, the advertising practices of tobacco companies in Victoria were curtailed by legislation prohibiting advertising of tobacco products, an action that has since been replicated around Australia. The implications of this for tobacco company profits are clear.

In 1990 the Victorian government announced that under the Tobacco Act 1987, tobacco advertisements could not be displayed at the Phillip Island motorcycle races. This was a major challenge to the tobacco companies, and one which the Victorian government seemed determined to see through. However, as the tobacco company concerned was trying to have this decision overturned, the New South Wales government announced that it would allow the races to be held in New South Wales, tobacco advertising being no problem. As a result, Victoria now risked losing the races. As it was in some financial difficulty and the races were an income-generating event, the Victorian government was backed into a corner. In October 1990, the premier of Victoria announced Parliament's decision that the races were exempt from the Tobacco Act 1987.

In 1991, when the Victorians succeeded in winning the event back to Victoria, the New South Wales Minister for Sport, Recreation and Racing publicly denounced the Victorian government for backing off its 'moral high ground'. The minister in question seemed oblivious to the fact that it was the actions of the New South Wales government some 12 months earlier that had led to this situation. We can only speculate whether or not the Victorian government would have won its stand against the tobacco industry if the New South Wales government had not interceded.

Since then, other states have developed their own health promotion foundations, with some variation in how they operate. Considerable opposition continues to come from tobacco companies, through the Tobacco Institute of Australia, which sees 'the introduction of Health Promotion Foundations as destructive of the free market economy which we understood existed in Australia ... We're very concerned about the future' (J. Welch, Spokesperson, Tobacco Institute of Australia, ABC TV, 30 October 1991).

Dealing with opposing values and conflicts of interest

In many respects, how people view health and health promotion reflects their broader views on the way the world works. As a result, many of the issues underpinning discussions of health promotion reflect the world views that people hold. It is therefore not surprising that some of the issues raised by health promotion create conflict between people with opposing views; after all, the difference is often not simply about an issue itself but also about the underlying philosophical framework. This is particularly so where health promotion action challenges profit or power.

Conflict can also occur with industries whose work has a negative impact on health, and for which profit has a higher priority than health. Because health promotion in many instances directly challenges these industries, the conflicts created may be intense. It is therefore not surprising that conflict can be an inherent part of health promotion work. Health workers need to develop skills to deal positively with potential conflict situations so that conflict is not created unnecessarily, and to deal constructively with conflict should it arise. This requires effective communication and negotiation skills, and skills in assertive communication.

It is not suggested, however, that all communication in health promotion is adversarial. Effective communication with many individuals and groups is an important part of working for health promotion, and the greater part of this is, or can be, positive and collegial rather than confrontational.

Health promotion requires communication and joint action with individuals, health workers from a variety of backgrounds, workers from a range of other sectors (e.g. local council workers, teachers, police, environmental workers, and road safety workers) and community groups. Much of this communication can involve building bridges between people. It is very important that barriers not be created unnecessarily between groups and that people collaborate as much as possible.

Personal value conflicts in health promotion

Value conflicts in health promotion do not occur just at the level of conflicts between individuals or institutions. They can also occur within individual practitioners as they make choices and adopt priorities as part of their normal working lives. Different aspects of health promotion may compete for priority, and choices made to support one aspect of health promotion may result in a worker feeling uncomfortable about the implications of this choice for other aspects of health promotion. These value conflicts can occur regularly in health promotion work, and you need to be able to recognise them and reconcile them within yourself to continue working effectively in health promotion.

Similarly, as we change and our ideas develop through experience, it is quite possible that actions that seemed acceptable in the past no longer seem appropriate. However, the past cannot be changed, and health workers may have to come to terms with their previous decisions. Developing a set of professional ethics, based on the principles of Primary Health Care, can provide a foundation on which ethical decisions can be made.

Working with change: the costs of healthy choices

Although making healthy choices does not always result in conflict, it can sometimes result in groups or individuals feeling ostracised or left out of a group that is important to them. For example, people who have tried to give up smoking report that they lose opportunities to socialise with friends who are smokers. Similarly, people eating a healthy or restricted diet may find it difficult to eat in restaurants they might previously have gone to. There are often such costs when people make healthy choices. These costs need to be acknowledged and prepared for as much as possible. Unless action is taken to overcome any barriers created by the

Value conflicts: 'Life. Be in it with a cat'

As part of its ongoing 'Life. Be in it' program, the New South Wales Department of Sport, Recreation and Racing produced a television and radio campaign encouraging pet ownership. 'Life. Be in it with a cat' is one part of this program. Certainly the health effects of companionship from pets are now well recognised and 'pets as therapy' programs continue to blossom and report success. However, 'Life. Be in it with a cat' highlights the value conflicts that can arise between health promotion programs which develop as a result of a focus on different aspects of health. For at the same time as cat ownership is being encouraged through the 'Life. Be in it' program, we are becoming increasingly aware of the damage that feral cats are doing to our natural environment. Many native animals are extinct, or severely threatened, as a result of the activities of feral cats.

Cats do not need to be dumped and left to fend for themselves, however, to threaten Australian wildlife. The night-time hunting activities of domestic cats, no matter how well fed they are, is also severely threatening our wildlife. So, while cat ownership is being encouraged as a way of providing companionship and support for lonely people, it is also potentially very health damaging because of its impact on the fauna in our environment.

A more critical perspective on the 'Life. Be in it with a cat' and 'Life. Be in it with a dog' campaigns raises the question of why the government is encouraging this stopgap measure to address the loneliness and alienation of people within our society, rather than dealing more directly with the problem by working to encourage a greater sense of community and breaking down the oppressive structures that put barriers between people and lead to alienation.

The above example demonstrates that even within health promotion work, value conflicts arise and need to be dealt with by health workers almost on a daily basis, and that even seemingly innocuous programs can present value conflicts that need to be considered and addressed.

costs of these healthy choices, people may not be able to keep to their decision and may revert to the behaviour they had hoped to change.

For example, in 1992, the teachers at Quakers Hill Primary School made the decision, supported by parents, that school sport in the summer would be played only in the mornings, before 11 o'clock, in order to protect the children from the risks of skin cancer (Mulcahey 1992, personal communication). The cost of this was that the children were unable to play in summer competitions with children from other schools, as these competitions are held in the afternoons, when the power of the sun is at its strongest. If it had not been for the strong support this policy received from parents, the cost of this healthy choice might well have been too great, and the decision might have been reversed. Of course, other schools have since adopted similar policies, so barriers to such a stance have been significantly improved.

Weighing up the good of the community versus the rights of the individual

In the discussion so far, we have examined the importance of people being actively involved in deciding what they want and health workers acknowledging the expertise that people have in the issues that impact on their lives. Unfortunately, there are times when this principle alone cannot guide health workers in their judgments. In many situations there are competing interests at stake, and health workers must choose between the wishes of different individuals, as well as between the wishes of individuals and their own professional judgment about what is 'best' for the community. At such times, health workers who are attempting to work by the principles of empowerment and community participation may experience intense personal conflict.

One related question that needs to be asked here is, who decides what is for the good of the community, and on what basis? As the discussion has demonstrated, imposition of decisions from above is problematic, but it is not always practical or possible to involve the whole community in decision making and prepare them with all the necessary information so that they can make informed decisions. When is it acceptable for decisions to be made on behalf of the community? Do health workers have the right to manipulate the environment 'for the good of the community'? Should current manipulation of the environment (for example, by companies) be counteracted by health workers? When different parts of the community have conflicts of interest on particular issues, whose interests should take precedence? These are just some of the ethical questions raised by community-wide health promotion.

Balancing responses to health problems — health promotion and illness management

As discussed in Chapter 1, Primary Health Care and the new public health movement represent a move to shift the emphasis from illness management to health promotion. This move does not sit comfortably with everyone, and will necessitate some shifts in power. The multimillion dollar medico-industrial complex, in particular, is likely to be significantly challenged by a reorientation of our approach to health.

The shift from illness management to health promotion philosophy needs to occur on more than the individual level. The most important changes are those that need to occur at the level of the health system, and it is here that the notion of 'doing yourself out of a job' is most powerful. Currently, the Australian health care system is one of the biggest public sector employers in the country, employing around half a million people (Australian Institute of Health and Welfare 1996, cited by Fawkes 1997, p. 392). The impact of this system on other related industries also accounts for a great many workers. Vast resources in bureaucracies, infrastructure and industry are tied up in the delivery of illness care. With the increasing privatisation of health services in Australia, this focus on an illness industry is set to increase. If the system is to change its emphasis and work to 'do itself out a job', a dramatic change of focus is needed. Moreover, many conventional health workers may have built careers around illness management and are reliant on research funds and high-technology institutions for their livelihoods.

One of the biggest value shifts facing workers when they move from an illness management philosophy to a health promotion philosophy is in how they see themselves and their role. A common reason health workers give for enjoying their work is that they are 'needed'. Unfortunately, there is a real trap in this because, if we are really to care for those who are sick or whose health we are hoping to promote, we would hope for them that they do not need us — that they can live their lives to the full without outside interference, or in an interdependent relationship with those around them. After all, this is what we would hope for ourselves. If we really are working for health promotion, then we are working to do ourselves out of a job. Working to do yourself out of a job is not an easy thing to come to grips with, but without awareness that this is what we are trying to achieve we may be unconsciously encouraging people to be dependent on us rather than independent of us, and while this might make us feel better, it does little to really help those we are meant to be working for.

Belief in the primacy of the illness management system is not limited to health workers. Because it has been part of the dominant ideology, many people believe that science and medicine will come up with a medical solution to just about any problem. We have come to expect this and to see it as more important than the prevention of illness and the promotion of health. The mass media's use of individual emotive cases in which the State does not deliver theoretically available high-technology care, supports the expectation that it should always be available, no matter the cost. In few of these instances is the opportunity cost of high-technology care mentioned, even though there may be situations where spending money on social services will do more for the health of a community than the provision of acute medical care (Labonté 1990).

Promoting your own health

It is not possible to survive for very long as a health promoter if you do not ensure that you promote your own health at the same time. As obvious as this may sound, it is often very difficult to do. Firstly, it can be difficult to take time out when you are working on an issue that is of great importance to other people's lives. This can be particularly so for community work campaigns. Secondly, health as an issue is never neutral, and at times this can make health promotion work stressful. Nevertheless, it is a challenge we must take up. Indeed, Baum urges us to remember that conflict is an inherent part of health promotion work (1990a) and urges us to be 'troublemakers for health' if we want to really be successful in health promotion (1990b).

It is therefore up to all health workers or community members involved in health promotion to develop healthy strategies to look after themselves and to support other members of the team with whom they are working. Unless we look after ourselves and each other, our impact on health promotion will be short-lived and more limited than we had hoped for when we first decided to take up the challenge.

Conclusion

This chapter has examined directly some of the key issues and concepts in health promotion, to provide a framework on which the following chapters will build. The concept of health was reviewed, with particular attention paid to the fact that health is more than a physical state and an individual phenomenon. The notions of individual, family, community and world health, and their interrelationships, were explored. Emerging from this was the importance of the interactivity of human beings, reflected through both the positive effects of social capital and social support, and the negative effects of inequity in personal relationships or social environments.

This paves the way for a broad definition of health promotion, endorsed in the *Ottawa Charter for Health Promotion* and the *Jakarta Declaration on Leading Health Promotion into the 21st Century,* and numerous other policy statements as identified in Chapter one. Some of the common potential conflicts of values in health promotion were touched on. These issues are complex and there are no easy answers to many of the dilemmas raised. Many more arise in practice. As health promoters, you are urged to examine the questions raised in this chapter and to be mindful of their implications for health promotion practice as you review the range of health promotion issues and strategies throughout the remainder of this book.

References and further reading

Arnstein, S. 1971, 'Eight Rungs on the Ladder of Citizen Participation', in Cahn, E. S. and Passett, B. A. (eds), *Citizen participation: effecting community change,* Praeger Publishers, New York.

Auer, J., Repin, Y. and Roe, M. 1993, *Just Change: the Cost-Conscious Manager's Toolkit,* National Reference Centre for Continuing Education in Primary Health Care, University of Wollongong, Wollongong.

Australian Bureau of Statistics 1997, *Labor Force Status and Other Characteristics of Families,* ABS catalogue No. 6224.0, ABS, Canberra.

Baum, F. 1990a, 'The new public health: force for change or reaction?', *Health Promotion International,* 5 (2), 145–50.

Baum, F. 1990b, 'Troublemakers for health?', *In Touch,* 7 (1), 5–6.

Baum, F. 1998, *The New Public Health: an Australian Perspective,* Oxford University Press, Melbourne.

Baum, F. and Sanders, D. 1995, 'Can Health Promotion and Primary Health Care Achieve Health For All Without a Return to their More Radical Agenda?', *Health Promotion International,* 10 (2), 149–60.

Beaglehole, R. and Bonita, R. 1997, *Public Health at the Crossroads: Achievements and Prospects,* Cambridge University Press, Cambridge.

Becker, M. H. 1986. 'The Tyranny of Health Promotion', *Public Health Review,* 14, 15–25.

Benn, C. 1981, *Attacking Poverty through Participation: a Community Approach,* PIT Publishing, Melbourne.

Bennett, M. 1986, 'A Developmental Approach to Training for Intercultural Sensitivity', *International Journal of Intercultural Relations,* 10, 179–96.

Bittman, M. and Pixley, J. 1997, *The Double Life of the Family: Myth, Hope and Experience,* Allen and Unwin, St Leonards.

Blaxter, M. 1990, *Health and lifestyles,* Tavistock/Routledge, London and New York.

Bowling, A. 1997, *Research Methods in Health: Investigating Health and Health Services,* Open University Press, Buckingham.

Brown, V. 1985, 'Towards an Epidemiology of Health: a Basis for Planning Community Health Programs', *Health Policy,* 4, 331–40.

Bryson, L. and Mowbray, M. 1981, 'Community: the Spray-on Solution', *Australian Journal of Social Issues,* 16 (4), 225–67.

Carlyon, W. H. 1984, 'Disease Prevention/Health Promotion: Bridging the Gap to Wellness', *Health Values: Achieving High Level Wellness,* 8 (3), 27–30.

Chapman, S. and Wong, W. L. 1990, *Tobacco Control in the Third World: a Resource Atlas,* International Organization of Consumers' Unions, Penang, Malaysia.

Clark, D. B. 1973, 'The Concept of Community: a Re-examination, *The Sociological Review,* 21 (3), 397–415.

Commonwealth Department of Human Services and Health 1994, *Talking better health: A resource for community action,* Department of Human Services and Health, Canberra.

Cox, E. 1996, *A Truly Civil Society,* ABC Books, Sydney.

Crawford, R. 1977, 'You Are Dangerous to Your Health: the Ideology and Politics of Victim Blaming', *International Journal of Health Services,* 7 (4), 663–80.

Dalton and Dalton. 1975, *Community and its Relevance to Australian Society: an Examination of the Sociological Definition,* Australian Government Publishing Service, Canberra.

de Vries, M. J. 1993, 'A Theoretical Model for Healing Processes: Rediscovering the Dynamic Nature of Health and Disease', in LaFaille, R. and Fulder, S. (eds), *Towards a New Science of Health,* Routlege, London and New York.

Douglas, T. 1983, *Groups: Understanding People Gathered Together,* Tavistock, London.

Downie, R. S., Tannahill, C. and Tannahill, A. 1996, *Health Promotion: Models and Values,* Oxford University Press, Oxford.

Doxiadis, S. (ed.) 1987, *Ethical Dilemmas in Health Promotion,* John Wiley and Sons, Chichester.

Doxiadis, S. (ed.) 1990. *Ethics in Health Education,* John Wiley and Sons, New York.

Dwyer, J. 1989, 'The Politics of Participation', *Community Health Studies,* 13 (1), 59–65.

Eckermann, A. K., Dowd, T., Martin, M., Nixon, L., Gray, R. and Chong, E. 1992, *Binan Goonj: Bridging Cultures in Aboriginal Health,* Department of Aboriginal and Multicultural Studies, University of New England, Armidale.

Edgar, D. 1992, 'Changing Families in Changing Societies', *Family Matters,* 31, April, 3–4.

Eng, E., Salmon, M. E. and Mullan, F. 1992, 'Community Empowerment: the Critical Base for Primary Health Care', *Family and Community Health,* 15 (1), 1–12.

Evans, R. G., Hodge, M. and Pless, I. B. 1994, 'If Not Genetics, Then What? Biological Pathways and Population Health', in Evans, R. G., Barer, M. L. and Marmor, T. R. (eds), *Why Are Some People Healthy and Others Not?,* Aldine De Gruyter, New York.

Ewles, L. and Simnett, I. 1999, *Promoting Health: a Practical Guide,* Bailliere Tindall in association with the Royal College of Nursing, Edinburgh.

Fawkes, S. 1997, 'Aren't Health Services Already Promoting Health?' *Australian and New Zealand Journal of Public Health,* 21 (4), 391–7.

Ferguson, B. and Browne, E. (eds) 1991, *Health Care and Immigrants: a Guide for the Helping Professions,* MacLennan and Petty, Sydney.

Fisher, K., Howat, P. A., Binns, C. W. and Liveris, M. 1986, 'Health Education and Health Promotion: an Australian Perspective', *Health Education Journal,* 45 (2), 95–8.

Fisher, R., Ury, W. and Patton, B. 1991, *Getting to Yes: Negotiating Agreement Without Giving In,* Arrow Business Books, London.

Freire, P. 1973, *Education for Critical Consciousness*, Sheed and Ward, London.

Glyn, A. and Miliband, D. (eds) 1994, *Paying for Inequality: the Economic Cost of Social Injustice,* IPPR/Rivers Oram Press, London.

Goeppinger, J. and Baglioni, A. J. 1985, 'Community Competence: a Positive Approach to Needs Assessment', *American Journal of Community Psychology,* 13 (5), 507–23.

Green, A. 1994, *An Introduction to Health Planning in Developing Countries,* Oxford University Press, Oxford.

Green, L. W. and Kreuter, M. W. 1991, *Health Promotion Planning: an Educational and Environmental Approach,* Mayfield Publishing Company, Mountain View, California.

Guttman, N., Kegler, M. and McLeroy, K. R. 1996, 'Health Promotion Paradoxes, Antinomies and Conundrums', *Health Education Research,* 11 (1), i-xiii.

Hawe, P. 1994, 'Capturing the Meaning of "Community" in Community Intervention Evaluation: Some Contributions from Community Psychology', *Health Promotion International,* 9 (3), 199–210.

Hayes, M. V. and Willms, S. M. 1990, 'Healthy Community Indicators: the Perils of the Search and the Paucity of the Find', *Health Promotion International,* 5 (2), 161–6.

Hill, S. 1991, *Who Controls Where the Health Dollar Goes?,* Health Issues Centre, Melbourne.

Honari, M. 1993, 'Advancing Health Ecology: Where To From Here?', in Newman, N. (ed.), *Health and Ecology — a Nursing Perspective,* Proceedings of the first national Nursing the Environment Conference, Australian Nursing Federation, Melbourne.

Hopkins, S. 1996, 'Foreword', in McSwain, R. *Culture and Health Care: Culture, Settlement Experience and Lifestyle of Non-English Speaking Background People in Western Australia,* Multicultural Access Unit, Health Department of Western Australia, Perth.

House, J., Landis, K. R. and Umberson, D. 1988, 'Social Relationships and Health', *Science,* 241, 29 July, 540–4.

Human Rights and Equal Opportunity Commission 1997, *Bringing Them Home: Report of the National Inquiry into the Separation of Aboriginal and Torres Strait Islander Children from their Families,* Human Rights and Equal Opportunity Commission, Sydney.

Jackson, T. 1985, 'On the Limitations of Health Promotion', *Community Health Studies,* 9 (1), 1–9.

Johnstone, M. J. 1994, *Bioethics: a Nursing Perspective,* W. B. Saunders/Bailliere Tindall, Sydney.

Kaplan, G. A., Pamuk, E. R., Lynch, J. W., Cohen, R. D. and Balfour, J. L. 1996, 'Inequality in Income and Mortality in the United States: Analysis of Mortality and Potential Pathways', *British Medical Journal,* 312 (20 April), 999–1003.

Kawachi, I. and Kennedy, B. P. 1997, 'Health and Social Cohesion: Why Care About Income Inequality?', *British Medical Journal,* 314 (5 April), 1037–40.

Kennedy, S., Kiecolt-Glaser, J. K. and Glaser, A. 1988, 'Immunological Consequences of Acute and Chronic Stressors: Mediating Role of Interpersonal Relationships', *British Journal of Medical Psychology,* 61, 77–85.

Kickbusch, I. 1994, 'An Overview to the Settings-Based Approach to Health

Promotion', in *The Settings Based Approach to Health Promotion: an International Working Conference in Collaboration with the World Health Organization Regional Office for Europe,* Conference report, Health Education Authority, London.

Kickbusch, I. 1997, 'Think Health: What Makes the Difference?', *Health Promotion International,* 12 (4), 265–72.

LaFaille, R. and Fulder, S. (eds), 1993, *Towards a New Science of Health,* Routledge, London and New York.

Labonté, R. 1989a. 'Community Empowerment: the Need for Political Analysis, *Canadian Journal of Public Health,* 80, 87–8.

Labonté, R. 1989b, 'Commentary: Community Empowerment: Reflections on the Australian Situation', *Community Health Studies,* 13 (3), 347–9.

Labonté, R. 1989c, 'Community Health Promotion Strategies', in Martin, C. J. and McQueen, D. V. (eds), *Readings For A New Public Health,* Edinburgh University Press, Edinburgh.

Labonté, R. 1990. 'Health Care Spending as a Risk to Health', *Canadian Journal of Public Health,* July/August, 251–2.

Marsick, V. 1988, 'Proactive Learning in Primary Health Care: an Adult Education Model', *International Journal of Lifelong Education,* 7 (2), 101–14.

Mathers, C. and Douglas, B. 1998, 'Measuring Progress in Population Health and Well-Being', in Eckersley, R. (ed.), *Measuring Progress: is Life Getting Better?,* CSIRO Publishing, Collingwood.

McMichael, A. J. 1993, *Planetary Overload: Global Environmental Change and the Health of The Human Species,* Cambridge University Press, Cambridge.

Minkler, M. 1994, 'Ten Commitments for Community Health Education', *Health Education Research,* 9 (4), 527–34.

National Aboriginal Health Strategy Working Party 1989, *A National Aboriginal Health Strategy,* Department of Aboriginal Affairs, Canberra.

National Health Strategy 1993a, *Healthy Participation: Achieving Greater Public Participation and Accountability in the Australian Health Care System,* Background paper 12, March, National Health Strategy, Canberra.

National Health Strategy 1993b, *Removing Cultural and Language Barriers to Health,* Issues paper No. 6, March, National Health Strategy, Canberra.

Pauwels, A. 1995, *Cross-Cultural Communication in the Health Sciences: Communicating With Migrant Patients,* Macmillan, Melbourne.

Raeburn, J. and Rootman, I. 1998, *People-centred Health Promotion,* John Wiley and Sons, Chichester.

Reid, J. and Trompf, P. (eds) 1990, *The Health of Immigrant Australia: a Social Perspective,* Harcourt Brace Jovanovich, Sydney.

Reid, J. and Trompf, P. (eds) 1991, *The Health of Aboriginal Australia,* Harcourt Brace Jovanovich, Sydney.

Research Unit in Health and Behavioural Change 1989, *Changing the Public Health,* John Wiley and Sons, Chichester, UK.

Rifkin, S. 1986, 'Lessons from Community Participation in Health Programmes', *Health Policy and Planning,* 1 (3), 240–9.

Rifkin, S. and Walt, G. 1986, 'Why Health Improves: Defining The Issues Surrounding "Comprehensive Primary Health Care" And "Selective Primary Health Care"', *Social Science and Medicine,* 23 (6), 559–66.

Rijke, R. 1993, 'Health in Medical Science: From Determinism Towards Autonomy', in LaFaille, R. and Fulder, S. (eds), *Towards a New Science of Health,* Routledge, London and New York.

Robertson, A. and Minkler, M. 1994, 'New Health Promotion Movement: a Critical Examination', *Health Education Quarterly,* 21 (3), 295–312.

Rodin, J. and Langer, E. J. 1977, 'Long-Term Effects of a Control-Relevant Intervention with the Institutionalized Aged', *Journal of Personality and Social Psychology,* 33 (12), 897–902.

Ryan, W. 1976, *Blaming the Victim,* Vintage Books, New York.

Sanders, M. R. (ed.) 1995, *Healthy Families, Healthy Nation: Strategies for Promoting Family Mental Health in Australia,* Australian Academic Press, Brisbane.

Sanderson, C. and Baum, F. 1995, 'Health and Social Welfare Councils', in Baum, F. (ed.), *Health For All: the South Australian Experience,* South Australian Community Health Research Unit in association with Wakefield Press, Kent Town, SA.

Saul, J. R. 1997, *The Unconscious Civilisation,* Penguin, Ringwood, Vic.

Saunders, P. 1998, 'Poverty and Health: Exploring the Links Between Financial Stress and Emotional Stress in Australia', *Australian and New Zealand Journal of Public Health,* 22 (1), 11–16.

Sax, S. 1990, *Health Care Choices and the Public Purse,* Allen and Unwin, Sydney.

Teshuva, K., Kendig, H. and Stacey, B. 1997, 'Spirituality, Health and Health Promotion in Older Australians', *Health Promotion Journal of Australia,* 7 (3), 180–4.

Turshen, M. 1989, *The Politics Of Public Health,* Rutgers University Press, New Brunswick, New Jersey.

Wadsworth, Y. 1988, *Participatory Research and Development in Primary Health Care by Community Groups: Report to the National Health and Medical Research Council,* Public Health Research and Development Committee, Consumers' Health Forum, Deakin, ACT.

Wallerstein, N. 1992, 'Powerlessness, Empowerment, and Health: Implications for Health Promotion Programs', *American Journal of Public Health,* January/February, 6 (3), 197–205.

Wass, A. 1995, 'Health Workers and Communities Working Together: Framework for a Meaningful Partnership', in *Primary Health Care: Working Together,* Proceedings of the sixth annual Primary Health Care conference, University of Sydney Cumberland Campus, Lidcombe.

Wearing, A. J. and Headey, B. 1998, 'Who Enjoys Life and Why: Measuring Subjective Well-being', in Eckersley, R. (ed.), *Measuring Progress: Is Life Getting Better?,* CSIRO Publishing, Collingwood.

Werner, D., Sanders, D., Weston, J., Babb, S. and Rodriguez, B. 1997, *Questioning the Solution: the Politics of Primary Health Care and Child Survival,* Healthwrights, Palo Alto, CA.

Wilkinson, R. 1994,, 'Health, Redistribution and Growth', in Glyn , A. and Miliband, D. (eds), *Paying for Inequality: the Economic Cost of Social Injustice,* IPPR/Rivers Oram Press, London.

Wilkinson, R. G. 1996, *Unhealthy Societies: the Afflictions of Inequality,* Routledge, London.

World Health Organization 1986, *The Ottawa Charter for Health Promotion,* World Health Organization, Geneva.

CHAPTER 3

Assessing community needs and resources

*T*he next two chapters will examine needs assessment and evaluation. These two areas have a great deal in common, being areas in which research skills form the basis of the process. Because of this, they have a certain mystique for many health workers, and people may feel that they do not have the skills to conduct needs assessment or evaluation. However, the idea that research is out of the reach of ordinary people is misleading. As you read through the next two chapters you will see that you already have a great many research skills, and that there are opportunities to further develop knowledge and skills. This will enable the development of a research base for health promotion in a way that both strengthens the relevance of health promotion work and enables health workers to be accountable for their practice. Before we examine the issues specific to needs assessment and evaluation, it will be useful to have a brief overview of some of the general issues involved in research in the context of the Primary Health Care Approach.

Research in Primary Health Care

The research process has an important role to play as an ongoing, integrated part of practice if it is to be meaningful to health workers and the community. When research is integral to practice, practice is strengthened in a number of ways. Firstly, health promotion practice will be built around the needs of the people for whom it is designed. It will be responsive to those needs and be based on a recognition that they are dynamic rather than static, and therefore change over time. Secondly, with a grounding in community needs, health workers are less likely to implement programs that do not meet these needs, thus preventing expensive mistakes. Thirdly, with this responsiveness and grounding in community needs, health workers are less likely to engage in activities that lead the community to lose confidence in health workers (Griffith 1992, personal communication). Such loss of confidence may take some time to repair and may result in further damage as community members ignore future health promotion work. Fourthly, when research is integral to practice, health promotion and other activities of health workers are routinely evaluated, and the findings used to improve the quality of health promotion work. This final point will be examined in Chapter 4.

The inextricable relationship between research and practice means that the additional resources required to carry out research may not be as great as expected. When research is an integral part of practice, it is as much a state of mind and an approach to working as anything else. Certainly there are times, for example, when a major community assessment may be required, and this may necessitate an additional commitment of time and resources and the active involvement of people with expertise in community assessment. However, not researching and improving practice may result in wasting the limited resources that are being allocated to health promotion.

Participatory research: the Primary Health Care approach in action

A Primary Health Care approach to health promotion emphasises the importance of health promotion work being socially relevant and conducted with people, rather than working on them. Research conducted as part of health promotion needs to meet this criterion also. If research is to reflect a Primary Health Care approach, the emphasis must be on working with people as equal partners, involving them in the research process and acknowledging their expertise. This will ensure that the research conducted is relevant to their needs and therefore useful.

This approach to research, known as participatory research, is growing in recognition. Several international reports have urged the acceptance and development of participatory research (e.g. Oakley 1989, p. 70). Within Australia, the Consumers' Health Forum, in particular, has urged the adoption of these principles, which it believes form the basis of true community research (Matrice & Brown 1990). Their importance in research into Aboriginal health has also been acknowledged (Houston & Legge 1992, pp. 114–15). There are an increasing range of publications exploring the principles of participatory research and providing examples of participatory research in action (e.g. Davies & Kelly 1993; Popay & Williams 1994). The participatory approach to research outlined in these books is an approach to working collaboratively with consumers or community members while drawing on a wide range of research methods of direct relevance to the problem at hand.

In such situations, planning committees comprised of researchers, practitioners and community members can work together to design, implement and evaluate the findings of research projects. Contributions of community members in defining the parameters of the research and reviewing issues that arise, from their perspectives as community members, add much to the value of the research.

Some research methods are of particular value in Primary Health Care because they actually have this participatory approach embedded in the research process. Of note here are participatory action research and feminist research. It is worthwhile examining them briefly in order to understand how these methods can be utilised in health promotion.

Participatory action research

Participatory action research is a dynamic process built on a foundation of working with people, enabling them to be the key developers of problem solving and change. Participatory action research has developed simultaneously in a number of fields, with slightly different styles, taking account of the different circumstances, but following similar general principles (Selener 1997). Of particular relevance for our purposes is participatory action research as it has developed in community development, and action research as it has developed in organisations.

Participatory action research in community development has been defined as 'a process through which members of an oppressed group or community identify a problem, collect and analyze information, and act upon the problem in order to find solutions and to promote social and political transformation' (Selener 1997, p. 17).

Participatory action research is based on a strong set of values relating to social justice and empowerment of oppressed groups, through working to change those things that constrain their lives, including dominating social structures (Selener 1997, p. 18). There are several characteristics of participatory action research:

- *The problem originates in the community itself and is defined, analyzed and solved by the community;*
- *The ultimate goal of research is the radical transformation of social reality and improvement in the lives of the people involved. The primary beneficiaries of the research are the community members themselves;*
- *Participatory research involves the full and active participation of the community in the entire research process;*
- *Participatory research involves a whole range of powerless groups of people: the exploited, the poor, the oppressed, the marginalised;*
- *The process of participatory research can create a greater awareness in people of their own resources and can mobilize them for self-reliant development;*
- *Participatory research is a more scientific method in that community participation in the research process facilitates a more accurate and authentic analysis of social reality;*
- *The researcher is a committed participant, facilitator, and learner in the research process, and this leads to militancy, rather than detachment.*

(Selener 1997, pp. 18–21.)

Participatory action research in community development clearly has many applications within health promotion, as it provides a process by which community members can identify and address problems by dealing with some of their root causes. Community development will itself be examined further in Chapter 6.

Two streams of action research have developed in an organisational context, based on the work of Kurt Lewin. These approaches, action research in organisations and action research in education, are very similar. What they offer health promotion is a framework for using an action research approach within an organisational context, which can be quite different to working at community level. These organisational approaches may be particularly valuable when working for health promoting settings (see p. 200).

Organisational action research is a continuing cyclical approach to work that involves an ever-developing 'self-reflective spiral of cycles of planning, acting, observing and reflecting' (Carr & Kemmis 1986, p. 162). It is likely to be a more consensual process than participatory action research in community development, because it is conducted within an organisational context to address problems at this level.

Like participatory action research in community development, organisational action research is a participatory process, although it may be instigated and led by an outside researcher. Its focus is on solving practical problems through organisational change and development (Selener 1997, pp. 65–8). It is therefore regarded as a learning process, both for the individuals involved in the action research process and for the organisation itself.

Because organisational action research is built on a recognition of the inextricable links between research and practice (Carr & Kemmis 1986), it has a great deal to offer health workers. It is ideal as an approach to working with community members, enabling them to reflect on their own experiences, plan how they can act to change their situation, act and then evaluate the impact of the changes in order to then re-plan, re-act and re-evaluate in a continuing cycle of change, development and learning. It can also be used to provide a framework for health workers to continually analyse and develop their own practice. That is, it provides a framework for good reflective practice.

Feminist research

While feminist research developed originally for work with women as an oppressed group, it has potential as a set of principles of use when working with any marginalised groups. Feminist research has been defined as:

> *research that relates to an understanding of women's position as that of an oppressed social group, and which adopts a critical perspective towards intellectual traditions rendering women either invisible and/or subject to a priori categorizations of one form or another.*

(Oakley 1990, pp. 169–70.)

Feminist research is therefore conducted in a way that is not oppressive to those involved in it and care is taken to ensure that the research findings can be used by the research participants (Acker et al. 1983; Roberts 1981, cited by Oakley 1990, pp. 169–70).

Feminist methodology is built on a recognition of the expertise of the people affected by a particular issue. Mies (1983, pp. 124–7) suggests several key issues to guide feminist research. These are:

1. There is a recognition that research is not value-free. Therefore, rather than attempting to remain totally distant from and uninvolved with research participants, feminist researchers identify with them sufficiently to see the problem from their perspective as well as their own.

2. The relationship between researcher and research participants is an equal partnership, not one where researchers are the 'experts' and the people being researched are mere subjects. This is reflected in the use of the term research 'participant', rather than 'subject'. Without this partnership approach to research, researchers contribute to the oppression of people they are attempting to help.

3. Research is inseparable from the wider actions for improvement of women's position in society. Therefore, researchers are also engaged in '*active participation in actions, movements and struggles* for women's emancipation' (p. 124 [author's italics]).

4. The interrelationship between action and research indicates that an inherent part of feminist methodology is '*change of the status quo*' (p. 125, author's italics). In particular, feminist methodology is built around changes to women's position in society and the fight for emancipation.

5. 'The research process must become a process of "conscientization"', or critical consciousness raising, for both researchers and research participants' (p. 127).

That is, through the research process, people are enabled to see the social, political and economic constraints on their lives and therefore recognise the context in which their lives are lived. This process also results in recognition of the experiences individual women share with each other; consequently, the power of the group becomes recognised and can be used for collective action (p. 127).

Towards a Primary Health Care approach to research

It is quite apparent that there are links between feminist research, participatory action research and the process of 'conscientisation', or critical consciousness raising developed by Paulo Friere (discussed in greater detail in Chapter 9). Together these form a powerful basis for dynamic relevant research that has the potential to promote the health of the people for whom it is designed. This Primary Health Care approach to research can be described by the following elements:

- Research is a dynamic cyclical process, inextricably intertwined with action. Its aim is to improve the conditions under which people live.
- The research process is guided by critical self-reflection on the part of the 'researcher' and the research participants. The values of researcher and research participants are acknowledged up front and are the subject of critical self-reflection as part of the research process. Conscientisation is a key feature of this process.
- The relationship between researcher and research participants is a partnership that itself acts to change the status quo by breaking down the traditionally 'top down' approach of researchers. Thus, all people involved in the research process are best described as research partners.

Developing participatory research in a way that is both rigorous and accepted by professional colleagues and funding bodies on the one hand, and meaningful and acceptable to community members participating in the process on the other, is a challenge that has been identified by several researchers committed to working in this way (Allison & Rootman 1996; Boutilier, Mason & Rootman 1997).

Involving community members as partners in the process means that the process may become unpredictable and uncontrollable, which may create difficulties for people if the framework in which they are working doesn't allow for that kind of flexibility, or if the community members want to take the process in a direction that is against the principles of Primary Health Care. This is by no means a simple issue. How do you balance the need to be flexible in your approach and to ensure community members are true partners in the process, with the need to remain committed to certain principles, which may mean being inflexible if those principles are transgressed? However, these are challenges worth grappling with if we are to see the Primary Health Care approach to research reach its potential. One of the key areas in which we may see this happen is in the area of community assessment.

Community assessment

Community assessment can be defined as a process that results in:

> *a comprehensive description of the needs of a population that is defined, or defines itself, as a community, and the resources that exist within that community, carried out with the active involvement of the community*

itself, for the purpose of developing an action plan or other means of improving the quality of life in the community.

(Hawtin, Hughes and Percy-Smith 1994, p. 13.)

This definition highlights several issues that are central to meaningful community assessment:

- Community assessment is a process of determining both the needs and the resources of a community. While considerable attention tends to be focused on the needs of communities, and these certainly are important, a focus on needs alone tends to paint a 'deficit' picture of communities. This itself can be a negative disempowering experience for communities and can ignore the positive characteristics and resources of that community. These community strengths can be a source of pride for the community, and may hold a key to successfully addressing the needs that arise.
- Community assessment should be carried out with the active participation of community members. As discussion in Chapter 2 noted, community members have the right and ability to be meaningfully engaged in determining what their needs and strengths are. Good community assessment is a participatory process.
- Community assessments are carried out for the specific purpose of achieving change that improves the quality of life of those living as part of that community. A community assessment is not an end in itself, but a guide to action. Unless community assessments are acted on, they are a waste of time and energy (Hawe 1996; Feuerstein 1986, p. 153). Community assessments that leave you with few resources for acting on what you find or for which there is no real commitment to act on after their completion are likely to do little to help those for whom the community assessment is purportedly being carried out and are likely to result in significant community frustration (Hawe 1996; Rissel 1991, p. 30).

Need — what is it?

While comprehensive community assessment examines both the resources and needs of a community, it is true that the notion of needs has a central place in community assessment. This is especially so when there is a focus on social justice and working to achieve equity for those who are disadvantaged. Any examination of community assessment should start, therefore, with an examination of just what need is, and a review of some of the issues surrounding the definition of something as a need.

Need has been defined as 'the condition in which something necessary, desirable or very useful is missing or wanted' (*Longman Dictionary of Contemporary English* 1987). This definition highlights the fact that the very concept of need itself is value-based and socially constructed. Whether something is identified as a need will depend on the perspectives and values of those involved. In addition, it is through the way in which issues are defined at a social and political level that individuals, groups and societies come to decide which issues are of concern to them and which things they need. Which issues are constructed as needs depends on the particular values in place in the society or group. Given the value-laden nature of need, it is important to be clear about which values should be driving the needs identification process in the Primary Health Care approach.

There are several different ways in which needs can be classified, according to the perspective used to identify need. Bradshaw (1972) has identified four types of need — felt need, expressed need, normative need and comparative need. The categories of felt and expressed need include need determined by people themselves, while the category of normative need represents need determined by experts, and comparative need represents need determined by past responses to similar problems. With an emphasis on equal partnership between professionals and community members in a Primary Health Care approach to health promotion, all these types of need have something useful to contribute to an assessment of need.

Felt need

Felt need is most easily described as what people say they need. For example, if a local community is surveyed regarding its highest priorities for health promotion action, people may say that they want more intensive-care beds, safer streets in which their children can play or less youth unemployment in the local area.

Felt need is important because it involves asking people themselves what their needs are. However, on its own it may not give a complete picture of need for a number of reasons. Firstly, people may limit what they tell you they need to what they think they can have (Walker & Dixon 1984, pp. 16–17). If they believe that meeting some of their needs is beyond their reach, they may not ask for it.

Secondly, people may only voice needs that they believe you are interested in. For example, if a health worker asks someone about their health needs, that person may interpret the question as referring to his or her illness problems alone, and may not think of health in its broad context.

Thirdly, powerful groups in the community can have a strong influence in determining how people see their needs. Community members' beliefs about what they need can, in fact, be socially constructed by interest groups, opinion leaders and the mass media. Groups and communities may 'adopt' certain needs as their own because these have been sold to them through the mass media. In many instances it is not the need alone but also one potential response to the need that is presented as the 'solution'. One example of this process can be seen in the recent establishment of the need for national mammography services. Because of a concerted media campaign, which actually 'sold' the importance of mammography screening rather than providing a balanced education about the issues, mammography screening units are increasingly seen as something every community should have. This has happened despite the limitations of mammography screening, which have not been widely discussed; for example, the risks of mammography screening, the problems of false negatives and false positives, and whether it actually makes a difference to people's lives or merely increases the length of time in which they know they are dying (Browning 1992; Wass 1990). Through the impact of the medical profession and medical insurance companies, which have advertised mammography as 'the only safe way to detect breast cancer', the need for appropriate breast cancer screening has been redefined for many people as the need for mammography.

Fourthly, the perspective of a small group of community members may not reflect the perspective of the whole community. Careful consideration needs to

---

Community participation or manipulation? The impact of dominant interests on a community's perception of needs

Stephanie Short (1989) has outlined a case study that demonstrates the power of dominant groups in society in structuring community needs. It describes the efforts of the Wollongong community to raise $1.5 million for the purchase of a linear accelerator, a piece of high-tech equipment for use in cancer treatment. The community took up the cause with gusto, and readily accepted that this was the thing that Wollongong most needed, despite the fact that the money could have been spent on a great many other health-related services, such as palliative care, cancer prevention and health promotion. It seems that beliefs about the primacy of high-tech medical care and the desire for all possible medical treatments to be available were dominant, and a lone attempt to question this, and the community's lack of real choice on the issue, was soon quashed.

As Short (1989, p. 34) argues, '"community needs" are easily manipulated or distorted by interest groups and … the political context within which community needs are recognized, articulated and mobilized is the most important issue for community participation in the health policy-making process'.

---

be made of whom a group of community informants represent — a section of the community, a small subsection or only themselves (Hawe, Degeling and Hall 1990, p. 19).

If we are to take the principles of Primary Health Care seriously, we need to work to promote health based on people's own assessment of their need — that is, felt need must be among the types of need present. However, because of the all-pervading forces that influence people's felt need, most particularly through the media, people may not have had a real opportunity to decide for themselves. In health promotion, as in any other area of health, workers need to ensure that people are able to make informed decisions and that they have access to the information they need to make those decisions. Of course, this process may require more than giving people information; it may require them to examine the forces that influence their decisions. That is, this process of helping people clarify their felt need may well involve the process of conscientisation.

Furthermore, the presence of felt or expressed need alone, without the presence also of normative or comparative need, raises some questions. What if a group or community wants something but there is no evidence to demonstrate the need for it? In such a situation, more information may be needed. Does the group or community know that it is comparatively well off in the area concerned? This may change the priorities that the group sets. Conversely, is it the case that there is a lack of formal evidence in this area because of the shortcomings of information collection, rather than that there is no objective need? For example, until relatively recently, few statistics on Aboriginal health were collected and the collection of these statistics continues to be poor (Thomson 1991, pp. 38–9). This means that there may still be inadequate formal evidence of the extent of Aboriginal health problems.

The problems of external funding and felt need

Currently, health promotion funding is available for specific projects, often aimed at particular diseases or risk factors. Frequently, funding may be granted and the project begun without any prior systematic assessment of the community's felt needs. The particular project being funded may be a long way down the community's list of priorities, and people may not be motivated to participate in the project. It is then imposed on the community, at 'best' with the community being educated about why they should want it. This approach to funding presents some very real dangers, as it encourages health workers and bureaucrats to ignore communities' own assessment of their needs or regard it as a simple 'add on' rather than an integral part of the project.

Expressed need

Expressed need is need that is demonstrated by people's use of services or demand for new or more services. That is, expressed need can be described as 'felt need turned into action' (Bradshaw 1972, p. 641). Examples of expressed need include waiting lists for services such as child care, nursing home places or public dental services. Needless to say, this expressed need has even more limitations on it than felt need, as people can only add their names to waiting lists for services that already exist or are about to come into existence. Indeed, waiting lists are limited to issues of service provision: it is not possible to join a waiting list for a new public policy, for example, although the number of letters written to a politician on a particular issue may be regarded as another form of expressed need.

The constraints on people's choices here are even greater than in felt need, since the specific service they are demanding must already be there. Moreover, expressed need can easily be misinterpreted. For example, a waiting list at the local dentist might be interpreted as the need for more dental treatment services, when in fact it could reflect inadequate oral health promotion or lack of awareness of school dental therapy services, to give just two examples. Another problem with expressed need is that in many situations people may add their names to all available waiting lists for a particular service, although in reality they would accept only one place (e.g. a nursing home placement). In such a situation, adding up the numbers of names on waiting lists is likely to give an inaccurate impression. In other situations, people may refrain from placing their names on waiting lists if they believe the waiting lists are already long and their chances of success low. In addition, people's beliefs about whether they have a right to particular services, or deserve to have access to them, will influence whether they act to formally express a need.

Naturally, there are strong links between felt need and expressed need. It may seem that expressed need is merely felt need written down. While to a certain extent this is true, there are also particular differences between them, and so they each may tell us slightly different things. However, you may find that some authors use these terms interchangeably.

Normative need

Normative need is need determined by 'experts' on the basis of research and professional opinion. Examples of normative need include safe levels of water pollution, recommended daily allowances of different food groups and unsafe levels of lead ingestion. Normatively determined need is often regarded as objective and unbiased because it has been determined by experts. That is, it often carries the assumption that it is value-free and beyond questioning or reproach, but this assumption needs to be called into question. In addition, professional opinion often changes over time, leaving the public confused (Bradshaw 1972, p. 641). For example, Becker (1986) cites the example of professionals' changing views of the dangers of cholesterol, and the consequent confusion among the public. As a result, the public is beginning to develop some healthy scepticism about professional opinion. Normative need may reflect some level of paternalism, and it certainly can provide conflicting information, depending on the values of the experts themselves (Bradshaw 1972, p. 641).

One crucial issue that influences normative need and that requires examination is the fact that many professional groups act, often unconsciously, as gatekeepers in society. Furthermore, they may be unable or unwilling to acknowledge publicly that something is occurring at an unsafe level if their judgment in this case has political implications. This, then, represents another possible limitation of normatively determined need. Finally, an over-reliance on epidemiological data to provide evidence of normative need is increasingly being called into question as the limitations of epidemiology are recognised (see pp. 106–10).

Comparative need

Comparative need is need that is determined by comparing the services available in one geographical area with those available in other geographical areas. Therefore, it may be argued that a particular area requires a certain service because other areas with similar demographic characteristics have one. Examples of comparative need are calls for neonatal intensive-care cots or smoke-free workplace policy on the basis of the argument that other areas have them.

Comparative need can be useful in highlighting relative deficiencies in some communities. However, it can also be problematic because it is based on the assumption that the service provided in the place of comparison was the most appropriate response to the problem (Bradshaw 1972: 641), and that the needs of the two areas are in fact the same.

Sources of information for community assessment

We can never assume that we know which needs exist in a particular situation. While our hunches about problems can often be sound, we cannot assume that they represent the problems as seen by those directly affected. We can use our hunches as a guide (and they usually lead us to notice particular issues in the first place), but it is vital that we take the time to find out how those affected by a problem interpret the situation and which priorities for action they set for themselves. We also need to determine what the external evidence suggests about the seriousness of the issues facing the community, and what resources are available within a community.

Sources of evidence of need can be classified into five key groups (developed from Ewles & Simnett 1985, pp. 61–2). As you read through these, consider how

'Teeth for Keeps'

The 'Teeth for Keeps' project was funded by the Commonwealth Department of Health, Housing and Community Services through the National Health Promotion Program in 1991 with $40 086. It aimed to promote oral health and prevent dental disease in school communities in the Moree Plains Shire of north west New South Wales. The shire is a wealthy agricultural area in which 10% of the rural population of around 20 000 is Aboriginal.

An oral health survey of about 1000 school children was conducted in 1990 by the New South Wales Department of Health. The resulting report, entitled 'Who caries?', showed a rate of decayed, missing and filled teeth that was 13% higher than the rate reported as the average throughout Australia in 1986 (Carr 1988, p. 206). Moreover, children in Moree (where the water is unfluoridated) were likely to require dental treatment at a rate 250% higher than children in Tamworth (where the water is fluoridated) (Patterson 1990, p. 2).

Fortunately, the 'Who caries?' report provided the quantitative data from which to argue a strong case to justify external funding. This situation was strengthened by the fact that dental disease was a high priority area and by Aboriginal communities being a targeted population for the current round of grant applications. On the other hand, the existence of the relevant dental data and the close fit with the external funding priority areas meant that a community needs analysis was not a requirement for the granting body, and so it is difficult to tell where oral health fitted with the community's list of priorities.

The issue of water fluoridation, however, was hotly debated by health professionals, environmentalists, civil libertarians and community members in the Moree Plains Shire between 1985 and 1990. In fact, it could have played a detrimental role in the adoption and success of the Teeth for Keeps project, as many community members associated oral health issues only with the water fluoridation debate. Individuals in the communities were reluctant to discuss oral health promotion because the long drawn-out debate over water fluoridation was turning them off the topic completely — they had had enough! Therefore, a great deal of effort went into transforming an emotional and divisive issue into a constructive and practical health promotion strategy.

From my point of view, the problems of external funding include working out the aims, objectives, strategies and outcome measures of a particular project well before it begins. This does not allow those working on the project the flexibility to respond to other needs that become apparent once one starts working with different sections of the community. A researcher never really knows what is going to happen during a research project because several factors are completely out of that person's control. It is that aspect that causes anxiety and panic in some researchers, but which makes 'real' research for me so dynamic and exciting!

Community meetings in Moree, Mungindi, Pallamallawa and Boggabilla revealed that community members wanted better access to public dental treatment. On a statewide basis, the New England region had a higher than average number of persons eligible for public dental care (NSW Department of Health 1991a). Furthermore, the number of dental therapists in the region was significantly lower than that recommended by the World Health Organization for non-fluoridated areas. Before the project began, only one fixed dental clinic with one dental therapist and one dental assistant was operational in Moree, so there was clearly a need for more public dental treatment.

The Teeth for Keeps project was, however, funded only for oral health promotion strategies for school children, so we were not able to respond directly to the community demands of public dental treatment for adults and children. Fortunately, as one of the project managers was the Principal Dental Officer for the New England Health Region, the community's requests in this regard were addressed by the allocation from regional dental funds for a dental officer, a dental assistant, goods and services ($75 000), a 'Molar Patroller' mobile dental clinic ($90 000) and oral health promotion posters ($18 000). If one of the project managers had not been the Principal Dental Officer, it would not have been possible to address community demands for dental services.

As the project developed, its redeeming feature was that it did not push the 'chemical fix' of water fluoridation but concentrated on activities within the control of school communities. These included classroom-based educational sessions, school 'brush-ins', school 'rinse-ins', healthy school canteens, salivary stimulation and posters promoting oral health.

Most important of all, the work begun by the Teeth for Keeps project did not finish with the end of the research. At the end of the official project, the two coordinators employed for it obtained full-time employment, while the project itself was continued for seven months by the Department of Health and then expanded for a further three years by the Moree Plains Shire Council and the Department of Health at a shared cost of $60 000 per year.

In the meantime, oral health was gaining increased attention at the state level. In 1996, after the appointment of an Oral Health Promotion Officer for NSW, a Dental Assessment and Prioritisation Program (DAPP) that was initiated in the Western Suburbs of Sydney was turned into a statewide program.

The $5m per year SOKS Program (Save Our Kids' Smiles) includes a quick clinical assessment of oral health and referral for public or private treatment. This takes place in kindergarten and years 2, 4, 6 and 8. On the same visit, dental therapists deliver classroom lessons in which a specially developed video on oral health is used.

SOKS subsequently replaced local oral health initiatives like Teeth for Keeps, despite the fact that Teeth for Keeps was a much more comprehensive program, developed in response to local needs and concerns. It is now very difficult to ascertain felt and expressed needs, as only those individual children referred for treatment are able to access oral health care through the public sector in NSW. SOKS is yet to be evaluated.

Leonie M. Short
former dental therapist and
Senior Lecturer in Oral Health
School of Public Health
Queensland University of Technology

they relate to the categories in Bradshaw's taxonomy of needs, and what sort of need is likely to be found from each source.

Listening to the community

Listening to the community is a vital part of needs assessment, and can be done through both formal and informal means. Informal opportunities to listen to what people have to say arise throughout daily interaction with community members. Twelvetrees (1987, pp. 25–6) suggests the following two ways to maximise informal opportunities to listen to the community.

Learn how to listen and take notice

As obvious as this may sound, so often we do not take full advantage of opportunities to listen to what people have to say. Every interaction that a health worker has with a community member or group is an opportunity to learn something about what that person or group thinks. Leaving space for people to talk and being ready to hear what they have to say enables every interaction with a community member or group to become an informal opportunity to learn about their needs.

Walk, don't drive

Take the time to walk around your community as a way of meeting people and getting a sense of how the community feels, where the difficult places to live are, and so forth. This is just as relevant if you have responsibility for an organisation rather than a community. For a health worker with a responsibility for the health of a geographical community, shopping where the locals shop and going along to important community events such as the local show may be useful. Here you can get a sense of some of the issues that are important to people and possibly meet some key people with whom you could work on health promotion projects. Increasing the number of times you are 'out there' in the community also increases your opportunities to listen to what people have to say. For an occupational health nurse, walking around the shop floor provides an opportunity to meet people, to be seen by people (and remind them that you are available) and to notice any potential problem areas or opportunities for implementing some positive change. As a general principle, taking steps such as this is a valuable part of getting to know your community and the people in it.

Formal ways to ask the community for their opinion, through community surveys, will enable you to assess people's needs more systematically. It is important that any formal needs assessment be carried out in a way that is supportive of the community and involves people as much as possible in the planning, implementation and analysis of findings. The specific details of how to conduct a community survey are beyond the scope of this book. Some valuable resources on this topic include those by the Southern Community Health Research Unit (1991) and Wadsworth (1997).

Social and economic indica tors

Social and economic indicators include a range of statistical information that helps to construct a picture of the community. Information such as proportion of people in each age group, income levels, number of people on each type of pension, number of single-parent families, number of single-income families and level of home ownership is useful in helping to construct a picture of the issues likely to be affecting this community. This information is available from Australian Bureau of Statistics data, which are often held by each local council for its own area and should be available for public viewing. In addition, information on such things as amount of land available for recreation, shopping facilities and availability

---

The importance of backing up requests for services with a needs assessment

I was involved in establishing a support group a few years ago but I didn't do the groundwork I normally do before establishing a support group. I responded to the needs of two people and I didn't find out if there was a community need for the group. We went through all the motions of establishing the group and after five or six meetings it was clear it wasn't working. The attendance was still limited to the two original people that had approached me. It then occurred to me to retrace my steps, and have a look at what went wrong. I realised I had responded to two people's needs, not the community's needs, and I hadn't done my usual homework.

Had I responded to this situation as I usually do, I would have identified a full list of the key people with a stake in this potential group and discussed the idea with them. Contacting other support agencies, including the local GPs, would have enabled me to discover that there were, in fact, only eight potential members of this support group in the entire region. Despite statewide epidemiological information giving the impression that there would be a significant number of people in our area with this problem, the reality was quite different. Local level information, at that stage only available through local GPs, presented a more accurate picture on which I could base a judgement.

Clearly, the individuals who approached me needed some kind of assistance and support, but it would not come in this situation through a community support group.

Sandy Brooks, Clinical Nurse Specialist
(Mental Health Promotion)
Mid North Coast Area Health Service (Southern Sector)

---

of public transport will also be useful to access. It should be available from your local council.

Epidemiological data

Epidemiology has been defined as 'the study of the distribution and determinants of disease in human populations' (Christie, Gordon & Heller 1987, p. 1). Epidemiological data provide information about the levels of death (mortality) and disease (morbidity) in the community and their distribution according to such criteria as gender, age and place of residence. They come from a number of sources (Christie, Gordon & Heller 1987, p. 8):

• death rates;
• cancer mortality and morbidity rates from State cancer registers;
• health surveys and studies, for example those conducted by the Australian Institute of Health and Welfare;
• hospital discharge records;
• reports of notifiable infectious diseases.

By providing information at a population level, epidemiology provides a useful tool against which to confirm or question the hunches of health workers or community members regarding health problems in an area. This can be valuable because assumptions about problems in an area may not always be correct. For example, when staff at Gloucester Soldier Memorial Hospital reviewed injuries to children in the area as part of the Rural Child Accident Prevention Program, they were surprised to discover that horse-related accidents, rather than injuries due to farm machinery, were the major cause of child injury. Epidemiological data and surveys of the local area provided the information that was needed and which in this instance did not support the beliefs of health workers or community members generally (Lower 1992, p. 10).

It is important to note that epidemiological data are not equally available for all health problems. Some health problems have well developed databases (for example, cardiovascular disease) while others, such as depression or family violence, do not (Hawe 1996, p. 474). Similarly, until relatively recently the seriousness of Aboriginal health problems was able to be ignored because data on Aboriginal health were not collected. Relying on pre-existing epidemiological data risks focusing further attention on conditions that are already well identified at the expense of those that may be serious but that have been ignored in the past.

Epidemiological data are available from the Australian Bureau of Statistics and the Australian Institute of Health and Welfare. The reports produced by the Australian Institute of Health and Welfare are of particular value in providing and analysing up-to-date epidemiological data. These include biennial reports, such as *Australia's Health 1998* (Australian Institute of Health and Welfare 1998). Many libraries and local councils may keep some of this material if it is relevant to the surrounding area. In addition, a growing range of this data is available on the worldwide web (see Appendix 5). Also, local public health units or health promotion units may prepare epidemiological data relevant to their own areas.

Beyond epidemiology: the need for a broader approach to health assessment

Until relatively recently, epidemiology was regarded as the only measuring stick of use in health work. For many workers this remains the case. A number of points are worthy of discussion here. If we were solely interested in preventing disease, rather than being interested in health promotion and a social view of health, we might be happy with the information we can gather from morbidity and mortality data. However, from a social health perspective, morbidity and mortality data are simply not sufficient to enable us to see the problems we are concerned about. In addition, epidemiological data are of limited use in situations where no simple cause-and-effect relationship exists or where delayed onset of symptoms occurs (Auer 1988, p. 41; Public Interest Advocacy Centre, cited by Brennan 1992: 18). This may particularly be the case, for example, with environmental health issues. Epidemiology also requires a fairly long time frame before there is 'evidence' of a problem, by which time a number of people will have already experienced illness or even death.

Nor is epidemiology sufficient to measure the extent of wellness of a community and of individuals in that community. We therefore need to look at other measures of community health. Brown (1985) has called for the development of an 'epidemiology of health' to overcome the shortcomings of current epidemiological data. This would need to recognise the multifaceted dimensions of health and

HealthWIZ

The *Health for All Australians* report, which was released in 1988, proposed that jurisdictions reorient their health promotion programs to ensure marked progress towards national goals by the year 2000. In 1991 the Commonwealth Minister for Health, in responding to the recommendations of this report, implemented a number of initiatives to aid health workers in targeting their initiatives in an appropriate manner. One of these initiatives was the establishment of a National Social Health Database. This database has since become known as 'HealthWIZ'.

HealthWIZ was, and still is, an ambitious project. The aim of the project is to develop and maintain a powerful but easy to use database system delivering a comprehensive and up-to-date range of Australian health statistical data to users in one application. The HealthWIZ data library is now the single most comprehensive collection of health data in Australia, with collections from Australia's major health and welfare agencies. Data collections that are to be found in the HealthWIZ data library include:

* six years of 'Hospital use' data, from 1992–93 to 1997–98, for every State and Territory;
* time series hospital use data for every State and Territory for the years listed above;
* population data from the last three censuses in 1986, 1991 and 1996;
* establishments data for residential hospitals 1995–96;
* ten years of mortality data 1985–95;
* Department of Social Security data 1996;
* cancer data for Australia 1982–93;
* cancer data from NSW 1972–90;
* cancer data from Victoria 1982-91;
* child care data 1995;
* Residential Aged Care Services data 1997;
* dementia estimates;
* Medicare use 1990–95; and
* data used specifically for the preparation of the *National Social Health Atlas,* 1st and 2nd Edition (1993 and 1999 respectively).

This is by no means an exhaustive list, but it illustrates the enormous wealth of data contained in HealthWIZ.

With HealthWIZ, users can build a comprehensive picture of the health of a target population, including patterns of health and illness, causes of hospitalisation, causes of death, referred and unreferred consultations, services used and even explore the links between ill-health and socio-economic status.

The data in the HealthWIZ library is presented in easy to understand data sets. Users are not confronted with a large and complex data collection that may be difficult to manage. Through a menu driven program, users select precisely the data they wish to study, and only this data is delivered to their screen. The program also has a full range of functionality that allows users to print the data they have selected, export the data to word processing or spread sheet packages and display the data in maps and graphs.

HealthWIZ is used by a wide range of users for an equally wide range of purposes including:

- planning and evaluation of health services;
- research to identify trends and associations, assessing the health status of specific populations;
- identifying unmet needs;
- providing 'evidence based' services;
- assessing service use;
  Users include:
- government policy makers in Commonwealth, State and local governments;
- health planning and administration agencies;
- divisions of general practice;
- health service provider organisations;
- universities;
- research organisations;
- pharmaceutical companies;
- health insurance companies.

HealthWIZ is the result of a significant and ongoing collaborative effort between a large number of national as well as State and Territory authorities and community health organisations. It represents a significant investment by the Commonwealth in its commitment to deliver easy access to accurate, reliable, comprehensive and up-to-date health information. HealthWIZ has been developed and is managed by Prometheus Information under contract to the Population Health Division of the Commonwealth Department of Health & Aged Care.

Further information is available from:

Prometheus Information Pty Ltd
PO Box 160
Dickson ACT 2602
Tel: 02 6257 7356
Fax: 02 6241 5284
email: healthwiz@prometheus.com.au
Web site: http://www.prometheus.com.au

Christopher Roberts
Business Manager
Prometheus Information

incorporate them into any analysis of health and health problems. It is important to note that this recognition of the value of measuring health rather than illness is relatively new, and so approaches to measuring community health are still being developed. Your own work in this area can be part of the ground-breaking work that is needed.

Another issue, closely related to this notion of an epidemiology of health, is the need for the development of positive health indicators (Catford 1983). If we want to measure more than disease processes or risk factors, we need to consider how we can do this. King (1990) has suggested one possibility that may provide a useful framework on which others can build. In considering the problem of social isolation, she suggests that the focus should be on examining social participation rather than social isolation. Not only will this enable us to examine the positive aspects of the issue, it may also enable us to see more clearly some of the barriers to social participation. King's framework also focuses on the community picture rather than just on the individual so that it enables a person to be seen within the context of the community in which they live.

The views of professionals

Health workers and other professionals working in areas related to the health of the community may contribute a great deal to the assessment of needs. In particular, other health workers may themselves have listened to community members or may have conducted formal needs assessments in the past, and your use of these can save valuable time and effort. Furthermore, several different health workers may discuss an issue and each bring to it a slightly different perspective, based on individual experience and professional background (Southern Community Health Research Unit 1991, pp. 52–4). Similarly, they may each notice slightly different issues in the same community. This can all be useful in gaining an understanding of problems and issues facing the community. Your own assessment, and the assessments of your colleagues, can be a valuable adjunct to information gained from other sources.

It is worthwhile briefly examining the relationship between health workers and their communities. Sometimes health workers suggest that, because they are a part of their community, there is little need to canvass community need: what they themselves see as problems is an adequate reflection of community need. However, although health workers may be members of the community, they cannot represent all groups in it. Indeed, as a result of their professional education and socialisation, they bring a particular perspective to health issues. Certainly this perspective is a valuable one that contributes much to the debate about health and health promotion. Nevertheless, it is but one perspective, and it should not be substituted for the opinions of other community members. Therefore, while professional opinion offers a great deal, it should not be assumed to reflect the views of the whole community or remove the need for listening to the community or checking external assessments of need.

National and State policy documents

National and State policy or strategy documents often provide material from a combination of sources, particularly epidemiological data, social and economic indicators and the views of professionals. They will also have been developed with varying degrees of community consultation, depending on political will and hthe 'need' for expediency. It is important to note that national and State policy documents are often reflective more of political priorities and processes than of the needs of the community. The politically determined nature of these documents must be acknowledged. They will also need to be compared with local evidence of need rather than be assumed to reflect the local picture. With a recognition of these issues in mind, such documents can be useful sources of information and should be used wherever possible as one component of identifying needs. Some examples of national and State policy documents of value are given below. Further information about the policy documents relevant to your State or region should be available from the State's health department or a regional public health unit, although sometimes these documents can be surprisingly difficult to locate.

Some useful Australian policy and strategy documents

This list provides just some examples of Commonwealth, State and Territory documents that have been produced since 1988 and that may prove useful in helping to assess the needs of your area or the priorities of government. Look around in your own State to identify other relevant documents. Copies are usually available through regional public health units or from the Department of Health in each State.

National

Australia's Health (1992, 1994, 1996, 1998)
Healthy Horizons: a National Rural Health Strategy for Regional, Rural and Remote Australians (1999)
The Health of Young Australians: a National Health Policy for Children and Young People (1995)
The National Health Plan for Young Australians: an Action Plan to Protect and Promote the Health of Children and Young People (1996)
Better Health Outcomes for Australians: National Goals, Targets and Strategies for Better Health Outcomes into the Next Century (1994)
Australian and New Zealand Guidelines for the Assessment and Management of Contaminated Sites (1992)
A Social Health Atlas for Australia (1992)
National Food and Nutrition Policy (1992)
National Road Safety Strategy (1992)
National Non-English Speaking Background Women's Health Strategy (1991)
National Aboriginal Health Strategy (1989)
National Women's Health Policy: Advancing Women's Health in Australia (1989)
Health for All Australians (1988)

New South Wales

Caring for Mental Health (1998)
The Health of the People Of NSW (1997)
NSW Aboriginal Mental Health Policy (1997)
Mental Health Promotion in New South Wales (1997)
Caring for Health: Caring for Young People (1996)
Caring for Health: The NSW Government's Vision for Rural Health (1996)
A Healthy Future in New South Wales: a Strategic Framework (1994)
Better Health, Better Living for Women in New South Wales (1994)
Promoting Health in the Workplace (1992)
Road Safety 2000 (1992)
Public Policy and Older People (1991)
Directions on Ageing in New South Wales (1990)
Health for All: Promoting Health and Preventing Disease in New South Wales (1989)

Victoria

Healthy Eating, Healthy Victoria: a Lasting Investment (1997)
Achieving Improved Aboriginal Health Outcomes: an Approach to Reform (1997)
Health: Taking Health to the People (1996)

Aged Care: a New Era (1996)
Victoria's Health: Second Report on the Health Status of Victorians (1995)
Achieving Better Health and Health Services (1992)
Promoting Health and Preventing Illness in Victoria: a Framework (1991)

Tasmania

Tasmanian Food and Nutrition Policy (1994)
Health Goals and Targets for Tasmania (1992)
Health Promotion in Tasmania: What Does it Mean for Health Workers? (1992)
Building Healthy Futures: the Public's View (1991)

South Australia

The Health of Older People in South Australia: Policy and Strategic Directions (1995)
Strategic Directions for Primary Health Care (1993)
The Health of Young People in South Australia: Policy and Strategic Directions (1993)
A Child Health Policy for South Australia (1990)
Social Health Strategy for South Australia (1988)
Primary Health Care in South Australia: a Discussion Paper (1988)

Western Australia

Aboriginal Food and Nutrition Policy for Western Australia (1998)
Our State of Health: an Overview of Health and Illness in Western Australia (1991)

Northern Territory

The Aboriginal Public Health Strategy and Implementation Guide 1997–2002 (1998)
Northern Territory Aboriginal Health Policy (1996)
Corporate Plan (1996)
Northern Territory Food and Nutrition Policy and Strategic Plan 1995–2000 (1995)
Northern Territory Health Outcomes: Morbidity and Mortality 1979–1991 (1995)

Queensland

Queensland Mental Health Policy Statement: Mental Health Services for Older People (1996)
Queensland Mental Health Policy Statement: Aboriginal and Torres Strait Islander People (1996)
Queensland Mental Health Policy Statement: Future Directions for Child and Youth Mental Health Services (1996)
Ten Year Mental Health Strategy for Queensland (1996)
Queensland Mental Health Plan (1994)
Towards an Ethnic Health Policy for a Culturally Diverse Queensland (1994)
Aboriginal and Torres Strait Islander Health Policy (1994)
Queensland Women's Health Policy (1993)
Primary Health Care Policy (1992)
Primary Health Care Implementation Plan (1992)
Rural Health Policy (1991)

In addition to national and State documents, some regions or areas may have their own policy and strategy documents. These may be even more useful because they are one step nearer to your community and so may reflect its needs more closely. However, it is worthwhile finding out about the process by which these documents were developed. Were they simply summarised from State and national documents, or were regional needs assessments carried out? The chances are that if you have not heard of them before, they may have been prepared without consulting the community members in the region. Their value may therefore be limited.

The process of community assessment

There are several principles that should guide the approach to assessing communities in the Primary Health Care approach:

- Community assessment should be an integral part of health promotion work;
- Community assessment should reflect the social view of health, which is so much a part of health promotion and Primary Health Care (Baum 1992, p. 83);
- Community assessment should involve both formal and informal assessment of needs and resources;
- Community assessment should recognise the partnership between people themselves and health workers in determining their needs and resources, planning action and evaluating any outcomes. Part of this process may involve negotiation between community members and health workers;
- Needs assessment should involve a combination of felt, expressed, normative and comparative need.

In preparing to assess the needs of any individual, group or community, it is vital that you keep in mind why you are doing this particular assessment. What is it you are trying to find out, and to what end? This will help to determine how you will go about finding out. It is rare that the resources, including your time and the time of others involved in the process, are so freely available that you can afford to conduct needs assessment without being clear about what the reasons for it are. You also need to ensure that you will have adequate resources, or are able to obtain them, to respond appropriately to the findings of any community assessment. As discussed above, uncovering needs, creating the expectation that something will be done about them, then not acting, is unlikely to develop confidence in those whose time has been wasted.

Presenting a step-by-step guide to conducting a community assessment is beyond the scope of this book but there are some excellent resources to help you to conduct such an assessment. Of particular value is *Planning Healthy Communities* (Southern Community Health Research Unit 1991) and *Do It Yourself Social Research* (Wadsworth 1997). It is worth noting the series of steps in community assessment indentified by the Southern Community Health Research Unit (SCHRU, 1991):

1. Identify the purpose of the community assessment;
2. Identify available resources;
3. Establish a project team and steering committee;
4. Develop a research plan and time frame;
5. Collect and analyse available information;
6. Complete community research;

7. Analyse results;
8. Report back to community;
9. Set priorities;
10. Determine responses to the needs identified.

These stages demonstrate that there is much more to a community assessment than collecting information, and the planning and development of a comprehensive community assessment can be an achievement in itself. This is one reason why there is the danger of assuming that once the assessment is completed, the job is done!

A community assessment can be considered as composed of two key components — a community profile and a community survey. The information for these two components may come from a variety of sources. This description is based on what may be useful for a geographical community, but the same principles apply when assessing the needs of a smaller community, such as a workplace or school.

Community profile

Every service that has responsibility to a community will need to have access to a relatively up-to-date profile of that community. This is necessary to have a sense of what needs there may be and what demographic and social issues are likely to be shaping the lives of people in the community. As a community health worker, you may be part of the team that sets about preparing or updating a community profile. It is worthwhile to examine what sort of information you need to include in a community profile and some of the general principles involved in preparing it.

Henderson and Thomas (1987, pp. 57–68) suggest that a community profile can be considered under six interrelated categories. However, these are meant as a guide only and, if they do not meet the needs of a particular community with which you are working, you can adapt the information you collect.

Taken together, the information in these categories will start to give you a picture of the community you are working with. Remember, however, that a community profile is not something that can be completed and then filed away. Communities are dynamic and changing, and so is your understanding of your community. Keep adding to your understanding of it as you live and work there.

History

An understanding of the history of an area may help you to understand a great deal about dominant values in the community and may help explain some of the current attitudes towards contemporary events.

Environment

The environment in which people live strongly influences the way in which they can interact with each other. It also may be the source of some health problems for the community (Henderson & Thomas 1987, p. 58). For example, a town that includes a number of dirty industries and is sited in a hollow may face serious environmental pollution; a community may have little recreational space within its boundaries; or a suburb may be designed around the needs of cars, often resulting in lack of access to services for those who do not own cars (as has been seen in new western Sydney suburbs).

Residents

Obviously, information about the people themselves is extremely valuable. The information you collect here will include information about demography, housing occupation, employment levels, numbers of people receiving single-parent benefits and pensions, residents' perceptions of the area, community networks, and the values and traditions that guide life in the area (many of these may take some time to discover). This will also include epidemiological data and any other information already available about health problems.

Organisations

Several organisations may operate in, and influence, an area. Their presence and the role they play in the community will be very useful to know about. Organisations can be classified under a number of categories, including local and State government bodies, industrial and commercial organisations, religious bodies and voluntary organisations. It is worthwhile finding out about the roles played by each of these organisations in the community. For example, is there a particular company that is the main employer? Is there a religious organisation that involves itself in a lot of community work?

Communication

Knowing which mass communication methods are used in the community will help the health worker keep in contact with many goings-on. For example, what radio and television stations are received in the area, and which stations seem to be listened to or viewed by which groups of people? Which newspapers are available locally? Is there a local newspaper? However, a number of other effective communications options may also be operating. For example, are there community noticeboards that are well used?

Power and leadership

Power and leadership can be both formal and informal, and an understanding of both are needed if you are to work in a community. Information of value here includes information about leaders of local political parties, local government and community groups as well as key influential people within those organisations. It may also include information about people who seem to have a strong voice in influencing public debate or a particular organisation but who may not necessarily hold a current position of formal power.

Community survey

This component of community assessment examines the needs of the community as they are defined by the community members themselves, as well as by professionals working in the area. However, the line between a community survey and a community profile may become quite hazy with the active involvement of community members themselves in planning and organising a community assessment.

Few communities are small enough for it to be possible to ask everyone to define their needs. Therefore, more often than not, a community survey will be conducted with only a sample of people. Determining which people to ask in order to obtain an appropriate sample is a key component of planning a needs survey, and may require the involvement of people with expertise in survey development.

An essential part of any needs assessment is reporting back its findings to the people involved (Southern Community Health Research Unit 1991, pp. 257–61). This should be done as a matter of course, to ensure that the information obtained accurately reflects what people said. It will then enable community members to be involved in the priority-setting process discussed below.

Separating the problem from the solutions

In analysing the findings of a community assessment, it is possible that the need will be expressed in terms of a solution to the problem, rather than the problem itself. Indeed, often when this occurs, the assumption is that the solution presented is the only solution to the problem. This point has also been made elsewhere (Baum 1992, p. 81). It is very important to develop a vision of the problem as separate as possible from any potential solutions, and so broaden the scope for solving the problem by coming up with a range of possible solutions. This process is one in which community members and workers together can be involved. It provides an excellent opportunity for consciousness-raising to occur. As people discuss the problems in their community, they may, layer by layer, be able to work their way through to alternative conceptualisations of them. This may broaden quite markedly the choices available to them in dealing with those problems.

Setting priorities for action

It is rarely the case that a community assessment identifies only one need. It will resources to be able to deal with all the needs at once. Sometimes a number of therefore be necessary to set some priorities, as it is rare to have the time or other needs may be able to be dealt with together if they all share a similar root cause and you have recognised this in your analysis, but this will not always be the case.

So, how do you set priorities for action? Some people suggest that you deal with the easiest or most 'winnable' issues first (for example, Minkler 1991, p. 272), but there are some problems with this approach. The easiest issues to deal with may not be the ones that make the biggest difference in people's lives. Indeed, the most difficult ones may well have the biggest impact if they are acted on successfully. Priority setting done in partnership with community members is most likely to be the most successful approach because of the community support for, and action on, any decisions made. Of course, there may be times when the health risks involved are great and time for community involvement may be limited. Even then, however, maximum possible involvement by community members should be built into the decision making.

Priorities set by national health documents can be taken up if they are identified also as local health needs. The advantage here is that if they are national priorities, it is more likely that funding will be available to support health promotion projects

Conducting a community needs assessment and coming to terms with addressing the issues you find

In 1989 a rural coastal community health centre was faced with the dilemma of identifying appropriate health promotion strategies to incorporate in its future policy document. The notion of assessing the community's health needs in order to plan action made good sense. This was the beginning of the centre's Health Needs Study.

The centre had expert assistance from a senior research fellow from a nearby university, the 'legwork' being done by one of its community health nurses. The progress of the study was overseen by a steering committee comprising members of the centre's Committee of Management and staff, as well as other local health service providers.

The health needs study

The study comprised four major sections:

1. Community profile

The community profile provided an overview of demographic characteristics, community and health-related services and recreation facilities. In essence, it set the stage for the study's later sections.

2. Community health survey

The second section was prepared by the senior research fellow. A self-report questionnaire, based on one developed by the Southern Community Health Research Unit, was used to survey a random sample of local residents. It asked questions about their recent illness experiences, health behaviours (exercise, weight, diet, alcohol use and smoking), use of health screening (cholesterol, blood pressure, breast self-examination and pap smears), social support and satisfaction with the community health centre's services.

3. Community opinion

The third section of the study was concerned with seeking the opinion of the local community regarding local health needs and concerns. Groups of community leaders were brought together to discuss their ideas about the health needs of the community, and groups of people representative of the community discussed their concerns, using nominal group process methods.

4. Patterns of illness and injury

This last section looked at rates of illness and injury using the centre's records, details of hospital admissions and Workcare data.

The role of the community health nurse

The legwork done by the community health nurse encompassed a range of tasks and responsibilities relating to all sections of the study and required perseverance, persistence and a healthy sense of humour. The following examples (affectionately known as the 'hassles and giggles' of the project) highlight some of the tasks involved:

- gathering data for the community profile, including information from the Australian Bureau of Statistics and interviews with staff from local agencies

and service providers;
- finding and coordinating volunteers to deliver the community health survey;
- accessing local community groups to investigate community opinion (it was difficult to access many groups);
- searching for client contact sheets that had been mistakenly 'spring-cleaned' and were required for the retrospective audit.

The findings

As the study attempted to look at health in its social context, it had the expected outcome of identifying some broad issues that people perceived as affecting their wellbeing, in addition to more traditional ill-health problems. The major issues identified were:
- poor local public transport;
- inadequate local child care services;
- dissatisfaction with the services offered by the community health centre;
- health and environmental concern regarding local ocean sewerage outfall;
- alcohol consumption by youth and the elderly;
- a significant amount of non-participation in women's health screening (compared with Anti-Cancer Council recommendations);
- lack of social networks;
- concern about additives and chemicals in food;
- concern about the quality of local domestic water.

The next step: tackling the findings

Identifying health problems is only the first step — addressing them in a way that is relevant and meaningful to the community is the next. The findings created several dilemmas for the community health centre. They challenged the notion of community health as just a geographical base for clinical services in the community. Some members of the centre's Committee of Management were keen to ignore many of the findings, as they were not seen as relevant to a community health centre. Others now felt some sense of accountability because the findings were public. The challenge was certainly there to address broader public health issues that had previously been ignored.

Two years later, despite some changes, many of the issues raised by the study, both traditional health issues and the broader social health problems, remained unaddressed. No clear strategies or implementation plan were developed by management and staff or formalised within the service plan of the agency. The minor findings that were seen to be easier to address were given priority; for example, asthma was one of the first issues to be addressed, not because it was a major finding but because it fitted comfortably within the medical model framework the centre operated from. The documented findings initially 'sat on the shelf' to be used during funding applications, rather than being used as a living document, providing guidelines for addressing the significant health issues in the community.

Poor attendance at some of the programs offered by the centre highlighted that simply addressing health needs identified by the community was not enough. In addition, how those programs are developed and delivered must be seen as appropriate and relevant by the community. If the centre was to develop appropriate relevant health promotion strategies, a change in approach was needed. This required rethinking the role of the community health centre and its staff.

Over a period of some 2 years, this is what occurred. Through a number of processes, including addressing the community's dissatisfaction with the centre's service, visiting other community health centres, working with organisational consultants and providing inservice education for staff, particularly in the area of community development, the centre shifted from a medical model to a social model of health as its operating framework.

One salient example of this shift in practice revolved around how the health service identified and worked with the community on an issue not directly identified in the health assessment, but that emerged in the community over several years. As a tourist town, the local community was faced with an increasingly difficult situation each New Year's Eve, as large numbers of young people came to the town to party. While injuries due to alcohol, fights and missile assaults grew, and safety became a prime concern, little had been done to address the cause of the problem. The health service assisted in facilitating a process through which the community could voice its concerns to local government, and a range of key players could come together to plan ways to turn New Year's Eve into a more positive event. A wide range of strategies resulted from this whole-of-community response, and the community health centre was seen as being actively involved in the process. Everyone experienced the benefits of taking a broad preventive approach.

However, since 1992 there has been increasing pressure on the community health centre to move away again from the social model approach. The new approach of the 1990s emphasised quantifiable outcomes at the exclusion of recognising any qualitative processes or benefits.

As both national and State governments developed their own health promotion priorities, the importance of locally based needs seemed to diminish. There seemed to be a passive acceptance that these centrally determined priorities were the major health promotion areas on which we *must* focus. In an environment where there were losses of health promotion positions, increasing one-to-one workloads, and evaluation based on outputs, it is easy to see how this could occur. However, it also meant that we were in danger of losing touch with our community and our expertise in developing new and responsive programs.

In addition, these national and State priorities, based on epidemiological data, result in a focus on issues that are by their very nature illness focused. This seems to be once again taking us away from the social issues that impact on health, and back to a medical model approach.

But as time moves on, it appears that the pendulum is once again swinging back. On a structural level, we now have regional health promotion officers, who serve to remind us of the importance and relevance of local needs and programs. Additionally in 1998, the State government's 'Primary Health Program Guidelines' indicated that community health staff need to spend at least 20% of their time on health promotion. At a staff level, frustrations with a purely medical model framework are again being expressed and active steps are being taken to develop locally relevant, innovative best practice programs.

Ten years ago, when we asked local people, 'what in your day-to-day life affects or troubles you?', we did not fully anticipate the path of change that this question would lead us on. Developing services that are responsive to community needs is not an easy process. It carries with it the responsibility of community needs is not an easy process. It carries with it the responsibility of not only involving the community at all levels of identification, development and implementation, but also the responsibility that, once we begin down the path of identifying community needs, we are committed to delivering on addressing them. The challenges of such a process are not to be underestimated, nor are the rewards and benefits of making a real difference to the health of the community.

Sue Lauder
Community Health Nurse

and health workers will be encouraged to take action in this area. Similarly, some areas may be included in the charter of the agency for which you work, and so these may need to be addressed first.

Furthermore, some issues may be able to be dealt with first because the necessary expertise is available in the team with which you are working or because you have ready access to it (Henderson and Thomas 1987, p. 101). While it would be a mistake to build an agency's work around the interests of the staff rather than the needs of the community, acknowledging and working with the expertise of the staff and other available expertise is a valuable use of resources.

There are several questions worth asking about each identified need in order to help to set priorities for action. Those in the following list are based on Lund and McGechaen (1981, cited by Gilmore et al. 1989, p. 22):

- What types of need are present? Does the individual, group or community consider this as a need?
- How many people are affected?
- What will the consequences be if this need is not met?
- Is this a critical need that should be met before other needs are addressed?
- How can this need best be met? Is it likely to be affected by health promotion action?
- Does the need coincide with your department's or agency's mission statement or policies? If not, why not? Can you influence the agency's policies?
- With which community members and other agencies do you need to work in order to address the issue?
- Are resources (funds, staff) available?

Determining the most appropriate response to a need

Once you have determined which needs there are and which need (or needs) you are going to address, the next step is to determine what the best response to the latter will be, before you can plan any action. A very useful framework within which to consider this issue is the *Ottawa Charter for Health Promotion*. Should the need be dealt with by working for healthier public policy and so creating supportive environments; by working to strengthen community action; by working

ORANGESEARCH — a community view of issues and needs in Orange

ORANGESEARCH was a dynamic process of research and community consultation carried out by a multidisciplinary team in Orange, a regional city of 33 000 people in the Central West of New South Wales. It began in 1989 and formally finished in 1991, although outcomes were ongoing.

The impetus for the study arose from the need for qualitative information on what makes the city 'tick' — the flesh on the bones of the statistical picture. The study took an action research approach using an innovative tool called Rapid Rural Appraisal, more commonly used at that time in agricultural areas of developing countries. It was based on personal interviews with a broad range of people in Orange and a quantitative community profile. The purposes of ORANGESEARCH were:

- to construct an integrated picture of community needs and issues as a basis for future planning, research and debate;
- to consult with a wide range of people in the city as a basis for community involvement, interaction and development;
- to develop an effective team approach as a basis for better intersectoral cooperation and 'ownership'.

The team working on the project was drawn from five local organisations whose decisions make an impact on citizens' lives and health (Orange City Council, Orange Base Hospital, the Regional Housing Department, Orange Community Health Centre and the Central West Regional Health Promotion Unit) and two universities (University of Western Sydney, Hawkesbury Faculty of Agriculture and Rural Development; and Charles Sturt University, Mitchell School of Nursing).

The process involved five different stages:

1. Planning and preparation (4 months). This first stage involved an intensive process of working out 'how to do it', with few guidelines for an urban context; negotiating for team members and training them; selecting respondents and interview techniques; organising 200 respondents and 12 team members to conduct interviews in different pairs each day over 5 days; and designing methods of analysis, documentation and feedback.

2. Community consultation (1 week). A total of 60 people were interviewed in August 1989 — some as key respondents in their field, many in special groups (demographic and occupational) and some as randomly selected householders in contrasting suburbs. The techniques used were focus groups and semi-structured interviewing.

3. Collation, analysis and documentation (8 months). This stage involved a lengthy process of sorting information, insights and ideas from written and tape-recorded material into patterns and themes, developing models and documenting findings in a user-friendly fashion. One full report and five smaller booklets for specific target groups were produced. Over 1300 copies were distributed around Orange, the Central West and other parts of Australia.

4. Community feedback (over a 5-month period). In 1990–91 a number of successful forums were held to feed back findings and develop priority issues and action strategies for youth, young families, older people and the future of Orange. Media coverage also stimulated discussion of issues.

5. Community action (ongoing). Various organisations and individuals have taken action on a range of issues, including:
- social isolation and loneliness (Friendly Visiting Service);
- youth issues, opportunities and a 'voice' (youth coordinator, youth council, newsletter, activities);
- poor youth nutrition (Fast Foods For Families project with high schools);
- lack of parenting skills (parenting programs);
- health needs of low-income people (health promotion through the Housing Department);
- falls among the elderly (Slip No More project);
- lack of parks and equipment for young children (Safe Park project);
- treatment orientation of health services (health promotion in health services).

Through its various stages, ORANGESEARCH has been a catalyst for people participating in planning to address their own community needs and issues. The process has been used extensively in the Central West and in other regions. Its main difficulties are in analysing a large amount of qualitative data and organising consultation. Its strengths lie in its flexibility and its capacity to involve people, improve understanding of complex issues and stimulate action related to community needs.

Margaret Carroll
(previously) ORANGESEARCH Coordinator

to further develop people's personal skills (through some form of health education); or by working to reorient the health system to a greater emphasis on health promotion? Or should it be dealt with by a combination of some or all of these approaches? You may decide that action will need to occur on some levels to address the problem in the short term, while you are attempting on other levels to address it over the longer term. For example, working for public policy change may take some time, and in the meantime you may need to help people to develop some of their own skills to deal with the situation they are in.

Individual needs assessment

You may be working with individuals in determining their needs. In that case, you are most likely to be useful as an assistant or consultant to the person concerned, rather than being the person making the assessment. As much as possible, you need to work with individuals to enable them to assess their situation, and help them to develop their own skills in assessment. However, remember that even self-assessments can be devised in a way that does not help people to gain control over their lives. Over-emphasising medical aspects in a health self-assessment may not be useful for people if they want to assess their health within the context of their whole lives, and may focus attention on individual behaviour changes alone. Individual needs may also be addressed by working for public policy change or other environmental changes, rather than focusing solely on the individual.

Group needs assessment

The principles to be considered when conducting an individual or a community needs assessment also apply when working with a group to assess its needs. An understanding of group dynamics will also help you to work with the group throughout the needs assessment process (see Chapter 8).

Conclusion

Research is an integral part of a Primary Health Care approach to health promotion. It has potential both to provide invaluable information for the understanding of major health issues and how best to address them, and to itself be a health promoting activity when it is conducted using participatory research processes.

One of the key uses of research in health promotion is in the community assessment process. Community assessment incorporates assessment of both needs and resources and provides a firm foundation on which health promotion priorities can be set and action undertaken. Community assessment may be both a formal and an informal process, but it is always a means to achieve health promoting change for community members; it is never an end in itself.

References and further reading

Alcorso, C. and Schofield, T. 1991, *The National Non-English Speaking Background Women's Health Strategy,* Australian Government Publishing Service, Canberra.

Allison, K. R. and Rootman, I. 1996, 'Scientific rigour and community participation in health promotion research: are they compatible?' *Health Promotion International,* 11 (4), 333–40.

Auer, J. 1988, *Exploring Legislative Arrangements For Promoting Primary Health Care in Australia,* Social Health Branch, South Australian Health Commission, Adelaide.

Australian and New Zealand Environment and Conservation Council and National Health and Medical Research Council 1992, *Australian and New Zealand Guidelines for the Assessment and Management of Contaminated Sites,* ANZECC and NHMRC, Canberra.

Australian Institute of Health and Welfare 1998, *Australia's Health 1998: the Sixth Biennial Report of the Australian Institute of Health and Welfare,* Australian Institute of Health and Welfare, Canberra.

Baum, F. 1992, 'Researching Community Health: Evaluation and Needs Assessment that Makes an Impact', in Baum, F., Fry, D. and Lennie, I. (eds), *Community Health: Policy and Practice in Australia,* Pluto Press/Australian Community Health Association, Sydney, NSW.

Baum, F. 1995, 'Researching Public Health: Behind the Qualitative-Quantitative Methodological Debate', *Social Science and Medicine,* 40 (4), 459–68.

Baum, F. 1998, *The New Public Health: an Australian Perspective,* Oxford University Press, Melbourne.

Becker, M. H. 1986, 'The Tyranny of Health Promotion', *Public Health Review,* 14, 15–25.

Billings, J. R. and Cowley, S. 1995, 'Approaches to Community Needs Assessment: a Literature Review', *Journal of Advanced Nursing,* 22, 721–30.

Boutilier, M., Mason, R. and Rootman, I. 1997, 'Community Action and Reflective

Practice in Health Promotion Research', *Health Promotion International*, 12 (1), 69–78.

Bradshaw, J. 1972, 'The Concept of Social Need', *New Society*, 30 March, 640–3.

Brennan, A. 1992, 'The Altona Clean Air Project', *Health Issues*, September, 32, 18–20.

Broadhead, P., Duckett, S. and Lavender, G. 1989, 'Developing a Mandate for Change: Planning as a Political Process, *Community Health Studies*, 13 (3), 243–57.

Brown, V. A. 1985, 'Towards an epidemiology of health: a basis for planning community health programs', *Health Policy*, 4, 331–40.

Brown, W. J. and Redman, S. 1995, Setting targets: 'A Three-Stage Model for Determining Priorities in Health Promotion', *Australian Journal of Public Health*, 19, 263–9.

Browning, C. J. 1992, 'Mass Screening in Public Health', in Gardner, H. (ed.), *Health Policy: Development, Implementation, and Evaluation in Australia*, Churchill Livingstone, Melbourne.

Carr, L. M. 1988, 'Dental Health of Children in Australia 1977–1985', *Australian*

Carr, W. and Kemmis, S. 1986, *Becoming Critical: Knowing through Action Research*, Deakin University Press, Victoria.

Catford, J. C. 1983, 'Positive Health Indicators: Towards a New Information Base for Health Promotion', *Community Medicine*, 5, 125–32.

Christie, D., Gordon, I. and Heller, R. 1987, *Epidemiology: an Introductory Text for Medical and Other Health Science Students*, New South Wales University Press, Kensington.

Commonwealth Department of Health and Family Services 1996, *The National Health Plan for Young Australians: an Action Plan to Protect and Promote the Health of Children and Young People*, Australian Government Publishing Service, Canberra.

Commonwealth Department of Health, Housing and Community Services 1992, *The National Food and Nutrition Policy*, Australian Government Publishing Service, Canberra.

Commonwealth Department of Human Services and Health 1995, *The Health of Young Australians: a National Health Policy for Children and Young People*, Australian Government Publishing Service, Canberra.

Crotty, M. 1998, *The Foundations of Social Research: Meaning and Perspective in the Research Process*, Allen and Unwin, Sydney.

Crowley, V. and Cruse, S. 1992, *Discussion Paper on Ethics in Aboriginal Research*, Aboriginal Research Institute, University of South Australia, Adelaide.

Davies, J. K. and Kelly, M. P. (eds) 1993, *Healthy Cities: Research and Practice*, Routledge, London and New York.

Ewles, I. and Simnett, L. 1985, *Promoting Health: a Practical Guide to Health Education*, John Wiley and Sons, Chichester, UK.

Federal Office of Road Safety 1992, *The National Road Safety Strategy*, Federal Office of Road Safety, Department of Transport and Communication, Canberra.

Feuerstein, M-T. 1986, *Partners in Evaluation: Evaluating Development and Community Programmes with Participants*, Macmillan, London.

Fitzsimmons, G. and Jorm, L. (eds) 1998, *The Health of the People of NSW: Report of the Chief Health Officer 1997*, Epidemiology and Surveillance Brach, Public Health Division, NSW Health Department, North Sydney.

Gilmore, G. D., Campbell, M. D. and Becker, B. 1989, *Needs Assessment Strategies for Health Education and Health Promotion,* Benchmark Press, Indianapolis, Indiana.

Glover, J. and Woollacott, T. 1992, *A Social Health Atlas of Australia, Volumes 1 And 2,* Australian Bureau of Statistics, Canberra.

Hawe, P. 1996, 'Needs Assessment Must Become More Change-Focused', *Australian and New Zealand Journal of Public Health,* 20 (5), 473–8.

Hawe, P., Degeling, D. and Hall, J. 1990, *Evaluating Health Promotion: a Health Workers' Guide,* MacLennan and Petty, Sydney.

Hawtin, M., Hughes, G. and Percy-Smith, J. 1994, *Community Profiling: Auditing Social Needs,* Open University Press, Buckingham.

Henderson, P. and Thomas, D. N. 1987, *Skills in Neighbourhood Work,* Allen and Unwin, London.

Houston, S. and Legge, D. 1992, 'Aboriginal Health Research and the National Aboriginal Health Strategy', *Australian Journal of Public Health,* 16 (2), 114–15.

Kane, P. 1991, *Researching Women's Health: an Issues Paper,* Australian Government Publishing Service, Canberra.

Kelly, J. G. 1988, *A Guide to Conducting Prevention Research in the Community: First Steps,* Haworth Press, New York.

King, L. 1990, 'Indicators of Social Participation', in *Healthy Environments in the 90s: the Community Health Approach,* Papers from the 3rd National Conference of the Australian Community Health Association, Australian Community Health Association, Sydney.

Labonté, R. and Robertson, A. 1996. 'Delivering the Goods, Showing our Stuff: the Case for a Constructivist Paradigm for Health Promotion Research and Practice', *Health Education Quarterly,* 23 (4), 431–47.

Lafaille, R. and Fulder, S. (eds) 1993, *Towards a New Science of Health,* Routledge, London and New York.

Lower, T. 1992, 'Town Survey: Horse Falls Top Injury List', *Better Health Briefing,* No. 5, January, 10.

Matrice, D. 1990. *'Fair-Play' Guidelines for Consumer Researchers,* Consumers' Health Forum of Australia, Curtin, ACT.

Matrice, D. and Brown, V. 1990, *Widening the Research Focus: Consumer Roles in Public Health Research,* Consumers' Health Forum, Curtin, ACT.

McTaggart, R. 1991, 'Principles for Participatory Action Research', *Adult Education Quarterly,* 41 (3), 168–87.

Mies, M. 1983, 'Towards a Methodology for Feminist Research', in Bowles, G. and Duelli Klein, R. (eds), *Theories Of Women's Studies,* Routledge and Kegan Paul, London.

Minkler, M. 1991, 'Improving Health through Community Organization', in Glanz, K., Lewis, F. M. and Rimer, B. K. (eds), *Health Behavior and Health Education: Theory Research and Practice,* Jossey-Bass, San Francisco.

New South Wales Consultative Committee on Ageing 1991, *Public Policy and Older People,* Office on Ageing, NSW Premier's Department, Sydney.

New South Wales Department of Health 1990, *Directions on Ageing in New South Wales,* Office on Ageing, NSW Premier's Department, Sydney.

New South Wales Department of Health 1991a, *Dental Health in NSW: a Strategic Plan (Draft),* Dental Health Unit, NSW Department of Health, Sydney.

New South Wales Department of Health 1991b, *Health Care at Any Cost?,* NSW

Department of Health, Sydney.

New South Wales Department of Health 1992, *Promoting Health in the Workplace,* NSW Department of Health, Sydney.

New South Wales Department of Health 1994, *A Healthy Future in New South Wales: a Strategic Framework,* New South Wales Department of Health, Sydney.

New South Wales Health Department 1998, *Caring for Mental Health: a Framework for Mental Health Care in NSW,* New South Wales Health Department, Sydney.

Oakley, A. 1990, 'Who's Afraid of the Randomized Clinical Trial? Some Dilemmas of the Scientific Method and "Good" Research Practice', in Roberts, H. (ed.), *Women's Health Counts,* Routledge, London and New York.

Oakley, P. 1989, *Community Involvement in Health Development,* World Health Organization, Geneva.

Office of Aboriginal Health, Health Department of Western Australia 1998, *Aboriginal Food and Nutrition Policy for Western Australia,* Office of Aboriginal Health, Health Department of Western Australia, Perth.

Ong, B. N. 1996, *Rapid Appraisal and Health Policy,* Open University Press, Buckingham.

Patterson, A. F. 1990, *Who Caries? A Report on the Dental Health Status of Children in the Moree District, New England, NSW,* unpublished report.

Plant, A., Condon, J. R. and Durling, G. 1995, *Northern Territory Health Outcomes: Morbidity and Mortality 1979–1991.* Northern Territory Department of Health and Community Services, Darwin.

Poland, B. D. 1992, 'Learning to 'Walk Our Talk': the Implications of Sociological Theory for Research Methodologies in Health Promotion', *Canadian Journal of Public Health,* Suppl. 1, March-April, S31–S46.

Popay, J. and Williams, G. (eds) 1994, *Researching The People's Health,* Routledge, London and New York.

Public Health Strategy Unit, Territory Health Services 1998, *The Aboriginal Public Health Strategy and Implementation Guide 1997–2002,* Territory Health Services, Darwin.

Queensland Health 1991, *Rural Health Policy,* Queensland Department of Health, Brisbane.

Queensland Health 1992, *A Primary Health Care Implementation Plan,* Queensland Department of Health, Brisbane.

Queensland Health 1992, *A Primary Health Care Policy,* Queensland Department of Health, Brisbane.

Queensland Health 1993, *Queensland Women's Health Policy,* Queensland Health, Brisbane.

Queensland Health 1994, *Aboriginal and Torres Strait Islander Health Policy,* Queensland Health, Brisbane.

Queensland Health 1994, *Queensland Mental Health Plan,* Mental Health Branch Queensland Health, Brisbane.

Queensland Health 1994, *Towards an Ethnic Health Policy for a Culturally Diverse Queensland,* Ethnic Health Policy Unit, Queensland Health, Brisbane.

Queensland Health 1996, *Future Directions for Child and Youth Mental Health Services,* Queensland Health, Brisbane.

Queensland Health 1996, *Queensland Mental Health Policy Statement, Mental health services for older people,* Queensland Health, Brisbane.

Queensland Health 1996, *Queensland Mental Health Policy Statement, Aboriginal and Torres Strait Islander People,* Queensland Health, Brisbane.

Queensland Health 1996, *Ten Year Mental Health Strategy for Queensland,* Queensland Health, Brisbane.

Rae, C. 1995, *Northern Territory Food and Nutrition Policy and Strategic Plan 1995–2000,* Territory Health Services, Darwin.

Rissel, C. 1991, 'The Tyranny of Needs Assessment in Health Promotion', *Evaluation Journal of Australia,* 3 (1) 26–31.

Roads and Traffic Authority, New South Wales 1992, *Road Safety 2000: the Strategic Plan for Road Safety in NSW, 1990s and Beyond,* Road Safety Bureau, Roads and Traffic Authority, Rosebery.

Scanlon, K., Williams, M. and Raphael, B. 1997, *Mental Health Promotion in NSW: Conceptual Frameworks for Developing Initiatives.* NSW Health Department, Sydney.

Selener, D. 1997, *Participatory Action Research and Social Change,* The Cornell Participatory Action Research Network, Cornell University, Ithaca, New York.

Short, S. 1989, 'Community Participation or Community Manipulation? A Case Study of the Illawarra Cancer Appeal-A-Thon', *Community Health Studies,* 13 (1), 34–8.

South Australian Health Commission 1988, *A Social Health Strategy for South Australia,* South Australian Health Commission, Adelaide.

South Australian Health Commission 1988, *Primary Health Care in South Australia: a Discussion Paper,* South Australian Health Commission, Adelaide.

South Australian Health Commission 1990, *A Child Health Policy for South Australia,* South Australian Health Commission, Adelaide.

South Australian Health Commission 1993, *Strategic Directions for Primary Health Care,* South Australian Health Commission, Adelaide.

South Australian Health Commission 1993, *The Health of Young People in South Australia: Policy and Strategic Directions.* South Australian Health Commission, Adelaide.

Southern Community Health Research Unit 1991, *Planning Healthy Communities: a Guide to Doing Community Needs Assessment,* Southern Community Health Research Unit, Bedford Park, South Australia.

Tasmanian Department of Health 1991, *Building Better Futures: the Public's View,* Background Paper No. 1, Health Policy Division, Department of Health, Hobart.

Tasmanian Department of Health 1992, *Health Goals and Targets for Tasmania,* Health Policy Division, Department of Health, Hobart.

Tasmanian Department of Health 1992, *Health Promotion in Tasmania: What Does It Mean for Health Workers?,* Health Policy Division, Department of Health, Hobart.

Tasmanian Department of Health and Human Services 1994, *Tasmanian Food and Nutrition Policy,* Department of Health and Human Services, Hobart.

Territory Health Services 1996, *Corporate Plan 1996/99,* Territory Health Services, Darwin.

Territory Health Services 1996, *Northern Territory Aboriginal Health Policy,*

Territory Health Services, Darwin.

Thomson, N. 1991, 'A Review of Aboriginal Health Status', in Reid, J. and Trompf, P. (eds), *The Health Of Aboriginal Australia,* Harcourt Brace Jovanovich, Sydney.

Twelvetrees, A. 1987, *Community Work,* Macmillan, London.

Waddell, V. P. and Lee, N. A. (eds) 1991, *Our State of Health: an Overview of the Health of the Western Australian Population,* Health Department of Western Australia.

Wadsworth, Y. 1982, 'The Politics of Social Research: a Social Research Strategy for the Community Health, Education and Welfare Movement', *Australian Journal of Social Issues,* 17 (3), 232–46.

Wadsworth, Y. 1992, *Hearing the Voice of the Consumer: an Annotated Bibliography of Consumer Research in Public Health,* Action Research Issues Association, Melbourne.

Wadsworth, Y. 1997, *Do It Yourself Social Research,* Allen and Unwin, St Leonards.

Walker, M. and Dixon, J. 1984, *Participation in Change: Australian Case Studies,* Mitchell College Of Advanced Education, Bathurst, NSW.

Wass, A. 1990, 'The New Legitimacy of Women's Health: In Whose Interests?', in Smith, A. (ed.), *Women's Health in Australia,* Angie Smith, Armidale, NSW.

CHAPTER 4

Evaluating health promotion

There is real value in health workers evaluating every aspect of their work, using appropriate methods and approaches. The daily practice of an individual health worker, the overall work of an agency or team, and specific health promotion activities or projects will all benefit from regular evaluation, either formal or informal. Each health promotion activity, whether it is community development, lobbying for public policy change or health education, will benefit from some form of evaluation.

In practice, good health promotion is guided by a recurring process of assessing, planning, acting, implementing and evaluating, followed by re-assessing, re-planning, re-implementing and re-evaluating, in a continuous cycle of reflection and action similar to action research. In such an approach, the lines between assessment, planning, action and evaluation become fine. Moreover, as this process continues and then recurs, the line between evaluation and assessment becomes particularly unclear. As a result, many of the issues discussed in the previous chapter are extremely relevant to evaluation.

This chapter will re-examine some of those issues as they relate to evaluation in health promotion and describe some of the important elements of evaluation applied to daily practice and the activities with which you are involved. It will also consider the importance of making evaluation itself a participatory, potentially empowering experience for both health workers and community members.

Approaches to research in evaluation

Evaluation in health care has traditionally been grounded in the positivist approach to research, with a focus largely on quantitative measurement of outcomes. In this approach, experimental techniques, and particularly randomised controlled trials, have been regarded as the most acceptable approach to evaluation.

However, this approach is clearly not appropriate for many health promotion activities, such as working for policy change or community action, when outcomes may not be amenable to statistical analysis. Even in more traditional health promotion, such as health education, focus on quantitatively measured outcomes may not always be appropriate because they cannot answer all the questions we need to ask. There is growing recognition of the importance of both qualitative and quantitative approaches to evaluation, as well as recognition of the importance of a wide range of outcomes not directly related to morbidity or mortality.

The limitations of a quantitative approach to evaluation have been recognised for some time (Furler 1979), although it seems that the primacy of the quantitative approach remains, particularly with many government decision makers. Certainly quantitative approaches to evaluation can contribute significantly to evaluation processes when they are used appropriately and in balance with other approaches. However, by their very nature, they are often unable to provide the answers to questions regarded as important in health promotion. Evaluating any activity needs to be built around evaluation methods appropriate to the program and enable it to maintain a level of flexibility sufficient to respond to the needs of the people for whom it is being implemented. There is a great deal of important work still to be done in this area to develop useful evaluation methods for health promotion.

Participatory evaluation

One of the key features of working with a Primary Health Care approach is that the evaluation process actively involves the people for whom the project is running, building on their active involvement in the assessment, planning and implementation of health promoting activities. It is for this reason that participatory evaluation fits most comfortably with a Primary Health Care approach — because it is built on this active involvement of community members in the evaluation process (Feuerstein 1986; Wadsworth 1997). Wadsworth points out that while non-participatory research may come up with useful outcomes, 'a non-participatory, non-democratic process of evaluation cannot *ensure* a user-appropriate outcome' (Wadsworth 1997, p. 16).

In addition to what you do to promote health, how you do it is very important and can have a positive or negative impact on the people with whom you are working. This is just as true for evaluation as for any other aspect of health promotion — the process of the evaluation activity can itself be a positive or negative experience for both community members and health workers. It is recognition of this fact, along with recognition of the expertise community members have on issues with which they are involved, that is behind support for participatory evaluation. Evaluation that makes conclusions about a health promotion activity but does so in a way that is disempowering will be of limited value for community members.

Of course, community members or program participants are not the only people interested in the outcomes of health promotion evaluation. Funding bodies, managers and other health workers may be keen to see health promotion evaluated, and their needs may be very different to those of community members participating in the program.

What is evaluation?

Evaluation has been described as 'the process by which we judge the value or worth of something' (Suchman 1967, cited by Hawe, Degeling & Hall 1990, p. 10). Despite the impression we are often given that evaluation is an objective process that will inform us of the 'best' way to proceed, it is clearly a process of judgment, and this judgment can never be value-free. On the contrary, evaluation is very much a value-driven process and in a Primary Health Care approach it is the values of Primary Health Care that drive the evaluation; that is, the needs of the people for whom the activity is carried out are foremost, as are issues of community control, social justice and equity. However, other evaluation requirements may not be reflective of these values and may be driven sometimes by competing values such as cost control or prior political decisions to close services.

Much detailed evaluation of the effectiveness of different strategies is beyond the scope of health workers in their everyday practice and more in the realm of special evaluation projects, conducted by either health workers or skilled researchers or a team of both (Hawe, Degeling & Hall 1990, pp. 10–11). Several books examine in detail how to plan and implement evaluation. Although this chapter will examine some of the principles of evaluation, you are advised to read elsewhere for more in-depth examination of the issues and skills (see, in particular, Wadsworth 1997; Feuerstein 1986; Hawe, Degeling & Hall 1990).

Why evaluate?

Whether you are working as a sole practitioner, in a team within a larger institution or as part of a small agency or centre, you will need to find out if your work addresses the needs of those to whom you are accountable. This raises the issue of the dual accountabilities that health workers usually face. On the one hand, health workers have a responsibility to their employer to work in accordance with any 'reasonable' demands made of them, while on the other hand they have a responsibility to the individuals and communities they are meant to serve. This dual responsibility has implications for each worker's practice, and the evaluation of the work of the agency.

In work done from a Primary Health Care approach, health workers' responsibility to the community is taken very seriously. If health bureaucracies and employers uphold a Primary Health Care approach, they are supportive of this primary responsibility and help health workers to respond to the needs of their own communities. Unfortunately, the Australian health care system has not reoriented to a Primary Health Care approach, and health workers may often find themselves experiencing some difficulty as they attempt to grapple with their dual accountabilities to central planning agencies and their communities. Evaluating against the principles of Primary Health Care on the one hand, and the sometimes competing requirements of bureaucratic expectation on the other, may present some challenges.

Evaluating activities carried out to promote health makes good sense, as a way of ensuring that people's needs are being met through those activities and that each activity is the best it can be. In recent years, however, there has been an increased expectation that health workers, particularly those engaged in community health or health promotion, evaluate their practice and justify how they spend their time by demonstrating the outcomes of their practice. Health workers therefore face two competing challenges in planning meaningful evaluation. The first is from the increased pressure to demonstrate efficiency and effectiveness as a result of reporting requirements to the health bureaucracy. The second is from communities and consumers wanting increased responsiveness and relevance to their needs.

The health outcomes movement has been growing in momentum with the growth of economic rationalism and managerialism. It is reflected in an increased expectation that strategies used in response to a health issue should be demonstrated to have a positive effect on health. This represents a serious challenge to much of medical and health care practice for, as the World Health Organization itself has identified, a significant proportion of medical technologies and treatments have not been evaluated for effectiveness.

The consequences of this for acute medical care could be far-reaching if there was an increased expectation of health expenditure making an improvement in people's health. Indeed, it would be expected that this itself may result in the health system shifting to a greater balance between illness treatment and health promotion.

However, it also raises some significant challenges for health promotion. Many health promotion activities are unevaluated, although in many situations there may be anecdotal reports from service users that they found the activity useful, or analyses by health workers that the environment seems to present less of a threat to health, for example. Also, because of the nature of much health promotion work, which may be long term, developmental and complex, much health promotion work is very difficult to evaluate, and attributing the cause of changes to specific activities almost impossible (see, e.g. Chapman 1993). This by itself is a serious difficulty when decision makers interpret this as a problem of the work itself rather than the realities of evaluation research.

With the increasing evaluation requirements placed on health promoters, there is a great danger that the short-term simple (and potentially less useful) health promotion activities will be encouraged over the more innovative, longer-term activities, which have potential to make a real difference to health, primarily because they are more easy to evaluate and outcomes can be reported in a short time frame (Baum 1996, p. 38). That is, in workers may be so driven to evaluate that programs are developed to match the evaluation methods available, rather than the other way round. 'Too often the evaluation tail wags the program dog as practitioners choose objectives amenable to evaluation' (Freudenberg 1984, p. 46).

This may also have the effect of discouraging health workers from taking up innovative health promotion work — because it is difficult to evaluate. It is not surprising that evaluation methods lag behind innovative strategies (Hawe, Degeling & Hall 1990, p. 9), but it is vital that this should not prevent innovation and experimentation. Hawe & Shiell (1995) suggest that we need to think of health promotion as an investment package, balancing innovative but high-risk (because we can't yet make definitive statements about outcome) programs with the more straightforward low-risk programs in which evidence of effect is provided in the research literature. Indeed, such an approach is needed if we are to implement health promotion across the range of strategies of the *Ottawa Charter for Health Promotion.*

For example, working to increase equity, to improve the health chances of the poor or Aboriginal and Torres Strait Islander people, would have to be regarded as the most important projects of health promotion. Such goals require long-term commitment and resources and face many barriers, but the outcomes if successful could be great. However, if outcome criteria revolve around whether or not a project is easily measurable, specific and achievable within a short funding cycle, a great deal of 'evaluatable' activity may be achieved but it may do little in the long term to improve health.

However, some concern has been expressed recently that government and other funding bodies expect health promotion to be evaluated to a much greater extent than is expected of the rest of the health system. This is not to suggest that evaluation of health promotion is a useless enterprise — clearly, it is very useful. However, those who express concern about evaluation at a greater level than that expected of the mainstream illness management system are concerned that health promotion is being set up to fail by being required to demonstrate its impact on people's health over a short period of time and after relatively minor activities. Furthermore, evaluating activities beyond a reasonable level acts as a drain on the very limited resources available for health promotion. For those reasons, evaluation activities need to be critically reviewed and carefully considered so that inappropriate evaluation does not become part of the problem.

There are several different reasons why you may be evaluating and these are important because they will determine to a large extent just what you will examine in your evaluation. For example, you might want to find out if your activities are meeting the needs of members of the community for whom they were designed. Also, you might need to find out how your activity measured up against the criteria set by your funding body to justify continuation of funding. Or you may want to evaluate the achievements of your agency or team in the process of working to promote health, to plan further staff development. The requirements of each of these types of evaluation are quite different, and may require you to evaluate the activity from a different perspective and to ask different questions. At any one time, you may be evaluating in order to address one or all of these issues. However, there may also be times when an evaluation is conducted to justify a decision already made, such as when an evaluation is used to justify closure of a service or a cutback of funds (Owen and Mohr 1986, p. 96). It is this kind of use of evaluation that has made health workers somewhat suspicious of evaluation.

One of the concerns of health workers is that the needs of these different evaluation perspectives often seem to conflict. Health workers may fear that if they evaluate their practice honestly and highlight areas for improvement, this information may be used to justify reduction of funding for their activities. This may realistically mean that evaluations should not be expected to be all things to all people, and evaluations conducted for different reasons can be conducted separately. The key here, of course, is to ensure that this does not result in too much repetition and excess energy being expended on evaluation. Another important point to be considered is that all these perspectives should share a concern for the needs of the people for whom the service or activity is performed. Evaluation from the point of view of whether or not the needs of the group for whom the service or activity is designed are being addressed should permit some common ground between evaluation from these various perspectives (Wadsworth 1997, pp. 15–16). Unfortunately, though, as government funding and services are withdrawn and the economy becomes all powerful, there is concern that this primacy of the needs of community members can no longer be assumed.

Thinking through the implications of all these perspectives at the planning stage will mean that much of the information that is required by the different perspectives can be built into the implementation of the activity, making even formal evaluation for the managers or funders of a project more easy than it might be if evaluation is regarded as an 'add on' activity.

A culture of evaluation

In discussing action research in Chapter 3, we described its potential use as a process for health workers' critical reflection of their own practice. Evaluating your own practice can be a part of every working day. It can also be part of a more formal process in which health workers, either individually or as part of the team with which they are working, take time out every so often to formally review the activities with which they have been involved and the priorities to which they have been working. Building informal and formal evaluation into your own practice will add greatly to the relevance and the power of your health promotion work.

No amount of formal evaluation will be able to make up for the quality of evaluative work that is possible when informal evaluation is a part of your way of working or that of your team. That is, if you keep an 'ear to the ground' and are receptive to learning about what other people think of your work and that of your agency as a whole, and if you informally evaluate your own practice on a daily basis, the quality of evaluation will be considerably higher than if you had considered your evaluation only at those times when a formal evaluation was being conducted. In addition, this ongoing evaluation will enable you to respond to problems that you see and needs that arise, and your resultant activity is likely to be so much more dynamic and in line with the needs you are attempting to address.

This process involves developing a 'culture of evaluation' (Wadsworth 1997, p. 57), and it is an essential part of Primary Health Care practice. Questions such as 'What went well there?', 'What would I like to do differently next time?' and 'What else would I like to experiment with next time?' are ones you can ask as a matter of course at the end of each activity. Such questions can easily be asked by every health worker on a regular basis throughout his or her working day as well as at various stages throughout health promotion programs. Colin and Garrow (1996) describe this process as 'thinking, listening, looking, understanding and acting as you go along'.

Planning to evaluate

Before planning any evaluation, you will need to address the question of whether you should evaluate the program, whether it is ready to be evaluated. This is described as evaluability assessment (Hawe, Degeling & Hall 1990). There are three questions to be considered here (Northern Community Health Research Unit 1991, p. 7):

1. Why is the evaluation being done?
2. Is the program able to be evaluated? Are aims and objectives for it clearly set down?
3. Do you have the time and resources to evaluate appropriately?

The evaluation itself needs to be realistic and achievable, within the budget (in terms of time and other resources) that you can afford. This may mean that you will need to prioritise your evaluation questions and ask those that will give you the most useful information at the most reasonable cost (Rissel 1991, p. 30).

Components of evaluation

There are three key components to evaluation — process evaluation, impact evaluation and outcome evaluation. Together, these components should paint a fairly comprehensive picture of your activity. Which elements fit into each of these categories will depend on just what your activity was aiming to do — something that forms the process of one activity may be part of the outcome of another.

Process evaluation

Process evaluation is about evaluating the way in which a health promotion activity was implemented. Because of the centrality of process in the Primary Health Care approach to health promotion, examination of the process of the activity is particularly important.

For a comprehensive evaluation of the process of health promotion, several issues need to be examined (Hawe, Degeling & Hall 1990, p. 61):
• Is the program or activity reaching the people for whom it was designed?
• What do the participants think of the program or activity?
• Is the program or activity being implemented as planned?
• Are all aspects of the program of good quality?

In addition, the particular process elements important in a Primary Health Care approach will include such things as how power was shared between health workers and participants — that is, what kind of participation occurred — and to what extent the direction of the project changed in response to the needs of the participants.

Impact and outcome evaluation

Impact and outcome evaluation consider what was achieved through the particular action being evaluated. Most commonly, impact and outcome evaluation occur when one is examining the extent to which the aims and objectives of the project have been met. In this case, impact evaluation measures the extent to which the objectives of the activity or project occurred, while outcome evaluation measures the extent to which the aim or aims of the project occurred (Hawe, Degeling & Hall 1990, p. 44). This form of evaluation is known as goal-based evaluation because you are evaluating against goals set for the activity or project (McKenzie & Jurs 1993, p. 204).

Evaluation will therefore be a matter of examining the extent to which the aims and objectives of the program or activity have been met. Objectives that are clearly stated will be relatively easy to evaluate, while it will be difficult to evaluate objectives which are not clearly stated because it may not be possible to work out just what was intended by the person or people who wrote the objectives. Of course, when people evaluate their own work and they were involved in setting the objectives, they may be able to compensate for unclearly written objectives to some extent.

However, evaluation carried out by comparing results with aims and objectives is not a complete evaluation of the outcome of a project because it does not provide an opportunity to note any outcomes that do not relate directly to the aims and objectives. These outcomes may either add greater benefit to the activity or undermine some of its other benefits. In either case, these unpredicted consequences are an important part of the program, and reliance solely on evaluation against aims and objectives would have caused them to be missed. For these reasons, some evaluation not directly linked to the aims and objectives is useful. This is described by some as 'goal-free evaluation' (McKenzie & Jurs 1993, p. 207).

Wadsworth (1997, p. 39) describes this goal-free evaluation as open-ended inquiry. She highlights the importance of conducting it before starting any examination of whether specific aims and objectives have been met. This is because this process of measurement against objectives is itself a fairly narrow process that does not encourage creativity. Doing this evaluation first may mean that it is then very difficult for people to think broadly and creatively. Open-ended inquiry will not, however, make it difficult to examine later the extent to which aims and objectives have been met, and, indeed, may help you to evaluate your aims and objectives themselves.

Another limitation of evaluating against aims and objectives is that the value of the evaluation is dependent on the quality and appropriateness of the aims and objectives, and therefore on the quality of the research on which they were based and the process by which they were developed (Wadsworth 1997, p. 48). Relying solely on aims and objectives that may not have been drawn up under optimum conditions severely limits the potential value of any evaluation.

Wadsworth (1997, pp. 48–9) suggests that the philosophical values that guide the development of an organisation may provide better guidance for an evaluation than the specific aims and objectives. This is because aims and objectives may not reflect the value base and long-term goals of the organisation, and the extent to which this has been implemented may in fact be the most important thing for you to evaluate.

Evaluating the work of your agency

Evaluating the work of your agency or team is a vital process to prevent it wandering from its original goals or away from addressing the needs of the community you are working for. Informal evaluation can be incorporated into the normal work of the agency or team, for example, through discussion and reflection at weekly staff meetings. It will be necessary, however, for the agency or team to take time out to evaluate itself more formally and to involve the community in this process. This can be done by setting time aside specifically for evaluation and strategic planning. Although much of this can occur as a regular internal process, such as yearly evaluation and planning days, it can also be done by involving the agency or team in formal evaluation processes that include external evaluators. In these situations, however, care must be taken to ensure that the process is a supportive and useful one for the health workers and community members concerned.

The Australian Health and Community Services Standards

One formal evaluation process that has developed in recent years and is built around the principles of Primary Health Care is the Australian Health and Community Services Standards. This program began in New South Wales in 1982 as the Community Health Accreditation and Standards Project (CHASP), under the auspices of the Australian Community Health Association, and was then developed into an Australia-wide accreditation project (Fry 1992, p. 132).

Although designed originally for community health centres, it quickly became apparent that CHASP provided a model on which evaluation and accreditation processes for other types of teams and services could be built to enable them to be evaluated against the principles of Primary Health Care. In addition, the fact that it not only reflects Primary Health Care in the issues it addresses, but also incorporates Primary Health Care principles into the accreditation process, means that the process can be an important developmental one, both for an agency as a whole and for individual workers.

When the CHASP review process was evaluated in 1992 to determine whether it was effective in improving community health services, the result was a largely positive evaluation by both the managers of services that have undergone a review and the internal reviewers from those services. Many unexpected benefits 'such as better team cohesion and more critical reflection amongst community health workers' were apparent in addition to the benefits derived from actual implementation of the CHASP recommendations (McDonald et al. 1993). Overall, CHASP provided an excellent framework against which health workers could evaluate their practice and set goals for future development.

Three editions of CHASP standards were developed as the process was refined through a decade of experience and the needs of various services, and some specific standards were developed for different contexts. As a result, the CHASP standards were used to review a wide range of services, including Aboriginal health services, women's health services, statewide health agencies, one-person remote and rural health services, Home and Community Care (HACC) services, mental health services and alcohol, tobacco and other drug services (Quality Improvement Council 1998a, p. vi).

Consequently, when the CHASP standards were reviewed in 1996, a new format was developed to better address the needs of the now wide range of services for which the process is used. The program was also incorporated and re-named as the Australian Health and Community Services Standards.

The development of the Australian Health and Community Services Standards also took into account the changes in the socio-political environment since the CHASP process had been developed. In particular, the new standards attempted to address the changing expectations of services as a result of managerialism, with its emphasis on customer focus and accountability against outcomes (Quality Improvement Council 1998a, p. vii). Changes to the ways in which services are delivered and administered also had implications for the new standards. Weighing these issues against continued commitment to the principles behind the Primary Health Care approach remains a continuing challenge in the development of evaluation processes such as these.

The process of evaluating against the Australian Health and Community Services Standards typically has four stages. Firstly, workers at a health service work together to conduct an internal assessment of their practice, reviewing it against the AHCS standards, and record their analysis in a workbook provided to the review team. Consumers and other services in the area are asked to comment on the service at this stage, and a report on this is also sent to the review team. Secondly, the review team (which includes a member of staff from the service being reviewed and two or three workers, managers or board members from other similar services) conducts an on-site review, examining records, interviewing staff, consumers and other stake

Principles for Effective Community and Primary Health Care Services
(Australian Health and Community Services Standards)

Management and Leadership
Consumer principle
Consumers and the community of interest receive high quality services and programs which are appropriate to their needs and are delivered in an efficient and effective manner.

Service principle
A service has accountable, efficient and effective methods of management and leadership which facilitate the achievement of its goals to improve outcomes for its consumers and community of interest.

Planning, Quality Improvement and Evaluation
Consumer principle
Consumers have opportunities to contribute to service planning, identifying priorities, quality improvement and evaluation to ensure services and programs are appropriate, of high quality and effective.

Service principle
A service plans its activities in accordance with consumer and community feedback, data analysis and needs assessment. It evaluates and continuously improves its services and other activities in partnership with its community of interest to ensure they are appropriate, of high quality and effective.

Training and Development
Consumer principle
Consumers receive high quality services consistent with the values, beliefs and attitudes of the service.

Service principle
The service provides a range of training and development opportunities to assist with the development of knowledge and skills of staff to enable them to provide high quality service.

Work and Its Environment
Consumer and service principle
The service provides a safe and healthy environment for staff, visitors and consumers attending the service.

Consumer Rights
Consumer principle
Consumers are aware of their rights and responsibilities.

Service principle
The service upholds the rights of its consumers.

Consumer and Community Participation
Consumer principle
Consumers and the community of interest are actively involved in debate and decisions about issues that affect their wellbeing.

Service principle
The service has a high level of mutual exchange and active involvement with the community it serves. The participation of consumers and the community of

interest in debate and decision-making about issues that affect their wellbeing is actively developed.

Assessment and Care
Consumer principle
Clients receive services which improve their health status and quality of life. The physical, social, emotional, cultural and environmental aspects of clients health needs are addressed in a multidisciplinary manner. Clients are informed and involved in decision-making about their care.

Service principle
Services take into account the physical, social, cultural, emotional and environmental aspects of people's health in a comprehensive way in order to improve their health status and quality of life. A multi-disciplinary framework with an emphasis on informing and involving clients in decision-making about their own health care is used.

Early Identification and Intervention
Consumer principle
The client, in partnership with the service, identifies and receives services that detect, monitor and intervene in early stage health problems to improve health and quality of life.

Service principle
A community/primary health care service identifies potential and early stage health problems of individuals and communities to enable effective early intervention and better management of health problems.

Health Promotion
Consumer principle
The client and community's capacity to protect and promote their health and wellbeing is enhanced through health promotion. Clients work in partnership with the community/primary health care service in planning, implementing and evaluating health promotion.

Service principle
The community/primary health care service is responsive to identified health issues using health promotion strategies. This develops community capacity to protect and promote the community's health and wellbeing. The community/ primary health care service works in partnership with its community of interest and other stakeholders to achieve improved population health.

Records
Consumer principle
Clients receive services and programs which are coordinated. This information is documented in records in a comprehensive, accurate and respectful manner which reflects the client's needs and progress.

    This information is made available to the client as required.

Service principle
Client and program activities are documented in a systematic and consistent way, to ensure effectiveness, accountability and evaluation.

(Quality Improvement Council 1998a; 1998b)

holders and inspecting the facilities. It also interviews those responsible for community health policy in the area. Thirdly, the review team then prepares a report, which includes suggestions for improving the service's operation. The report is discussed with staff at the service while still in draft form, to obtain additional feedback. Recommendations for action may then be negotiated. Fourth, the service being evaluated then plans how it will respond to the report's recommendations. A further review can then be conducted 12–18 months later if the centre wishes to gain accreditation (Quality Improvement Council 1998a, pp. ix–x).

The Australian Health and Community Services Standards are built around a set of six core sections for all services. In addition, several sets of service delivery modules, each designed for different kinds of services, such as community and primary health care services, home based care services, integrated health services, maternal and infant care services, and alcohol, tobacco and other drugs services, are provided to address the specific issues relevant to each of these services (Quality Improvement Council 1998a, p. v).

A set of core concepts provides the framework around which each module is developed. Each of the sections then begins with a consumer principle and a service principle, which identify the important elements of that section, and a set of key outcomes against which that section can be evaluated. These principles are then examined by means of a set of standards, each of which is then evaluated against a number of specific indicators (Quality Improvement Council 1998a, p. viii). The result is a comprehensive set of indicators against which a service can be evaluated. The principles that guide the evaluation process for community and primary health care services are provided in the box on pages 130–31.

Towards best practice in Primary Health Care

If we are to see the principles of the Primary Health Care approach effectively implemented, we need to encourage and reward best practice in Primary Health Care. Best practice provides an opportunity for practitioners to critically evaluate their own practice in the light of how others are dealing with similar issues, to determine how they might strengthen their own responses (Legge et al. 1996a, p. 14). Best practice guidelines may therefore be a very useful tool in the evaluation and continued development of Primary Health Care and health promotion. And, with their focus on creating 'organisational cultures which are directed at the pursuit of excellence' (Lansbury 1994, cited by Legge et al. 1996a, p. 13), best practice principles have potential as a mechanism for developing the infrastructure and processes to support individual best practice in the workplace.

What is best practice in Primary Health Care? Clearly it is practice in which the principles of social justice, equity, community participation and responsiveness to need are implemented. But what does this actually mean in the context of the daily practice of health workers? Legge et al. (1996a; 1996b) attempted to find this out through a process of analysing practice as it was reflected in documented case studies. They examined 185 examples of published Primary Health Care practice, 99 of which were then evaluated by peer reviewers and rated on a number of aspects identified by the research team as important to good practice. The most highly rated 25 examples were then analysed in greater detail through interviews with those who were well acquainted with the projects.

Towards best practice in Primary Health Care

Elements of good practice in Primary Health Care

- consumer and community involvement;
- collaborative local networking;
- strong vertical partnerships;
- intersectoral collaboration;
- integration of the macro and micro;
- organisational learning;
- policy participation;
- good management.

(Legge et al. 1996b, p. 8.)

Preconditions for best practice in Primary Health Care

- clarity of need;
- strong and well resourced communities;
- supportive policy and program environment;
- supportive organisational environment;
- well prepared and committed workforce; and
- inspirational leadership.

(Legge et al. 1996b, p. 9.)

The project identified eight elements of good practice and six preconditions for best practice (see box above). These provide a clear set of principles against which other examples of Primary Health Care practice can be evaluated or towards which developing practice can aspire. They present a valuable opportunity for us to deepen our understanding of what makes for excellence in Primary Health Care practice.

The Best Practice in Primary Health Care project paid particular attention to the question of outcomes in Primary Health Care. Considering the increasing attention given to evaluation of outcomes in recent years and the questions that have been raised about how to meaningfully evaluate the outcomes of activities that aim to make long-term social change, this aspect of the project is of particular value. The Project Team concluded that, for it to be meaningful, three levels of outcomes in Primary Health Care were worth examining:

- *the outcomes we value for today (immediate health gains);*

- *the outcomes we value for tomorrow (including improvements in the social conditions for health and the strengthening of identified health care programs and services; and*

- *the outcomes we value for 'the day after tomorrow' (community, institutional and professional capability-building).*

(Legge et al. 1996b, p. 8.)

These three levels of outcomes provide a useful framework around which further evaluation work can be developed.

The Best Practice in Primary Health Care Project has highlighted many important features of good practice, and points the way forward for how this issue may be further explored. The documents produced by this project should be of value and interest to practitioners wishing to critically evaluate their own practice. They also serve to highlight the importance of proper resourcing and management support if effective Primary Health Care is to flourish and develop.

Conclusion

Evaluation should be an integral component of good health promotion practice and therefore an integral component of the daily practice of health workers. It enables us to ensure the relevance and appropriateness of practice, enabling health promotion practice to contribute to important long-term goals.

There are several challenges in evaluation for health workers aiming to work using a Primary Health Care approach. Firstly, the pressure to demonstrate success should not discourage innovation in health promotion practice. Secondly, the accountability demands of funders should not prevent meaningful evaluation enabling the active participation of community members and health workers learning how activities may be improved. Thirdly, evaluation should not be regarded as an 'add on' activity considered separately from other aspects of health promotion planning. Finally, evaluations should rarely, if ever, be an end in themselves. The ultimate value of any evaluation will be determined by what improvement in health promotion practice resulted.

References and further reading

Australian Community Health Association 1993, *Manual of Standards for Community Health,* Australian Community Health Association, Sydney.

Baum, F. 1992, 'Researching Community Health: Evaluation and Needs Assessment that Makes an Impact', in Baum, F., Fry, D. and Lennie, I. (eds), *Community Health: Policy and Practice in Australia,* Pluto Press/Australian Community Health Association, Sydney.

Baum, F. 1995, 'Researching Public Health: Behind the Qualitative–Quantitative Methodological Debate', *Social Science and Medicine,* 40 (4), 459–68.

Baum, F. 1996, 'Community Health Services and Managerialism', *Australian Journal of Primary Health Care* – Interchange, 2 (4), 31–41.

Baum, F. and Brown, V. 1989, 'Healthy Cities (Australia) Project: Issues of Evaluation for the New Public Health', *Community Health Studies,* 13 (2), 140–9.

Beattie, A. 1995, 'Evaluation in Community Development for Health: an Opportunity for Dialogue', *Health Education Journal,* 54, 465–72.

Bichmann, W., Rifkin, S. B. and Shrestha, M. 1989, 'Towards the Measurement of Community Participation', *World Health Forum,* 10, 467–72.

Birrell, C. 1993, *The Health Promotion Evaluation Kit for Community Health Staff,* Inner South Community Health Centres Project Group, Melbourne.

Braw, J., Sheldon, J. and Gaffney, D. 1991, *Self Evaluation Kit;* Drug and Alcohol Services, NSW, Rozelle, NSW.

Chapman, S. 1993, 'Unravelling Gossamer with Boxing Gloves: Problems in Explaining the Decline in Smoking', *British Medical Journal,* 307, 429–32.

Colin, T. and Garrow, A. 1996, *Thinking, Listening, Looking, Understanding and Acting As You Go Along*, Council of Remote Area Nurses of Australia, Alice Springs.

Community Development in Health Project 1988, *Community Development in Health: a Resources Collection*, District Health Council, Preston/Northcote, Vic.

Copeman, R. C. 1988, 'Assessment of Aboriginal Health Services', *Community Health Studies*, 12 (3), 251–5.

Davies, J. K. and Macdonald, G. 1998, *Quality, Evidence and Effectiveness in Health Promotion: Striving for Certainties*, Routledge, London and New York.

Ewles, L. and Simnett, I. 1999, *Promoting Health: a Practical Guide*, Bailliere Tindall in association with the Royal College of Nursing, Edinburgh.

Feuerstein, M-T. 1986, *Partners in Evaluation: Evaluating Development and Community Programmes with Participants*, Macmillan, London.

Freudenberg, N. 1984, 'Training Health Educators for Social Change', *International Quarterly of Community Health Education*, 5 (1), 37–52.

Fry, D. 1992, 'Quality Assurance and Community Health Services', in Baum, F., Fry, D. and Lennie, I. (eds), *Community Health: Policy and Practice in Australia*, Pluto Press in association with the Australian Community Health Association, Sydney.

Furler, E. 1979, 'Against Hegemony in Health Care Service Evaluation', *Community Health Studies*, 3 (1), 32–41.

Green, L. W. and Kreuter, M. W. 1991, *Health Promotion Planning: an Educational and Environmental Approach*, Mayfield, Mountain View, California.

Guba, E. and Lincoln, Y. 1989, *Fourth Generation Evaluation*, Sage, Newbury Park.

Hawe, P. 1994, 'Capturing the Meaning of "Community" in Community Intervention Evaluation: Some Contributions from Community Psychology', *Health Promotion International*, 9 (3), 199–210.

Hawe, P. and Shiell, A. 1995, 'Preserving Innovation Under Increasing Accountability Pressures: the Health Promotion Investment Portfolio Approach', *Health Promotion Journal of Australia*, 5 (2), 4–9.

Hawe, P., Degeling, D. and Hall, J. 1990, *Evaluating Health Promotion: a Health Workers' Guide*, MacLennan and Petty, Sydney.

Legge, D. 1999, 'The Evaluation of Health Development: the Next Methodological Frontier?' *Australian and New Zealand Journal of Public Health*, 23 (2), 117–18.

Legge, D., Wilson, G., Butler, P., Wright, M., McBride, T. and Attewell, R. 1996a, 'Best Practice in Primary Health Care', *Australian Journal of Primary Health – Interchange*, 2 (1), 12–26.

Legge, D., Wilson, G., Butler, P., Wright, M., McBride, T. and Attewell, R. 1996b, *Best Practice in Primary Health Care*, Centre for Development and Innovation in Health and Commonwealth Department of Health and Family Services, Northcote, Vic.

McDonald, J., Michels, D. and Ryan, P. 1993, 'National Evaluation of CHASP', in Clarke, B. and MacDougall, C. (eds), *The 1993 Community Health Conference, vol. 1, Papers and Workshops*, Australian Community Health Association, Sydney.

McKenzie, J. F. and Jurs, J. L. 1993, *Planning, Implementing, and Evaluating Health Promotion Programs: a Primer*, Macmillan, New York.

Moodie, R. 1989, 'The Politics of Evaluating Aboriginal Health Services', *Community Health Studies*, 13 (4), 503–9.

Northern Community Health Research Unit 1991, *Research and Evaluation in Community Health Kit*, Northern Community Health Research Unit, Adelaide.

Nutbeam, D. 1996, 'Health Outcomes and Health Promotion – Defining Success in Health Promotion', *Health Promotion Journal of Australia*, 6 (2), 58–60.

Nutbeam, D. 1998, 'Evaluating Health Promotion – Progress, Problems and Solutions', *Health Promotion International*, 13 (1), 27–44.

Ovretveit, J. 1998, *Evaluating Health Interventions*, Open University Press, Buckingham.

Owen, A. and Mohr, R. 1986, 'Commentary: Politics and Pitfalls in Evaluation', *Community Health Studies*, 10 (1), 95–9.

Quality Improvement Council 1998a, *Australian Health and Community Services Standards: Health and Community Services Core Module,* Quality Improvement Council Limited, Bundoora, Vic.

Quality Improvement Council 1998b, *Australian Health and Community Service Standards: Community and Primary Health Care Services Module,* Quality Improvement Council Limited, Bundoora, Vic.

Rauch, A. 1992, 'The Development of Community Health Accreditation and Standards Project (CHASP)', in Courtney, M. (ed.), *Issues in Rural Nursing: Proceedings of the 1st National Conference of the Association for Australian Rural Nurses,* University of New England, Armidale, NSW.

Rissel, C. 1991, 'The Tyranny of Needs Assessment in Health Promotion', *Evaluation Journal of Australia,* 3 (1), 26–31.

Rovers, R. 1986, 'The Merging of Participatory and Analytical Approaches to Evaluation: Implications for Nurses in Primary Health Care Programs', *International Journal of Nursing Studies,* 23 (3), 211–19.

Ryan, P. 1992, *Cases for Change: CHASP in Practice,* Australian Community Health Association, Sydney.

Shiell, A. and Hawe, P. 1996, 'Health Promotion, Community Development and the Tyranny of Individualism', *Health Economics,* 5, 241–7.

Sinclair, A. 1993, 'Reorienting to Primary Health Care: a Case for National Standards', in Clarke, B. and MacDougall, C. (eds), *The 1993 Community Health Conference, Vol. 1, Papers and Workshops,* Australian Community Health Association, Sydney.

Smithies, J. and Adams, L. 1993, 'Walking the Tightrope: Issues in Evaluation and Community Participation for Health For All', in Davies, J. K. and Kelly, M. P. (eds), *Healthy Cities: Research and Practice,* Routledge, London and New York.

South Australian Community Health Research Unit. 1994, *Health Outcomes in Community Health,* South Australian Community Health Research Unit, Bedford Park, SA.

Stewart-Brown, S. L. and Prothero, D. L. 1988, 'Evaluation in Community Development', *Health Education Journal,* 47 (4), 156–61.

Tones, K. and Tilford, S. 1994, *Health Education: Effectiveness, Efficiency and Equity,* Chapman and Hall, London.

Wadsworth, Y. 1997, *Everyday Evaluation on the Run,* Allen and Unwin, Sydney.

Wilson, G. and Wright, M. 1993, *Evaluation Framework: Women's Health Services and Centres Against Sexual Assault,* Centre for Development and Innovation in Health, Northcote.

CHAPTER 5

Using the mass media

*T*he mass media can be a powerful influence on health, attitudes to health issues and accepted definitions of what constitutes the good life. Its impact on our views of the world can be profound. We are increasingly dependent on the mass media for information on the world around us and influenced by it in the development of our attitudes, expectations and beliefs about life. This chapter will review the ways in which the mass media can be used to lead or support health promotion work and examine some approaches to working with the mass media. This will involve examining both the ways in which the mass media can be used by health workers on a broad social level to present information about health issues, and how different forms of mass media can be used on a smaller scale in developing health education materials for use with individuals and groups.

Media representation of health issues

Over the last few years there has been growing media interest in health issues that has been largely welcomed by health promoters. However, it is interesting to examine the media's coverage of health issues, and the approach they take. Media coverage of health issues has been classified into four groups (Karpf 1988, pp. 9–22):

- the medical approach, in which the focus is on disease and the marvels of modern medicine in curing disease, with the doctor as the linchpin in this process;
- the consumer approach, in which problems in the doctor–patient relationship and unfair treatment of people in the health system are examined;
- the look-after-yourself approach, in which the focus is on the behaviour of individuals in preventing ill-health (this could also be called the lifestyle approach);
- the environmental approach, in which the focus is on the social and environmental causes of ill-health and the need to make changes at those levels if we are to create health in individuals and groups.

In examining the health related stories that appear in the mass media, it is apparent that the greater proportion of media coverage of health issues fits into the first three groups, where the focus is on individuals and individual cure, prevention and responsibility for disease. In the USA, it is estimated that 80% of stories are framed around short-term individual issues (Wallack et al. 1993, p. 72), and it is unlikely that the picture in Australia is significantly different. The mass media play a substantial role in maintaining a focus on individual responsibility for and treatment of disease, which helps maintain the invisibility of social determinants of health.

Health promoters have an important role to play in trying to reorient the mass media's coverage of health issues so that due recognition is given to the environmental and social issues that impact on health. Otherwise, the media's growing interest in health issues will serve to further support public belief in high-technology curative medicine at the expense of health promotion in its broadest sense. Furthermore, health workers using the mass media have a role to play in ensuring that they use them in a more balanced way, presenting the environmental and structural issues related to health as much as the individual issues.

When health messages are presented in the media, they may be used in a number of ways: they may be used alone, as the sole form of health promotion; they may be used to support other health promotion activity; they may be used to advertise services available; or they may be used to encourage the maintenance of healthy behaviours and to keep health issues on the agenda (Flora & Cassady 1990, pp. 143–8). Which of these approaches is used will depend on the aim of the health promotion activity. While a well developed media campaign may be useful in raising awareness or influencing public opinion, use of the mass media alone is unlikely to be successful in helping people develop new skills and behaviours (Nutbeam & Blakey 1990, p. 237). It is important to bear this in mind when considering use of the mass media.

There are two key approaches to using the mass media in health promotion, stemming from different approaches to health promotion. They are media advocacy, in which the mass media are used to raise the profile of particular health issues in a manner that changes the way in which the community, including decision makers, sees them; and social marketing, in which the mass media are used to 'sell' health through a particular health behaviour or health product. These two approaches reflect quite different ways of using the mass media. However, they are by no means mutually exclusive. Both approaches may be valuable in health promotion work, though the aims for which they are used vary considerably (Wallack 1990a, p. 143).

Media advocacy

Media advocacy is the use of the mass media to influence the development of healthy public policy through changing the nature of public debate on issues that impact on health. In media advocacy the mass media is used as a political tool to influence the decision making of policy makers, both directly and through pressure from community members (Wallack & Dorfman 1996, p. 296).

Media advocacy is based on the recognition that health is a result of the social and environmental conditions in which people live. It is also based on a recognition that community participation in the policy-making process is invaluable (Wallack & Dorfman 1996, p. 295). For these reasons it fits well with the Primary Health Care approach to health promotion. Through advocating the development of healthy public policy, media advocacy works to change the environment in which people live their lives. This focus on policy addresses health problems in their political context (Wallack et al. 1993, p. 77).

Media advocacy involves both influencing the mass media to identify certain topics as newsworthy and influencing the nature of the debate on these topics. Media advocacy therefore often involves challenging public perceptions about health issues and refocusing public attention away from individual responsibility for health problems and onto the broader environmental issues influencing individual choice. This change in focus, or reframing of issues, is a central component of media advocacy.

Framing, or reframing, of the debate involves presenting the issue being discussed differently from the way it is normally presented in the mass media, thus creating a quite different view of the situation. Wallack describes the way in which anti-smoking media advocates began discussing tobacco companies' exploitation of women, children and minority groups, to change the public image of tobacco companies (Wallack 1990a, pp. 151–2). Greenpeace has used the same approach through its public events and media campaigns to draw attention to environmental pollution. By drawing attention to pollution caused by large chemical companies in Sydney, for example, Greenpeace works to break down the image of these companies as environmentally responsible and demonstrates their pollution of Sydney waterways. This reframing of issues is an important precursor to lobbying for public policy changes on these issues.

There are three key steps in media advocacy — setting the agenda, shaping the debate and advancing the policy. Setting the agenda involves framing a story in a way that captures the attention of journalists and demonstrates to them that it is newsworthy. That is, rather than focus on discussions in community noticeboard space, media advocacy involves presenting information in such a way that it will run as a news item (Wallack 1990a, p. 152). The second step, shaping the debate, involves telling the story the way you want it told, with the focus on the broad social issues rather than on the individual issues so commonly of interest to journalists. This may require some explanation, since it runs contrary to common sense assumptions about the causes of health problems. The third step, advancing the policy, then involves putting forward the policy solution that you are aiming to achieve (Wallack et al. 1993, p. 79).

Effective media advocacy is not simply about health workers taking on the role of advocate for public policy issues — community participation plays a central role in media advocacy. Media advocacy often involves concerted campaigns over a relatively long period of time. A ground swell of pressure is often needed to get a new perspective on issues represented in the media. Therefore, successful media advocacy is based on coalition building — bringing together a range of community groups who can work together to maintain an issue in the public debate (Wallack et al. 1993, pp. 74–5). Health workers therefore have a central role to play in enabling and supporting community groups and other agencies with a concern about health issues to join together to lobby for public policy change.

An example of such collaborative action occurred after the Port Arthur massacre in Tasmania — several individuals, community groups and professional associations that had been working for gun control instigated a concerted campaign to keep gun control in the public attention and focus on the necessary public policy changes (Chapman 1998). The resultant political and public support for new gun control legislation was a major achievement.

Working to have health issues regarded as newsworthy, taken up by media outlets and then presented with the public policy perspective advocated is a major challenge for health workers. It takes considerable time, energy and planning. It is not surprising that health workers may then feel a great sense of achievement when their story is taken up by the mass media in an appropriate manner. However, Wallack and Dorfman (1993, p. 308) remind us that this media coverage is not an end in itself. Rather, the aims of media advocacy include the development of community support and action to work for the change, mobilisation of key decision makers, and actual public policy change, and it is against these yardsticks that media advocacy should be measured.

Social marketing

Social marketing aims to influence people's behaviour by encouraging individuals to make healthy choices. It therefore uses the mass media as an educational tool to inform or motivate individuals. Social marketing is built on recognition of the powerful influence of the mass media on the choices that people make: not only does television provide the images and role models on which people may model themselves, but also advertising influences people to identify products as available and desirable. Social marketing aims to use the principles on which advertisers work, but to use them to 'sell' a healthy message and therefore undo some of the work of advertisers who sell products and lifestyles that create ill-health.

This is a major task. Millions of dollars are spent annually on advertising unhealthy, but profitable, products. Health promoters, even when they are supported by national media campaigns, are in no position to match the extent to which unhealthy products are marketed — they simply do not have the same financial resources at their disposal (Eisenberg 1987, p. 110).

One recent attempt to help balance the influence of unhealthy and healthy advertising in Australia has been the banning of some unhealthy advertising, most notably, tobacco advertising. However, for an impact to be made on unhealthy advertising overall, there would need to be considerable legislative control of advertising. This would be likely to be vigorously opposed, because it would be regarded as seriously eroding people's expectations about freedom of speech and freedom of choice. It would also raise ethical questions about the right of the State to take over the life of the individual. This is by no means a simple issue; after all, it is argued that mass media advertising itself manipulates people's free choice, often beyond recognition (Connell 1977, pp. 195–6).

It is to be expected, then, that advertising is here to stay, but within this framework social marketing may have some influence. Those who support social marketing in health promotion believe that it can contribute positively if it is part of an integrated health promotion program and if too much is not expected of it, given the context in which it is being used.

It is important to bear in mind that the advertising industry itself conducts considerable market research and targets its advertising very specifically to the groups it wishes to convince. Health workers simply do not have the resources or the skills to match these activities. This is an important point because it alerts health workers to the problems inherent in trying to emulate (and undo) the larger campaigns run by the advertisers. Two issues arise here: the need to draw on the expertise of those in the field when planning major advertising campaigns, and the need to work very carefully when running small social marketing campaigns or using the social marketing approach to support other health promotion work.

A question of ethics in social marketing

The whole notion of social marketing does not sit comfortably with everyone. The tactics advertising companies themselves use are often held to be unethical

Replacing unhealthy messages with healthy ones: the Victorian Health Promotion Foundation

The Victorian Health Promotion Foundation was established as a result of the Tobacco Act 1987. One of the key elements of its work is tobacco replacement in sport sponsorship and billboard advertising. Billboards previously used for advertising tobacco products are now being used to present healthy messages. Many of these are 'quit smoking' messages, while others are healthy messages supporting other health promotion programs (for example, the 'Active at any age' campaign).

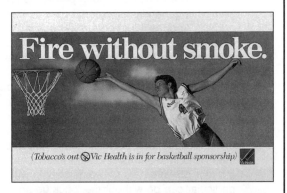

(Tobacco's out ⊗Vic Health is in for basketball sponsorship)

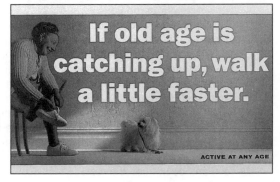

ACTIVE AT ANY AGE

This billboard advertising is financed by the 5% levy imposed on tobacco products under the Tobacco Act 1987. It is only because of this unique arrangement that a public health promotion foundation is able to afford the costs of billboard advertising and tobacco replacement messages.

because they are based on the idea of influencing people's choices, often without their awareness. Using the same tactics, and therefore trying to beat advertisers at their own game, does have some ethical problems.

Much media advertising is built on unhealthy stereotypes of people, and much social marketing seems to accept these unquestioningly, rather than challenge them. There is therefore much work to be done in challenging these stereotypes, which themselves can contribute to narrow views of health and normality and reduced feelings of self-worth in individuals. If social marketing builds on these stereotypes, rather than challenging them, the overall health benefit from any messages may be limited.

Proponents of social marketing argue that it can be used effectively in a way that supports Primary Health Care work and is empowering for those it is designed to assist. For example, it can be used as a reminder of healthy behaviours and can therefore be supportive of other health promotion strategies. It can educate the public about the importance of new healthy policy or legislation at the same time

Do media campaigns motivate people or put additional pressure on them?

The practice of using famous people as role models in media campaigns on arthritis is generally accepted, but does their use motivate those of us who have arthritis, or does it just put unnecessary pressure on us? I think the latter is the case and, as an arthritis activist, researcher and lobbyist with a long personal experience of rheumatoid arthritis, I believe the practice needs to be questioned.

There is a lack of awareness of the impact on people with arthritis, when the achievements of television personalities or sportsmen are continually emphasised during fund-raising campaigns. Their achievements certainly help to raise funds, but with the reports of these 'Super Cripps' doing remarkable things despite their arthritis, comes the implication that we should be emulating them, and that is impossible for many of us. Getting out of bed in the morning is a major achievement for some people with arthritis, and these people in particular can do without the 'buck up and go out' treatment presented by current media campaigns.

Our society's obsession with competition and achievement is inappropriate when people are sick. It is also inappropriate to use male role models when arthritis predominantly affects women. In the Arthritic Women's Task Force's video 'Women with rheumatoid arthritis: don't take us at face value', one of the women talks about the arthritis posters, which depict the achievements of a famous AFL footballer, and the resulting pressures on her also to be an achiever. Those pressures are usually exerted by well-meaning relatives, friends and neighbours, who are impressed by the media campaigns. They do not understand the difference between rheumatoid arthritis and the milder forms of arthritis and fail to realise the seriousness of her illness. They just look at her face and do not see the rest.

This is probably an even greater problem for women whose arthritis has not yet reached the obvious stage. They do not look sick and, if their husbands do not understand what rheumatoid arthritis is like, or if their husbands have deserted them, the pressures to achieve, according to male perceptions of achievement, are especially distressing. These women are already aware that they are considered to be inadequate underachievers; having media pressure put on them, particularly when they are trying to cope with a major flare-up of their arthritis and care for their homes and children at the same time, only increases their problems.

There is another aspect of the practice of using famous people in media campaigns that should be questioned. That is the failure of the media and the fundraising organisations to recognise the fact that some of these people are doing irreparable harm to their bodies in their determination to achieve stardom and that they are not, in fact, good role models for people with arthritis to emulate. The pressures on television personalities and sportspeople to perform to a very high standard are just as destructive as the pressures on us to emulate them, and it is distressing to see how soon famous people are forgotten when they are no longer able to perform.

It is extremely difficult for people with arthritis to object to or challenge the way media campaigns are carried out because the famous people, the fund-raisers, the media and the community at large all believe that they are helping us. The concept of charity is deeply rooted in our culture, and we are seen as ungrateful when we question the way it is dispensed. The fact that no one asked us whether we wanted that sort of media campaign or whether we want to be treated as objects of charity is overlooked in a sea of hurt feelings.

The needs of a great many people are met when they participate in a media fund-raising campaign. It makes them feel good and, until they question the real impact of their actions on us, or until we, the people with arthritis, become politically active consumers, I think the failure of media campaign organisers to recognise the difference between motivation and pressure (the latter exemplified by the threatening slogan 'Move it or Lose it') will persist.

Joan Byrne
Consumer and arthritis activist

that those changes are being developed. The principles of Primary Health Care, however, are not an inherent component of social marketing, and so it is up to each individual health promoter to ensure that he or she uses social marketing in a way that supports the principles of Primary Health Care. This may require considerable effort, for, as Joan Byrne's discussion of the use of media campaigns demonstrates (see box), a great many assumptions are made in media health messages.

Skills in using the mass media

Working effectively with the mass media requires skill. As with any other specialty, it is wise to seek out the support and advice of experts when planning a major media campaign. The following hints are suggested to help you develop an effective working relationship with local media outlets.

Preliminary work

An important first step in using the mass media is establishing contact with the people who make the decisions in local newspapers, radio stations and television stations, as well as the writers and production people (Weiss and Kessel 1987, p. 40). Getting to know all these people may increase the chance of your articles or stories being accepted. Furthermore, speaking to them will enable you to find out more about how you need to present your stories so that they are more likely to be accepted. They may also be able to provide you with some valuable advice on how to improve your presentation skills.

When you are in touch with any of these people, find out about the deadlines for copy. You will need this information if you are planning on having articles or stories support other work you are doing. It can be very frustrating if you miss the deadline and your story runs too late for other elements of your work.

Check the local paper and radio station to see if particular journalists or interviewers seem to have an interest in health issues, and then establish a working relationship with them. Working with those people will be much more useful, since they are the ones most likely to be interested in your stories. They may also be more inclined to call you for information about other issues should they need it. Establishing an ongoing relationship in this way can be useful for both health workers and media people.

A word of warning, however. You will need to check the protocol of the institution for which you are working. Many hospitals and health services require all contact with the mass media to be approved and overseen by the chief executive officer. If that is the case in your area, make sure you use the correct channels and prepare your material sufficiently in advance to enable it to be reviewed and passed on.

What makes an item newsworthy?

If you are hoping to present stories as news, it is important to present them in a manner that is newsworthy. Elements that help make an item newsworthy (Levey 1983, cited by Weiss & Kessel 1987, p. 40) include:

* information — the item will need to give information that is new to people or provides a new angle on what they know;
* timeliness — the item will need to be presented at a time that fits in with other local or national events. Indeed, part of the skill in producing newsworthy items is in taking advantage of other events that have already proved newsworthy by 'dovetailing' into them. If your item is to be timely, it will also need to be presented far enough ahead of any action in which you are encouraging people to become involved, so that they have the opportunity to become involved if they wish to;
* significance and relevance— the item will need to present material that is significant and relevant to the lives of the audience. If the relevance is not likely to be obvious to the whole of the audience, the item should outline the significance of the issues discussed;
* scope — the item will need to be relevant to many community members or a significant group in the community;
* interest — the item will need to be interesting to the audience. Weiss and Kessel (1987, p. 40) suggest that items can be made more newsworthy by involving a famous person, linking the story to a national or historical issue, or presenting the story with interesting photographs or cartoons. It is important to note, however, that these things need to be done with some sensitivity or they may backfire. Joan Byrne's discussion of the use of famous sports people in media campaigns directed at people with arthritis (see pp. 140–1) is a good illustration of this point;
* human interest — the item is more likely to be newsworthy if it is made directly relevant to the lives of ordinary people or the life of the community;
* uniqueness — the item is more likely to be newsworthy if it presents an angle not found in other stories about the issue

The more of the above elements present in your item, the more likely it is that it will be accepted for publication. Remember, however, that these are a guide only, and an item that really stands out on one or two of these points may be more newsworthy than an item that just satisfies each point. Since decisions about newsworthiness are made more on the 'feel' of the editor than the application of any equation, the way in which your story is presented and how it appeals to the editor will be a key factor.

Another key factor will be when your story is submitted and what other stories have come in that day. An excellent story may be rejected if it arrives on the editor's desk at the same time as stories about a forthcoming political battle, a bus crash and a rags-to-riches lottery win. In such a case, you may need to wait a few days and resubmit your story. Furthermore, some days are easier for having stories accepted because they are less likely to be days when the media have many stories to deal with. Beauchamp (1986, p. 76) suggests that Fridays are invariably bad days to submit items, and so should be avoided unless you think you have something that will stop the presses.

One additional technique that has been used with success, particularly in regional areas, is to arrange sponsorship of health promotion activities by mass media outlets. The Taree Community Health Centre in rural New South Wales, for example, had its 'Walk Oz' program well publicised because the local television station was a sponsor of the program (Sunderland 1993, personal communication).

Writing to persuade: writing letters and media releases

Rather than merely letting a journalist know that an important event is soon to occur or that a particular issue warrants discussion, and hoping that he or she will

---

Working with the local press

When I became a community mental health nurse at Kempsey Community Health Centre, I discovered that 10% of my time was to be devoted to health promotion. I decided to offer articles for the 'Go Health' column in the local paper. The health promotion nurse had had a column running for several years and was delighted to acquire an extra writer. As she was so encouraging, I wrote more and more often, and eventually took over responsibility for the column, with her blessing. I wrote about many areas of health, both physical and mental, always in the form of a short story, simply written, with a lot of conversation, and always with some facts, or some information about where to get more facts or seek help.

The editor of the paper was particularly helpful and supportive. He always used the stories, was adept at writing a good headline, and made sure they were set up so that they caught the reader's eye and read well. Our successful working relationship contributed much to the quality of the articles published.

Unfortunately, good editors move on to better things and, in time, he left. There was an interim period when a senior journalist functioned as editor. The stories continued to be used, but without such good headlines, and without so much care being given to presentation. Eventually, a new editor was appointed. It was not possible to develop a positive working relationship with this person, who was prepared to run my stories only if I provided him with 'inside information' about the hospital and photos of newborn babies. I wasn't prepared to do either, and said so politely but firmly. My next story appeared, but it was the last to do so!

Through these experiences, I really came to appreciate the value of a good editor, and if I'm ever in a similar situation, I will always put energy into developing a good working relationship with an editor or journalist.

Anna Treloar
Registered Nurse
Kempsey District Hospital

Hints for writing letters to the editor

- check the newspaper to which you are writing for any guidelines on presentation of letters;
- type or write clearly, using double spacing and leaving a wide margin;
- be as brief as possible, examining the length of letters previously published may be a useful guide;
- keep your sentences short and sharp;
- present constructive criticism, rather than simply being critical;
- avoid using too much emotional language;
- if you wish to have your letter published anonymously, you can request this, but you will still need to supply your name and address, explaining why you want your name withheld;
- if your letter does not appear, you can contact the Letters Editor to find out why. It is not unusual for letters to take a number of weeks to be published.

[Based on Beauchamp (1986, pp. 64–7)]

---

write an article about it, you can submit a media release. This increases the chance that the story will run, because most of the work has already been done for the journalist. Moreover, the media release itself may provide the information that convinces the journalist that the issue is a valuable one and a newsworthy item. There may have been many times when journalists have rejected potential news items simply because they did not have enough information at their fingertips.

Similarly, you may want to present your views on an issue to members of a community. Writing a letter to the editor of a local or major newspaper may be a useful way to get your message across. If you can present a good argument, and present it in a way that is interesting, the letter is more likely to be published.

Whether you are writing a media release, a letter to the editor of a newspaper or a letter to a member of parliament, the key to success is to write persuasively. This takes some practice but there are a few simple steps to follow to increase the chance that your written material will present a persuasive argument. Keep in mind, also, the elements of a newsworthy item. Firstly, you will need to write clearly and simply, so that your message is understood. Robert Gunning (cited in Anderson & Itule 1988, p. 39) has suggested 'ten principles of clear writing', which provide a useful guide to help you express yourself:

1. *Keep sentences short, on the average.*
2. *Prefer the simple to the complex.*
3. *Prefer the familiar word.*
4. *Avoid unnecessary words.*
5. *Put action into your verbs.*
6. *Write the way you talk.*
7. *Use terms your reader can picture.*
8. *Tie in with your reader's experience.*
9. *Make full use of variety.*
10. *Write to express not impress.*

As well as being clearly written, your media release or letter will need to be well structured. Wrigley and McLean (1990) suggest four steps in the development of persuasive writing. They are: get the reader's attention, arouse the reader's interest, motivate the reader to take action, then tell the reader what action to take.

Get the reader's attention

Wrigley and McLean (1990, pp. 238–9) suggest two ways in which to get the reader's attention: use an attractive layout, and make the content relevant to the reader. The layout of the document will give the reader an idea of whether he or she wants to read it, and this is therefore very important. It includes a title that grabs the reader's attention, together with the use of headings and white space to help break up the document. These will be discussed in more detail below. Making the content relevant to the reader starts with being clear about whom you intend the article for and writing with that audience in mind. Writing to the reader (by saying 'you' and 'your'), focusing on people, using graphics where appropriate and keeping your message simple and clear will all help.

Arouse the reader's interest

You will need to arouse the reader's interest through your title and the first paragraph of your document, which, like any good introduction, should summarise what the document will tell the reader.

Motivate the reader to take action

You will need to present a succinct summary of the issues in a way that helps the reader to work through the facts and come to an opinion. You can do this by arranging information in a logical order, explaining where necessary and documenting any new or contentious information you present.

Hints for preparing media releases

- present the release in typewritten form on A4 paper, double spaced, typed on one side only and with a wide margin;
- use letterhead paper, so that the organisation presenting the release is clearly identifiable;
- ensure that the release is clearly dated, or that the date for publication of the material is given;
- clearly mark the document with the heading 'Media Release';
- use plain language, and short sharp sentences;
- put the most important information first;
- keep the release short — no more than two pages;
- suggest an attractive title;
- include quotations from relevant people;
- include a contact name and phone number (and be prepared to be contacted).

[Based on Flood and Lawrence (1987, pp. 84–5) and Beauchamp (1986, pp. 71–2)]

Tell the reader what action to take

Although putting all the above into practice may have convinced the reader that your message is valid, your aim is often to do more than that. If the aim is to encourage people to act on an issue, you need to tell them what action they can take. If you do not do so, they may feel more informed when they have finished reading, but no more sure of what to do. It is important, then, that you tell them clearly what they can do to make a difference.

Using photographs

Whether you are submitting a press release to a journalist or simply asking him or her to cover a particular issue, providing a photograph, or advising of a photo-opportunity, will help your story in two ways. Firstly, it will increase the chance that your story will be published, because it will be a more interesting piece for the newspaper to print with a photograph nearby. Secondly, because your story has visual appeal, more people are likely to read it when it appears in the paper. Photographs, then, can attract a reader and persuade just as successfully as words, and sometimes even more so. If you are providing a photograph, it will need to be of high quality and preferably black and white, although a sharply contrasted colour photo may be acceptable.

Preparing for a radio or television interview

Radio and television interviews are useful means of getting across a message to a wide audience. However, since the pace is usually fast, complex issues are often not given the depth they may require. Because of the fast pace, preparation for such an interview is important.

Wherever possible, present your interviewer with a list of the questions you believe should be asked to cover the topic. You may need to explain to this person why the questions you have chosen are important, but it is well worth the effort. There is nothing worse than a two-minute interview disappearing without having got your message across because the interviewer did not understand a basic point (which you could have clarified beforehand) and subsequently asked an irrelevant question.

In addition to presenting your interviewer with questions, prepare your answers, even if you will be talking on a topic that you feel you know very well. It is very easy to become nervous and forget what you wanted to say. Also, because you will not have very long to answer the interviewer's questions, you need to make sure you say the most important things first. Preparing answers in advance will help you to do that. There is no shame in not doing totally off-the-cuff interviews; indeed, only very experienced interviewees can usually get away with them.

If you are not able to provide your interviewer with a list of questions, you should be able to discuss with that person beforehand the questions he or she plans on asking you. Use this discussion as an opportunity to suggest other questions if you feel they are appropriate. Remember, you are likely to know more about the topic than the interviewer, and he or she will usually appreciate any suggestions that will improve the quality of the interview. Once again, take the time to plan your answers, making sure that you give your most important information first.

Martin Street story in the news

When the residents of the Martin Street subdivision in Armidale, New South Wales, began dealing with environmental pollution in the land on which their homes were built, they made sure that the local media knew about all the important things as they happened. They presented their perspective, being careful not to overstate the facts so that people were not turned against the issue, and worked for three and a half years to keep the story in the media. Many of their actions were newsworthy because of the way in which they presented the story. For example, a year after the environmental pollution was discovered, they constructed a large cross inscribed 'Martin St subdivision died 15.1.90. R.I.P.'. This had great visual and emotional impact, and a photo of it appeared on the front page of the local newspaper as the lead story. Throughout their fight for environmental health, many such stories have appeared in the local paper. Residents were aware of the value of visual impact, and made sure that they informed the local media whenever an opportunity to take a good photo arose.

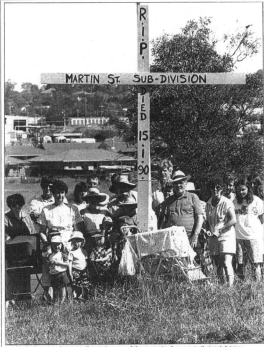

Martin St residents mourn the anniversary of the creosote discovery in their subdivisions.

Martin St residents' unhappy anniversary

It is 12 months today since creosote contamination was discovered on a block of land fronting Martin St.

One year after this discovery residents of the contaminated subdivision are bewildered, angry and concerned that they appear to be no closer to a solution than they were in January 1990.

Spokeswoman for the residents Mrs Irene Thompson said that there was general concern that they were awaiting results of a second report on the subdivision.

Mrs Thompson said: "It is time that something positive was done to resolve the problems facing residents.

"Over the past 12 months we have heard a great many words but witnessed very little action.

"Why is it that our children are still forced to play on land contaminated by copper chrome arsenate and creosote

"All available information indicates that the components of creosote are all either known or highly suspected of being carcinogenic."

Mrs Thompson said that many people were now questioning why the present consultants AGC Woodward-Clyde had not carried out further tests.

She said that the 25 metre grid used by Sinclair Knight and Partners was always intended as a base for further testing.

"Every report we have seen indicates there was a strong possibility of further hot spots"

"Residents have faced 12 months of worry and concern about our health and financial future.

"One resident has recently been retrenched but cannot accept an offered transfer because of the impossibility of selling the family home in Martin Street."

● Support for residents, Page 2

Find out if the interview is going to be pre-taped or live. If it is pre-taped, there will be an opportunity for it to be edited if necessary. You may be able to request that your interview be pre-taped if you are nervous and being interviewed for the first time; many interviewers will be happy to oblige if it is possible. However, be careful in such situations that you treat all of the interview as though it will be used — never assume that something you say is 'off the record'.

One valuable hint when being interviewed, even on radio, is to ensure that you make eye contact with the interviewer. Maintaining eye contact with the interviewer, rather than continually reading notes, is enough to help keep your voice sounding conversational. If you read from something, your voice can very

---

Using television to discuss health and illness issues

My first television interview! Yes, I was nervous, but I was also looking forward to it. I was to talk on the local television station about the need for a hostel for the frail aged in Hervey Bay, Queensland, and to encourage the community to support it financially. It was a subject I knew well, so it held no fears for me. After the first session I spoke with the show's compère (Melissa Davies) and we found that we shared a concern about the community's lack of access to information on health issues. We decided to start a regular health issues segment. We agreed that the range of topics was probably infinite, and so we decided to start on a small scale. I was to do a four-minute segment once a month.

It sounded so simple. I would send the compère a topic and the sort of information that I wanted to cover, and she would do the rest. But I started to feel frustration! Four minutes went so quickly and I found that I was not covering all of my subject. We discussed the problem and I offered to write my own questions, with brief notes on the answers I would give. That proved much more successful, although I was still surprised at how quickly four minutes went by.

In 1991, with the restructuring of television services, Melissa was given a daily show and I was given the opportunity to have a four-minute segment every week. We tried to tie these in with nominated health weeks, such as National Heart Week or Diabetes Awareness Week. We covered many topics, but the ones that created most public response were a series of three on continence. In the first segment I discussed continence promotion and then followed up with two segments examining the impact of continence education and the aids available to people who are incontinent. The response was heart-warming — many people (mainly women) had just not known that there was an alternative to incontinence and being confined to the house.

During 1992 we covered many subjects, from childhood immunisations to Alzheimer's disease, from asthma and its treatment to caring for someone who has suffered a stroke, from healthy eating to HIV infection, from breast self-examination to management of diabetes. We also had sessions on relaxation, medication and women's issues.

Putting subjects into plain language that people would listen to and understand was an exciting challenge. The informal feedback we received from the general public indicated that having a nurse talking about health issues was well received. Presenting health discussions to local people using a local television station and local health staff provides an excellent opportunity to give people access to the information they need if they are to make the most of their lives and make informed decisions.

Judyth Collard
(previously) Director of Nursing
Blue Nursing Service
Tablelands, Queensland

often become a monotone. However, talking directly to the interviewer as much as possible will help keep your voice interesting.

Controversial issues and media interviews

You may find yourself being interviewed on a controversial topic. If so, you may find an interviewer who asks you a question for which you are unprepared. This may be part of a deliberate strategy by the journalist to create some controversy. The important thing to remember in these situations is to stay focused on the issue and not get caught up in the controversy that is being created. This takes some self-discipline but is well worth it if you do not want to cloud the issues. Since health issues can so often involve differences of opinion, it is a good idea to go into every interview expecting the unexpected!

Preparing health education materials

Using the media to support or strengthen a personal health message is increasingly part of health promotion work. It is vital, therefore, that you understand enough about their use so that you can critically review any materials you are considering using, to determine whether they are appropriate to the needs of the people you are hoping to use them with. With some skills in this area, you will also be able to develop your own material if nothing suitable is available. Below are some general principles to guide the way in which these materials are produced for maximum effect.

Written materials

Written materials such as brochures, posters and booklets can provide useful re-inforcement for other health education materials and enable people to take information home with them. With any written materials, a few key elements can make the difference between a readable appealing document and one that does not invite the potential reader to go beyond a casual glance. These are the use of white space, a variety of print sizes, readable language, and drawings and photographs to help any words used come alive.

White space

White space is simply the amount of empty space left in the document. It is very important because, without adequate white space, a document can seem crowded and difficult to read. Space between words and paragraphs helps potential readers to see that the document is unlikely to swamp them, and will help them to work their way through it.

Variety of print sizes

Varying the print size and style, through the use of headings and different type fonts, makes the words on the page interesting and again helps to break text up. Headings that stand out also act as a summary of the document for people flipping through it, and so enable them to see if they would like to continue reading.

Readable language

Of course, no amount of variety in print size will counteract words that are difficult to understand or unreadable by the people your materials are supposedly designed for. So many written materials produced for health education contain language that makes the information in them inaccessible to many people. Several formulas for assessing the readability of education materials have been suggested (see, for example, Hawe et al. 1990, pp. 70–2).

Involving some of the people you are designing the materials for in the development process will ensure that they are readable. It will also ensure that they are appropriate and acknowledge the expertise of these people in issues related to their own lives. Schwab et al. (1992) and Neuhauser et al. (1998) provide an example of how this process was implemented in the preparation of a Wellness Guide. Through involving a group of potential consumers of the Wellness Guide in reviewing a draft of the guide, and responding when these community members identified a range of problems from a consumer's perspective, the developers were able to produce a final product whose impact far exceeded their original idea, and which had real meaning for the community.

On clarity in using diagrams

Some time ago two student nurses, gaining experience in health education and promotion as part of their studies, were asked to talk to a group of older people on arthritis and self-help strategies. They worked hard preparing their materials, which included a number of posters to use as teaching aids. One of these posters showed a knee joint, to help demonstrate the physical impact of arthritis.

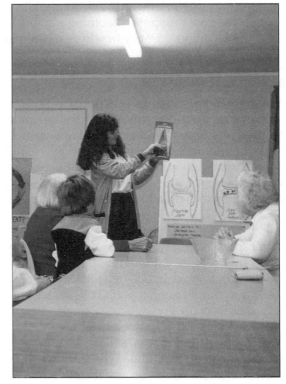

One student was explaining the process of arthritis, using the poster of a knee joint to assist her. After about 5 minutes of discussion, a member of the group inquired, 'That's a stomach, isn't it?'

Although any student of human bioscience has been trained to recognise a synovial joint at 50 paces, members of the public clearly do not have the same mind-set! Pictures of the human body, particularly its internal functions, need to be put in context if they are to help, rather than confuse, people trying to learn a little more about how their bodies work.

Drawings and photographs

Drawings and photographs are key ingredients in written health education materials. Indeed, there are times when they may appropriately represent all the 'writing' in the document. The old saying 'A picture is worth a thousand words' is relevant here. Drawings and photographs may tell the reader a great deal more than words alone could do, and this is the case not only for people who have difficulty in reading, but for all readers. Drawings and photographs help to make sense of any words, and may clarify things that are expressed with difficulty in words. They also give the document appeal and break up any writing in much the same way as white space does.

A word of caution about drawings, however. Ensure that they make sense to the people you are presenting the material for. Drawings, like words, have readability levels. Health workers have a range of knowledge about matters of health and illness, and it is easy to forget how much of this is not shared by members of the community. This point is demonstrated by the example opposite.

Audiovisual materials

Videos and audio tapes can provide useful health education in a form that is often more interesting than written materials and accessible to people who do not have good literacy skills. They may also be preferred by those people who learn more readily through listening and watching than through reading.

If you wish to make a video, it is well worth having the expertise of an experienced producer; otherwise, you may waste valuable resources, including time. Producing a video is expensive, but it is possible to keep the costs down by engaging a producer to take on the role of consultant.

The process of making a video can itself be a valuable educational experience if you involve community members in developing it. In addition, materials produced by community members themselves are more likely to address a group's needs and be acceptable to it. In fact, amateur videos may be quite successful if made by members of the group whose needs you are addressing, and can be very useful teaching tools.

Adapting material from State or national campaigns to your local area

There may be times when your agency is implementing a campaign developed at a level somewhat removed from that of your workplace. For example, the region's Public Health Unit or the State Health Promotion Unit may plan a health promotion program to be implemented in a number of areas. You may be provided with health education materials as part of the program. Once you are satisfied that the need addressed is relevant to your local area, you will have to assess the materials to decide whether they are relevant to your community or group. If they are not, you may be able to adapt them to suit the specific needs of your group, or you may need to put them aside and develop your own materials.

Conclusion

The mass media have a powerful influence on people's lives and the manner in which they view the world. Using the mass media to promote health is therefore of considerable potential value and importance. Whether it be attempting to

'With Ears That Hear, Koorie Kids Can Fly' — using videos as part of an evolving Primary Health Care Project

The Aboriginal Hearing Program in Griffith was developed in the early 1990s. It was designed after a needs assessment highlighted hearing loss as a significant problem among Aboriginal children. It focuses on a single problem and uses resources in the local community to help address it.

The needs assessment took the form of a mass audiometry and questionnaire screening of Aboriginal children at a local public school. It revealed that 20% of the children tested had a significant hearing problem. Evaluation of the parent questionnaire revealed that while parents recognised that their children had signs of ear problems and hearing loss, they did not realise that these could be significant or have serious sequelae.

Following the needs assessment, the local Koorie community was consulted in an attempt to design a program that would be effective, accessible and culturally appropriate. The result of this consultation was a three-pronged program based on awareness and education, screening and treatment.

It was decided that a video should form the basis of the awareness and education program. Local Aboriginal workers felt that storytelling was still the most acceptable means of relaying information in the community and that a video featuring local community members would provide the community with reliable information in a 'storytelling' format.

Based on the results of the needs assessment, the video did not focus on detecting signs of ear and hearing problems, but rather on their significance and what could be done. It was hoped that the video would increase community development within the Koorie community and that families would be encouraged to own the issue and seek help rather than be told what to do by a health worker.

The first step was to plan the video. Its length had to be decided in advance, as this determined how much information was to be included, how it would be presented and, of course, how much the video would cost to make. It was decided that the video should be relatively short, to encourage people to view it. It was felt that 8–10 minutes would enable enough information to be presented but still be easy for all to watch.

Before the script was written, a rough plan of who should be involved in the video was drawn up. At this stage, the Aboriginal health education officer gauged community support and asked many members of the community to take part. Everyone was eager to have their children involved and the local Aboriginal preschool was chosen as the most appropriate location for shooting. Finding adults to appear on the video was much more difficult. Most were reluctant to tell the stories of generations of their families who had experienced difficulties with hearing, but came along on shooting day to lend support. The Aboriginal health education officer acted as presenter. He introduced the topic, interviewed parents and provided the voice-over for visual shots. All his lines were carefully scripted to ensure that accurate information was conveyed in an appropriate manner that would be easily understood. All the Koorie parents and children spoke spontaneously, as it was felt that they would feel more comfortable this way and their own words would mean more to those watching the video than any script could.

Members of the Koorie community also arranged and played culturally acceptable music to open and close the video. The video has many shots of children laughing, playing and singing. It was important to the community that Koorie people be portrayed in a very positive manner, and there was some apprehension that this would not happen.

From the earliest planning stages, it had been our aim to produce a video that would be positive, enthusiastic and informative. The resulting video, 'Koorie Booris Need Ears That Hear', was extremely well accepted by the community and formed the cornerstone of the Aboriginal Hearing Program for several years.

Towards the mid 1990s, however, it became obvious that the program needed to shift its focus if it was to continue to meet the needs of the community. Awareness of the problem had been heightened considerably by the initial campaign but attendance at school screening and follow-up continued to be problematic.

In response to this situation, it was decided that a second video should be produced. This video would highlight the positive outcomes of children who had taken part in the program and emphasise the bright future that was possible with good hearing. In contrast to the first video production, when many had been to shy to participate, it was easy to find both adults and children who were eager to be involved.

The title, 'With Ears That Hear, Koorie Kids Can Fly' was chosen to present a very positive picture of how much had been achieved. Children who had been on the program told their stories of how better hearing had helped them learn to read and parents told their stories of how poor hearing had affected them, and how things were improving for their children. The video was again unscripted, and people told their own stories. Information on how children could access the program was included and parents were encouraged to send their children to school on testing day. Again, the emphasis was on the positive outcomes that the community had already achieved and how these could be continued.

By 1999, the Aboriginal Hearing Program had been running in Griffith for almost ten years. Thanks to adequate planning, implementation, evaluation and modification, it has become increasingly accepted and used. It continues as an excellent example of what can be achieved when video is used as part of a complete program, rather than an end in itself, and when health workers work with the community to achieve a goal.

Karen Williams
(previously) Paediatric Clinical Nurse Specialist
Griffith Community Health Centre

reframe health issues in the public eye to raise awareness of public policy issues through media advocacy, or working to encourage a positive health idea or behaviour through social marketing, the mass media offers considerable scope in the promotion of health. As with other health promotion strategies, there is much to be gained by working in partnership with community members when working with the mass media, and being mindful of the fact that media coverage of health issues, even successful media coverage, is not an end in itself, but a means to achieve health promoting change.

References and further reading

Anderson, D. A. and Itule, B. D. 1988, *Writing the News,* Random House, New York.

Beauchamp, K. 1986, *Fixing the Government: Everyone's Guide to Lobbying in Australia,* Penguin, Ringwood, Vic.

Buchanan, D. R., Reddy, S. and Hossain, Z. 1994, 'Social Marketing: a Critical Appraisal', *Health Promotion International,* 9 (1), 49–57.

Chapman, S. 1998, *Over Our Dead Bodies: Port Arthur Australia's Fight for Gun Control,* Pluto Press, Annandale.

Chapman, S. and Lupton, D. 1994, *The Fight for Public Health: Principles and Practice of Media Advocacy,* BMJ Publishing, London.

Chesterfield-Evans, A. 1988, 'Why the Media Makes You Sick: Aspects of the Relationship Between the Media and Public Health', *Australian Journal of Communication,* 14, 34–47.

Connell, R. 1977, *Ruling Class, Ruling Culture,* Cambridge University Press, Cambridge.

Cunningham, S. and Turner, G. (eds) 1997, *The Media in Australia: Industries, Texts, Audiences,* Allen and Unwin, Sydney.

Egger, G., Donovan, R. and Spark, R. 1993, *Health and the Media: Principles and Practice for Health Promotion.* McGraw-Hill, Sydney.

Eisenberg, L. 1987, 'Value Conflicts in Social Policies for Promoting Health', in Doxiadis, S. (ed.), *Ethical Dilemmas in Health Promotion,* John Wiley and Sons, Chichester, UK.

Flay, B. R. 1987, 'Mass Media and Smoking Cessation: a Critical Review', *American Journal of Public Health,* 77, 153–60.

Flaysakier, J. D. 1990, 'The Journalist as Health Educator', in Doxiadis S. (ed.) *Ethics in Health Education,* John Wiley and Sons, Chichester.

Flood, M. and Lawrence, A. 1987, *The Community Action Book,* NSW Council of Social Services, Sydney.

Flora, J. A. and Cassady, D. 1990, 'Roles of Media in Community-Based Health Promotion, in Bracht, N. (ed.), *Health Promotion at the Community Level,* Sage Publications, Newbury Park, USA.

Hastings, G. and Haywood, A. 1991, 'Social Marketing and Communication in Health Promotion', *Health Promotion International,* 6 (2), 135–45.

Hawe, P., Degeling, D. and Hall, J. 1990, *Evaluating Health Promotion: a Health Workers' Guide,* MacLennan and Petty, Sydney.

Hevey, D. 1992, 'Fear for Sale', *New Internationalist,* July, 20–22.

Karpf, A. 1988, *Doctoring the Media,* Routledge, London.

Neuhauser, L., Schwab, M., Syme, S. L., Bieber, M. and Obarski, S. K. 1998, 'Community Participation in Health Promotion: Evaluation of the California Wellness Guide', *Health Promotion International,* 13 (3), 211–22.

Novelli, W. D. 1990, 'Applying Social Marketing to Health Promotion and Disease Prevention', in Glanz, K., Lewis, F. M. and Rimer, B. K. (eds), *Health Behavior and Health Education: Theory Research and Practice,* Jossey Bass, San Francisco.

Nutbeam, D. and Blakey, V. 1990, 'The Concept of Health Promotion and AIDS Prevention: a Comprehensive and Integrated Basis for Action in the 1990s', *Health Promotion International,* 5 (3), 233–42.

Palmer, D. 1992, 'Mass Media for Health Promotion: Health Leninists or Change

Agents?', *Australian Journal of Public Health,* 16 (2), 206–7.

Research Unit in Health and Behavioural Change 1989, *Changing the Public Health,* John Wiley and Sons, Chichester, UK.

Schwab, M., Neuhauser, L., Margen, S., Syme, S. L., Ogar, D., Roppel, C. and Elite, A. 1992, 'The Wellness Guide: Towards a New Model for Community Participation in Health Promotion', *Health Promotion International,* 7 (1), 27–36.

Spark, R. and Mills, P. 1988, 'Promoting Aboriginal Health on Television in the Northern Territory: a Bicultural Approach', *Drug Education Journal of Australia,* 2 (3), 191–8.

Tones, K. and Tilford, S. 1994, *Health Education: Effectiveness, Efficiency and Equity,* Chapman and Hall, London.

Wallack, L. 1990a, 'Two Approaches to Health Promotion in the Mass Media', *World Health Forum,* 11, 143–64.

Wallack, L. 1990b, 'Media Advocacy: Promoting Health through Mass Communication', in Glanz, K., Lewis, F. M. and Rimer, B. K. (eds), *Health Behavior and Health Education: Theory Research and Practice,* Jossey Bass, San Francisco.

Wallack, L. and Dorfman, L. 1996, 'Media Advocacy: a Strategy for Advancing Policy and Promoting Health', *Health Education Quarterly,* 23 (3), 293–317.

Wallack, L., Dorfman, L., Jernigan, D. and Themba, M. 1993, *Media Advocacy and Public Health: Power for Prevention.* Sage, Newbury Park, CA.

Weiss, E. H. and Kessel, G. 1987, 'Practical Skills for Health Educators on Using Mass Media', *Health Education,* June/July, 39–41.

Windschuttle, K. 1984, *The Media,* Penguin, Ringwood, Victoria.

Wodak, A. 1991, 'I Feel Like an Alcohol Advertisement', *Australian Journal of Public Health,* 15 (3), 170–1.

Wrigley, J. and McLean, P. 1990, *Australian Business Communication,* Longman Cheshire, Melbourne.

CHAPTER 6

Community development

*W*orking at the level of the community, and community development in particular, has become very popular in the health field since the Declaration of Alma-Ata highlighted community development and community participation as important strategies for health promotion. Before that, many health workers were unfamiliar with the concept of community development although it had been used in other fields and by health workers in developing countries for some time.

An essential component of the Primary Health Care approach to health promotion is the recognition that it is necessary to change the structures that influence people's lives in order to improve their health. There is also recognition that people themselves have a right to work for changes to those structures. A key challenge in health promotion work is to put these ideas into practice by encouraging and supporting community-led and community-controlled activities, rather than only those activities that are led and controlled by health workers or the health system.

In community-level work, the environment, rather than the individual, is defined as the target for change (Labonte 1986, p. 347). As a result, community-level work is appealing because it has the potential to address some of the structural issues that lead to poor health. In addressing those issues, community-level work is more obviously political than other health work, since it means working for change to create social justice. While any form of health work is political in nature, as it involves either acting for social change or as social control (Connell 1977, p. 219), in community-level work the political nature of the health worker's action is usually more explicit. It is perhaps because of this that there has been a significant reduction in government support for community development in recent years with the move to more conservative government in Australia, despite the endorsement of community development as a key strategy in the promotion of health by the WHO. This chapter will examine the potential of community development as a way of working with communities, on issues they identify with, to achieve changes to the environment and enable community empowerment.

What is a community?

In Chapter 2, we briefly examined the question of what a community is and reviewed some of the key issues in considering community and community health. Important points discussed include the multiple ways in which community has been defined and the value-laden nature of the term, which is often used in an 'add-on' way to help create a positive bias for government programs or to help disguise the exploitative nature of such things as community care. We also examined definitions of 'community', which are often geographically based, and 'community of interest', which recognises that communities may be built around a common interest or concern. We noted further that, importantly, communities often include groups with conflicting interests, and that this fact is often hidden behind the romantic connotations of the term 'community' (see pp. 50–1).

These issues are of particular importance in considering community development, as these aspects of community may really come to the fore in the community development process. Indeed, workers using the community development process may have to regularly consider the implications of these issues for their work.

We also noted that community can mean a variety of different things, some specific and others very broad and general. In community development, emphasis is placed on community as a social system, bounded by geographical location or common interest, recognising that community is 'a "living" organism with interactive webs of ties among organizations, neighbourhoods, families, and friends' (Eng, Salmon & Mullan 1992, p. 1).

A sense of community

Several writers describe what they call a 'sense of community'. This is an ideal state in which everyone affected by the life of the community participates in community life. The community as a whole takes responsibility for its members and respect for the individuality of the members is maintained (Daly & Cobb 1989, p. 172). It is described by Clark (1973, p. 409) as a 'sense of solidarity and a sense of significance'. This sense of community can be an important component of people feeling as though they belong to a community, and it also has implications for the process of community development. However, two points are worth making here. Firstly, this description of an ideal sense of community is reminiscent of romantic descriptions of community life, and we need to take care not to oversimplify the consequences of human beings living in communities. Secondly, we must be careful not to assume that this sense of community is an ideal state for everyone, because some people may not choose living in a community as their ideal.

What is community development?

Community development is increasingly recognised as the process by which health workers are most able to work *with* communities. It is quite a complex concept, and one not easily captured in a simple definition. It is also fraught with ambiguities and is often described in a simplistic manner and applied uncritically. Like the notion of community participation, community development can be used in ways that manipulate people, through co-opting them to take a predetermined action, or in ways that encourage true community control and community development. However, as with participation, its thoughtless or manipulative use is likely to create distrust among community members. This could also be described as a process of building social capital (Cox 1996). It is therefore a process that must be treated with great respect.

Community development has been described as a process of moving towards the state of 'community' described above (Dixon 1992, p. 2). That is, community development aims to increase people's participation in the life of their community and the interdependence of community members. This could also be described as a process of building social capital (Cox 1996). It has been defined as a process of 'working with people as they define their own goals, mobilize resources, and develop action plans for addressing problems they collectively have identified' (Minkler 1991, p. 261).

While the latter definition was coined by Minkler to refer to community organisation, it actually describes community development. The terms 'community development' and 'community organisation' are both defined variously, and often overlap in their definition. Rothman (1987) describes community development as one form of community organisation. Egger, Spark & Lawson (1990, p. 87) have described the difference between the two terms as one of directiveness, because they regard community organisation as being a process more directed by workers, while community development is more directed by members of the community.

Sanders' four views of community development

Sanders (1958, cited by Dixon, 1989, pp. 86–7) argued that community development may be seen as a process, a method, a program and a movement. You will notice the similarity here to the different ways in which Primary Health Care is conceptualised. You will also notice the way in which these four aspects are inextricably linked.

The community development process

The community development process is the series of steps that an outsider would normally take in establishing community development. These steps have been listed as 'establish felt needs, use local leadership, foster self-help and follow up with an institution to carry forward the gains' (Walker 1982, cited by Dixon 1989, p. 87).

The community development method

The community development method is described as community development as 'a means to an end' (Dixon 1989, p. 86). As a method, community development is used to increase the autonomy and competence of the community, through its involvement in decision-making and problem-solving processes (Dixon 1989, p. 87).

Community development programs

Community development programs are programs that use the community development method and process in their implementation.

The community development movement

The themes of collectivity and empowerment that run through community development represent a particular philosophical approach that sits comfortably within Primary Health Care. This community development philosophy can guide the way in which people work, even when they are not working on community development programs, and is likely to sensitise them to times when community development is appropriate. Sanders (1958) argues that widespread support for this philosophy represents a community development movement.

Principles of community development

At this point, it will be valuable to examine in more detail the key principles of community development. Together, these help construct a picture of what community development practice is about. Perhaps the two most important

principles are the community's identification of its own needs and the importance of the process as well as the outcome of the participation of community
members in the community development process. Other important concepts are
empowerment, creating critical consciousness, the development of community
competence and the careful selection of issues to be dealt with (Minkler 1991, pp.
267–74).

Felt need

In working with need in the community, community developers are particularly
concerned with the needs of those who have little power, as it is these people
who are most likely to be suffering ill-health as a result of their lack of access to,
and influence over, the structures that are impacting negatively on their health. If
these people are not skilled in articulating their needs or do not believe they are
likely to have them met and so do not express them, finding out what they believe
they need may be a slow (but important) part of the community development
process.

You will recall that in Chapter 3 we examined Bradshaw's taxonomy of needs,
which emphasised that needs may be identified either by people themselves or
by 'experts'. This is a particularly useful framework in community development
because, unless we start from where people are at, we are unlikely to succeed, as
people will not be committed to act on issues they do not see as relevant to them.
Therefore, community members must identify with the needs being addressed if
they are to involve themselves in working for change or to support it in any other
way. That is, using Bradshaw's taxonomy of need, felt or expressed need must be
present.

Although the presence of felt need is a prerequisite for community development,
relying on its presence alone may mean that communities will act on problems
they see without fully understanding the issues. The presence also of comparative
need or normative need will increase the likelihood that the work will be successful.
For example, if a community is working for increased public housing in its area,
evidence of a low rate of public housing or a high rate of people on low incomes
(comparative need) will provide valuable support for increased housing, and will
be a stronger argument than if residents' demand for more housing was the only
rationale.

Participation — process and outcome

In Chapter 2, we discussed the range of approaches to participation. In examining
the importance of participation by community members in community
development, it is apparent that approaches to participation that are appropriate
in Primary Health Care are generally also the approaches to participation necessary
in community development. In other words, for the process of participation to be
empowering, it must be one of true participation in which decision-making power
is shared by community members. Control over decision making by community
members is encouraged and supported by health workers with a community
development philosophy. Participation that fits into the upper rungs of Arnstein's
Ladder of Citizen Participation (see pp. 60–1), in which power is shared between
workers and community members, or even completely handed over to community
members, is a fundamental part of community development.

As mentioned above, the process of participation in change is often considered to be just as important as the outcome. This is particularly so in community development. By participating in community development, people gain skills in such things as negotiation, submission writing, organisation, working with the mass media and working as part of a group. These skills, the networks people establish with others in the community and their sense of being able to negotiate the system and achieve something are regarded as valuable, and sometimes as more valuable than any outcome of the group's activity.

Although the process elements of community development are extremely important, giving more importance to them than to the outcome elements has some limitations. There is a real danger of this being paternalistic towards community members, for it effectively says that, even though they worked long and hard and lost, it was good for them. Community members themselves may not define this as success, but rather may be quite horrified by the suggestion (although they may acknowledge that they learnt from the process). Certainly the process of involvement may be very important for community members, but they may regard it as such only if they are successful in achieving what they set out to achieve.

The particular process and outcome (or objective) elements of community development have been described by Butler (1993, p. 10) as follows:

Process elements

- **Control of decision-making** – *community members participate to control the project and particularly to control the identification and definition of the issue;*

- **Involvement in action** – *the project involves the people concerned with the issue in action for change;*

- **Development of community culture** – *the project contributes to a culture of groups of individuals taking responsibility for improving and protecting their area and services;*

- **Organisational development** – *the project builds a new organisation or improves an existing one;*

- **Learning** – *the participants are acquiring new skills, information and/or new perspectives on themselves, their community and their concerns.*

Objective elements

- **Concrete benefit** – *the project sees the achievement of some new or improved service or facility, or the protection of something valued by the community;*

- **New power relationships** – *the project changes the social landscape of the community so that new and more equitable power relations are formed (this is also a process aspect).*

Empowerment and the creation of critical consciousness

Central to community development is the importance of empowerment of those people for whom the activity is occurring. Empowerment within the community development context has been defined as:

a social action process that promotes participation of people, organizations, and communities towards the goals of increased individual and community control, political efficacy, improved quality of community life, and social justice.

(Wallerstein 1992, p. 198.)

This notion of empowerment has been described as not designed to achieve power over others, but instead to achieve power to act *with* others and achieve change (Wallerstein & Bernstein 1988, p. 380).

Three important points about empowerment are worth noting. Firstly, empowerment is a term that is currently popular and tends to be used quite frequently, often in a band-aid fashion without consideration of the real implications of the term. Secondly, empowerment is not about people simply feeling better about themselves, but rather about people improving their control over issues impacting on them (Hawe, Degeling & Hall 1990, p. 115). Thirdly, empowerment is not something that can be 'done to' someone. Rather, people can only empower themselves (Labonte 1989b, p. 87) — if empowerment is forced upon people, can it rightly be called empowerment?

If people are to gain greater power over their lives, they need greater access to information, supportive relationships, decision making and resources (Benn 1981, p. 82). Health workers can play an important role in creating a climate for empowerment by enabling access to these things through the community development process.

Workers using the community development process focus on the people who have the least power, and endeavour to improve their level of control over the situations impacting on their lives. Often the first step in this process of empowerment is critical consciousness raising (Friere 1973). In other words, people need to see the causes of their problems as they are rooted in the social, political and economic structures that constrain their lives before they can be ready to work to change those structures.

This empowerment needs to occur through both the process and the outcome of community development activity. That is, it is not acceptable to take over from community members in order to achieve a positive outcome for them, when in the process they are left feeling no more capable, or even less capable, of acting more independently next time. While there may be times when quick action on issues by workers is warranted, this action cannot be described as community development.

Minkler (1991, p. 267) suggests that empowerment needs to occur on two levels: individuals need to be empowered by the process; and the community as a whole also needs to be empowered. If empowerment occurs at the individual level only, we would have to question whether community development has been occurring (Dixon 1992).

One last point is worth emphasising: empowerment is about increasing people's power over things influencing their lives, but power is rarely a neutral concept. An increase in the power that one person or group has over something in their lives will often result in someone else losing that power. This fact is extremely important because it reminds us that as long as community development concerns itself with the empowerment of people, those involved in the process risk experiencing conflict. Although consensus building is an important part of community development, conflict may sometimes be an unavoidable consequence.

Development of community competence

The concept of community competence is very much linked to community empowerment (Minkler 1991, p. 268). A competent community is one that is able to recognise and address its problems. If a community learns to better solve its own problems, then it is being empowered and becoming a more competent community.

Hawe, Degeling & Hall (1990, p. 114) suggest that an increase in a community's competence can be examined by considering 'changes in the community itself, its networks, its structures, the way in which people perceive the community, ownership of community issues, [and] perceived and actual "empowerment" in health and social issues'.

Careful selection of issues

Several writers suggest that the choice of issues used in community development is important. Minkler (1991, p. 272) suggests that if an issue is to be a good one for community development, the community must feel strongly about it, and it must be 'winnable, simple and specific'. She argues that this is particularly the case early in the community development process. Once people have started to develop a sense of their ability to effect change, they may be less easily swamped by resistance from others, or by lack of success on a particular issue. In the early stages, however, failure or resistance may lead the group to give up, so starting with winnable issues while people develop some skills can be productive. Other more difficult issues can then be tackled, with people building on the skills that they have already developed through these experiences.

In practice, however, this idea of starting with winnable issues may not be possible, as it may well be a difficult, even almost unwinnable, issue that brings a community to the point of wanting to act. In that case, the idea of starting with winnable issues goes out the door! This is more likely to be so where the community development process begins spontaneously, as a result of people responding to an issue crucial to their lives.

The role of the health worker in community development

> *Go to the people*
> *Live among them*
> *Love them*
> *Start with what they know*
> *Build on what they have*
> *But of the best leaders*
> *When their task is accomplished*
> *Their work is done*
> *The people all remark*
> *We have done it ourselves*

(Chabot 1976, cited by Ashton 1990, p. 8.)

The approach described by the poem above is the approach taken by a health worker using a community development approach. However, the community development process may also begin without the assistance of employed health workers. Local people and community leaders are often committed to using that process and may work away quietly in their own areas or groups, attempting to build consensus and initiate collective action to address people's needs.

Health workers have an important role to play in supporting the people involved in community development, whether the community development process began through the efforts of strong local leaders or was instigated by health workers themselves. There are a number of reasons for this. Firstly, it is quite clear that the *Ottawa Charter for Health Promotion* urges health workers to take up community development strategies if they are to promote the health of the people they are working for. This may mean that their work becomes uncomfortable because it has political implications, but it is not sufficient reason for us to ignore this way of working. Secondly, health workers are well placed to work for community development because they come into contact with members of marginalised groups as part of their everyday work. Indeed, because of the special relationship that develops between many health workers and their clients, the context in which they work and the 'crisis' situations in which they often meet their clients, health workers are often already in a position of trust with regard to these community members. In addition, their close involvement with people in crisis situations means that they see quite clearly the health implications of poverty and dis-empowerment. On the other hand, however, health workers may still need to break free from some community perceptions that they should be dealing directly with ill-health through clinical services only.

Health workers need to join in the life of the community, making the most of opportunities to listen to the community and develop relationships with community members, if they are to identify opportunities for community development (see p. 80). Henderson and Thomas (1987) and Twelvetrees (1991) both discuss in further detail the approach to take when 'entering the community'.

A health worker using a community development approach places particular emphasis on the roles of enabler, catalyst, coordinator, teacher of problem-solving skills, small-group facilitator and advocate (Rothman & Tropman 1987, p. 17). You can see once again how well this fits in with the particular roles of advocate, enabler and mediator that the *Ottawa Charter for Health Promotion* highlighted as important roles for health workers in health promotion action.

How might these roles be translated into everyday practice?

There are several things that health workers or health centres can do to effectively resource and support a community if they are to take up their responsibility for community development and health promotion. These can be valuable whether the community development activity in progress began spontaneously or as a result of worker 'encouragement' (although greater support may be needed if the activity did not begin spontaneously, as it is possible that the community involved is less prepared to act). Some of the political nature of community development work may become apparent as you consider the health worker activities described below.

Providing resources

Workers can support the community by providing necessary resources in their campaign. These might include access to photocopying and typing facilities and the use of meeting rooms if this is necessary. Negotiating to find accessible, neutral meeting places that are comfortable for group members will be an important component of this process. Assisting with applications for funding for some projects may be necessary also.

Assisting with skills development

Community members may need assistance with developing skills in such things as communicating with the media, writing press releases and writing letters to members of parliament, the public service or local companies involved in a particular issue. Health workers can be active in teaching people how to carry out these tasks effectively in order to get the message across.

Assisting with research

Health workers may have better skills than community members in researching information, and better access to databases holding useful information. They can therefore assist communities in developing their research skills where appropriate and can themselves conduct research through information systems to which members of the public may not have easy access.

Planning action

If health workers have a better knowledge than community members of the bureaucratic process and other useful channels to follow and approaches to take, they can provide valuable information that will help the community group to plan an effective campaign. This can save it much worry and uncertainty, as well as a great deal of valuable energy that might have been wasted if the group had acted inappropriately owing to lack of knowledge.

Supporting localism

While not all communities are locality-based, many of them are. Health workers can support opportunities for community development through actions that support the local community. For example, encouraging the establishment of local credit cooperatives will help keep local money in the local area and will make more money available for financial support of local endeavours (Williams 1986). Endeavours such as local food cooperatives will also help strengthen the resources available to people in the local community. For example, staff at the Fitzroy Community Health Centre in Victoria organised a regular fresh food market to increase the availability of cheap, fresh food in the local area. Local employment initiatives, too, present valuable opportunities to support local economic development (Sindal & Dixon 1990, p. 246). A variety of community enterprises are explored by Pearce (1993) and Morehouse (1997).

Supporting community members

Community development is hard work and can be exhausting, physically and emotionally, for those involved. Unless support is provided when necessary, community members involved in the process can end up burnt out, unable to continue and feeling disempowered. Health workers therefore have a key role to play in supporting and encouraging community members involved in community development.

Community development work may also be a tiring process for health workers, and so it is valuable for health workers using this approach to support each other. This can be particularly so when progress seems slow, and when community development is not endorsed enthusiastically by some health decision makers.

Encouraging community development: in whose interests?

'Pure' community development can be described as a process by which members of a community are enabled to work together to solve a problem they face and, through their involvement, perhaps develop skills and greater power over some of the issues that impact on their lives. However, community development is not always used to empower communities and increase their access to a range of choices. In many instances, some of its principles may be used to increase the compliance of community members with a program being imposed on the community, as a means of increasing the success of that program.

Tones and Tilford (1994, p. 271) suggest that there is a continuum of approaches to the use of community development strategies, ranging from community development as empowerment at one end through to the use of community development strategies to impose the beliefs of professional groups or politicians at the other end. In between these extremes lie a number of variations. As can be seen from Figure 6.1, this continuum of approaches parallels the range of approaches to participation in Arnstein's Ladder of Citizen Participation (discussed on pp. 55–6).

Community health projects (Tones and Tilford 1994, p. 271)

Type 1   Innovators' goals for the community are primarily self-empowerment and improvement in socioeconomic status. Self-empowerment = Health.

Type 2   As with type 1 but during the process of developing a community profile and identifying felt needs, the community itself acknowledges needs which are consistent with standard preventive medicine goals — e.g. a need for better primary care service, accident prevention, dealing with child health problems.

Type 3   Characterized by 'community health projects'. Innovators' goals are to enhance health and prevent disease. They aim to do this by raising the profile of health but are prepared to help the community work through other more pressing 'felt needs' prior to their acknowledging a need to improve cardiovascular health, for example.

Type 4   Innovators' goals are primarily those of the preventive medicine. This type is epitomized by the various CHD prevention programs. It is more top-down than types 1-3 but it emphasizes the importance of enlisting the support of the community and utilizing community dynamics such as networks.

Type 5   More limited 'outreach' programs; limited community participation but uses mix of agencies, e.g. media plus schools, plus drop-in centres and delivery of services to housing estate or workplace.

Figure 6.1 a. A continuum of approaches to community health projects. Note how the continuum of approaches to community work mirrors the approaches to participation demonstrated by Arnstein's Ladder of Citizen Participation (opposite).

Werner (1981, p. 47) describes the two extremes of this continuum as the difference between community-supportive programs and community-oppressive programs:

> **Community-supportive** *programmes or functions are those that favourably influence the long-range welfare of the community, that help it stand on its own feet, that genuinely encourage responsibility, initiative, decision-making and self-reliance at the community level, that build upon human dignity.*

> **Community-oppressive** *programmes or functions are those which, while invariably giving lip-service to the above aspects of community input, are fundamentally authoritarian, paternalistic or are structured and carried out in such a way that they effectively encourage greater dependency, servility and unquestioning acceptance of outside regulations and decisions, and in the long run cripple the dynamics of the community.*

In terms of community development, this difference can be described as the difference between community development *as* health promotion and the use (or abuse!) of community development *in* health promotion.

When a more limited form of community development is used, it is worth asking whose interests are being served. To what extent is this type of community development likely to serve the needs of the disempowered in the community? As Werner's definition of community-oppressive programs suggests, some uses of community development may serve more the needs of the workers or bureau-

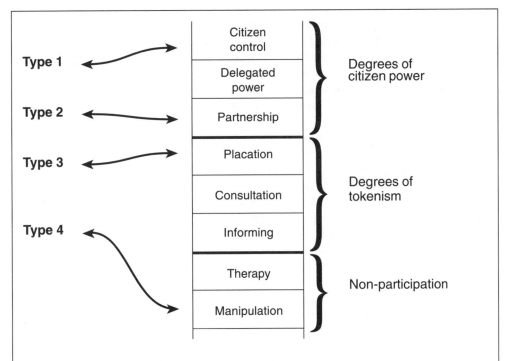

Figure 6.1 b. Relationship of the the continuum of approaches to community health projects (opposite) to Arnstein's Ladder of Citizen Participation (Arnstein 1971, p. 70).

cracies whose decisions are being imposed than the needs of the people they are meant to assist. There may be times when the community may benefit from the imposition of good ideas, but this may be the case only in the short term. In the longer term, the community may have become more, rather than less, dependent on the health workers, and so the principles of Primary Health Care may not be operating. It is only when 'pure' community development is being implemented that community development can live up to its reputation for addressing the structural causes of ill-health. While it may be argued that some of the projects that use the more limited form of community development are useful, they will not result in structural change or change in the power relationships between health workers and community members, and so they cannot rightly be regarded as community development.

Walker (1986) has described the aim of community development as being to 'establish a dialogue between people and the system, so that people can demand things from the system, and the system can be responsive to their needs'. If community development activities result in people being more obedient to health workers, rather than making the system more aware of and responsive to the needs of the community, then we have a fair indication that the aims of community development and the principles of Primary Health Care are not being addressed.

Critical evaluation of community development practice is therefore vital. It often needs to include critical evaluation of the way in which the employing agency or funding body sees community development being applied. If they have unrealistic or manipulative uses of community development in mind, you may need to provide some clarification, because administrators and bureaucrats, like others, do not always understand the intention of the approach to community development endorsed in the Primary Health Care approach.

With the reduced support for community development in health work by government in recent years, a critical review of the reaction by governments is in order. Community development places emphasis on people working together as a group to achieve things for themselves, and changing the structures that influence their lives at the local level. Governments might therefore support community development because it takes the focus of responsibility away from government, public policy and broad social change. Community development also provides a cheap option for government. In supporting community development for those reasons, governments may have little regard for its goals of empowerment and increased community competence. This may mean that they support community development in theory, but in practice support only those limited forms described by Tones and Tilford (1994). Indeed, this is reflected in recent government expectations that community development will be used to meet specific disease-related goals and targets — for example, to improve nutrition or reduce cardiovascular disease.

On the other hand, governments may reject community development as an approach to community health work because of their recognition that it emphasises drawing people together to work for common problems. As government services that government may be nervous of an approach that encourages people to work for social change, as it is possible that people may start demanding increased accountability from government.

The consequence of these two perspectives has been a somewhat fickle relationship between Australian governments and community development programs, with support waxing and waning and practitioners reliant on their own commitment to the philosophical assumptions underlying community development in order to continue working in this way. However, rather than making the notion of community development obsolete, McArdle (1999, p. 4) argues that the growth of economic rationalism and move away from nation building by government actually makes the need for community development even greater. Health workers with a commitment to the Primary Health Care approach cannot afford to lose their focus on community development.

The limits of community development

As community development has been endorsed with great gusto in recent years by those working in health, there has been a tendency to expect from it much more than it is capable of achieving. It is important to recognise that while community development can have some impact on power relationships and equity at a local level, it cannot shift power relationships on a broad scale (Dixon 1989). That is, even with the best intentions in the world, it cannot by itself change widespread social, economic and political conditions that are creating inequality and ill-health. Change of this nature requires broad social movements beyond the boundaries of community development, though community development may well form the stepping stones for some of these broader processes (Tesoriero 1995, p. 270). Work on this level is certainly an important part of health promotion, but it will not come from community development alone.

Conclusion

With the endorsement of community development as a health promotion strategy in the *Ottawa Charter for Health Promotion,* and recognition that it reflects the Primary Health Care approach due to its focus on working with people and enabling them to take a leadership role, health workers need to develop their skills in community development and make it a central part of their practice philosophy. However, if we are to work with community development realistically and optimistically, we need to recognise its limits as well as its potential. We also need to develop skills in those forms of action that may help bring about social change on a broader level. The next chapter will address these issues.

References and further reading

Arnstein, S. 1971, 'Eight Rungs on the Ladder of Citizen Participation', in Cahn, E. S. and Passett, B. A. (eds), *Citizen Participation: Effecting Community Changes,* Praeger Publishers, New York.

Ashton, J. 1990, 'Healthy Cities: an Overview of the International Movement', in Australian Community Health Association (eds), *Making the Connections: People, Communities and the Environment, Papers From the First National Conference of* have been significantly rolled back in some Australian States, it is little wonder *Healthy Cities Australia,* Australian Community Health Association, Sydney.

Benn, C. 1981, *Attacking Poverty Through Participation: a Community Approach,* PIT Publishing, Bundoora, Vic.

Blakely, E. J. and Bowman, K. 1986, *Taking Local Development Initiatives: a Guide to Economic and Employment Development for Local Government Authorities,* Australian Institute of Urban Studies, Canberra.

Bryson, L. and Mowbray, M. 1981, 'Community: the Spray-On Solution', *Australian Journal of Social Issues,* November, 255-67.

Butler, P. 1993, 'Introduction' in Butler, P. and Cass, S. (eds), *Case Studies of Community Development in Health,* Centre for Development and Innovation in Health, Northcote, Vic.

Clark, D. B. 1973, 'The Concept of Community: a Re-Examination', *Sociological Review,* 21 (3), 397–415.

Community Development in Health Project (eds), 1989, *Community Development in Health For All: Proceedings of a National Workshop, 12–14 July, Melbourne University,* Community Development in Health Project, Northcote, Vic.

Community Development in Health Project 1988, *Community Development in Health: a Resources Collection,* District Health Council, Preston/Northcote, Vic.

Connell, R. 1977, *Ruling Class, Ruling Culture,* Cambridge University Press, Cambridge.

Copeman, R. C. 1988, 'Assessment of Aboriginal Health Services', *Community Health Studies,* 13 (3), 251–5.

Cox, E. 1996, *A Truly Civil Society,* ABC Books, Sydney.

Daly, H. E. and Cobb, J. B. 1989, *For the Common Good: Redirecting the Economy Toward Community, the Environment and a Sustainable Future,* Beacon Press, Boston.

Dixon, J. 1989, 'The Limits and Potential of Community Development for Personal and Social Change', *Community Health Studies,* 13 (1), 82–92.

Dixon, J. 1992, The Logics Inherent in Evaluating CD: Evaluating Community Development Programs, the Community Development Approach and Community Interventions, paper presented at the Fourth Annual Health Promotion Workshop, Adelaide, 16–18 February.

Dixon, J. and Sindall, C. 1994, 'Applying Logics of Change to the Evaluation of Community Development in Health Promotion', *Health Promotion International,* 9 (4), 297–309.

Dwyer, J. 1989, 'The Politics of Participation', *Community Health Studies,* 13 (1), 59–65.

Egger, G., Spark, R. and Lawson, J. 1990, *Health Promotion Strategies and Methods,* McGraw-Hill, Sydney.

Eng, E., Salmon, M. E. and Mullan, F. 1992, 'Community Empowerment: the Critical Base for Primary Health Care', *Family and Community Health,* 15 (1), 1–12.

Freire, P. 1973, *Evaluation for Critical Consciousness,* Sheed and Ward, London.

Hawe, P., Degeling, D. and Hall, J. 1990, *Evaluating Health Promotion: a Health Workers' Guide,* MacLennan and Petty, Sydney.

Hazlehurst, K. M. 1996, *A Healing Place: Indigenous Visions for Personal Empowerment and Community Recovery,* Central Queensland University Press, Rockhampton.

Henderson, P. and Thomas, D. N. 1987, *Skills in Neighbourhood Work,* Allen and Unwin, Sydney.

Hoatson, L, Dixon, J. and Sloman, D. 1996, 'Community Development, Citizenship and the Contract State', *Community Development Journal,* 31 (2), April, 126–36.

Hunt, S. 1990, 'Building Alliances: Professional and Political Issues in Community Participation, Examples from a Health and Community Development Project', *Health Promotion International,* 5 (3), 179–85.

Ife, J. 1995, *Community Development: Creating Community Alternatives – Vision, Analysis and Practice,* Longman, Melbourne.

Kenny, S. 1994, *Developing Communities for the Future: Community Development in Australia,* Thomas Nelson, Melbourne.

Labonté, R. 1986, 'Social Inequality and Healthy Public Policy', *Health Promotion* 1 (3), 341–51.

Labonté, R. 1989a, 'Community and Professional Empowerment', *Canadian Nurse,* March, 23–8.

Labonté, R. 1989b, 'Community Empowerment: the Need for Political Analysis', *Canadian Journal of Public Health,* 80, March/April, 87–8.

McArdle, J. 1998, *Resource Manual for Facilitators in Community Development,* Vista Publications, Melbourne.

McArdle, J. 1999, *Community Development in the Market Economy,* Vista Publications, Melbourne.

McIntyre, J. 1995, *Achieving Social Rights and Responsibility: Towards a Critical Humanist Approach to Community Development,* Community Quarterly, St Kilda, Vic.

Minkler, M. 1991, 'Improving Health Through Community Organization', in Glanz, K., Lewis, F. M. and Rimer, B. K. (eds), *Health Behavior and Health Education: Theory, Research and Practice,* Jossey Bass, San Francisco.

Morehouse, W. (ed.) 1997, *Building Sustainable Communities: Tools and Concepts for Self-Reliant Economic Change,* The Bootstrap Press, New York, and Jon Carpenter Publishing, Charlbury, UK.

Pearce, J. 1993, *At the Heart of the Community Economy: Community Enterprise in a Changing World,* Calouste Gulbenkian Foundation, London.

Roberts, R. and Pietsch, J. 1996, 'Community Management and Social Action: Politicisation or Parochialism'?, *Community Development Journal,* 31 (2), 143–52.

Robertson, A. and Minkler, M. 1994, 'New Health Promotion Movement: a Critical Examination', *Health Education Quarterly,* 21 (3), 295–312.

Rothman, J. with Tropman, J. E. 1987, 'Models of Community Organization and Macro Practice Perspectives: their Mixing and Phasing', in Cox, F. M., Erlich, J. L., Rothman, J. and Tropman J. E., *Strategies of Community Organization,* F. E. Peacock, Itasca, Illinois.

Ryan, P. 1992, *Cases for Change: CHASP in Practice,* Australian Community Health Association, Sydney.

Sanders, I. T. 1958, 'Theories of Community Development', *Rural Sociology,* 23, 1–12.

Scott, D. 1981, *Don't Mourn for Me – Organise,* Allen and Unwin, Sydney.

Short, S. 1989, 'Community Participation or Community Manipulation? A Case Study of the Illawarra Cancer Appeal-A-Thon', *Community Health Studies,* 13 (1), 34–8.

Sindal, C. and Dixon, J. 1990, 'Creating Supportive Economic Environments for Health', in Australian Community Health Association (eds), *Healthy Environment in the 90s: The Community Health Approach,* papers from the 3rd National

Conference of the Australian Community Health Association, Australian Community Health Association, Sydney.

Tesoriero, F. 1995, 'Community Development and Health Promotion', in Baum, F. (ed.), *Health For All: The South Australian Experience,* South Australian Community Health Research Unit in association with Wakefield Press, Kent Town, South Australia.

Thorpe, R. 1992, 'Community Work and Ideology: an Australian Perspective' in Thorpe, R., Petruchenia, J. and Hughes, L. (eds), *Community Work or Social Change? – an Australian Perspective,* Hale and Iremonger, Sydney.

Tones, K. and Tilford, S. 1994, *Health Education: Effectiveness, Efficiency and Equity,* Chapman and Hall, London.

Twelvetrees, A. 1991, *Community Work,* Macmillan, Basingstoke.

Walker, M. 1986, Community Development Lecture, Mitchell College of Advanced Education, Bathurst, 12 August.

Wallerstein, N. 1992, 'Powerlessness, Empowerment, and Health: Implications for Health Promotion Programs', *American Journal of Public Health,* January/ February, 6 (3), 197–205.

Wallerstein, N. and Bernstein, E. 1988, 'Empowerment Education: Freire's Ideas Adapted to Health Education', *Health Education Quarterly,* 15 (4), 379–94.

Webster, K. 1993, 'Australian Case Studies in Community Development 1972– 1992: an Annotated Bibliography', Centre for Development and Innovation in Health, Preston/Northcote, Vic.

Werner, D. 1981, 'The Village Health Worker: Lackey or Liberator'?, *World Health Forum,* 2 (1), 46–68.

Williams, S. 1986, 'Community Based Finance', *Community Quarterly,* 8, 4–10.

CHAPTER 7

Working for change in communities and organisations

*W*ork to develop healthy public policy and create more supportive environments *has been identified as central to effective health promotion practice since the development of the* Ottawa Charter for Health Promotion. *Developing public policy that supports healthy choices may also be one of the most challenging areas of health promotion, as it requires health workers to move beyond their traditional sphere of work. At the same time, this approach to work offers scope for developing effective long-term change with wide-ranging impact.*

The challenges presented by working to build healthy public policy and create supportive environments have resulted in development of the settings approach, in which work for structural change, in partnership with community members and people working in other sectors, whose work impacts on health, aims to improve people's health chances at the local level. The settings approach has much potential for change in a variety of settings and these are currently being explored by practitioners around the world.

This chapter explores the key issues in the development of healthy public policy and more supportive environments, at both a broad social level and within organisations. It also examines some of the main strategies for change when working to create more health promoting environments.

Working for communities

Although community development is an important means of working with communities to deal with issues that impact on their lives, it is clearly not the only form of community-level work. Chapter 6 identified that not all work attempting to address needs at a community level can be correctly labelled 'community development'. This section will briefly review a number of ways in which you can work *for* communities while maintaining, as much as possible, the spirit of Primary Health Care.

The distinction between working *with*, working *for* and working *on* communities is a useful one, because it provides a framework in which we can critically examine the perspective of community-level work. Working *with* communities is reflected in 'pure' community development, where the focus is on the developmental process and on the partnership between health workers and community members as they work for change. Working *for* communities describes those instances where health workers are more directive in planning action and implementing it, but where they continue to act with the philosophy of Primary Health Care to involve community members as much as possible and to work for changes that increase people's control over their health. Working *on* communities describes those activities where health workers impose on communities interventions they believe are important, but do this with little reference to the way in which communities define their needs.

The distinction between these three sets of activities is by no means clear: there may be overlap between these areas and a fine line often separates them. Nevertheless, the distinction can be a useful framework for assessing community-level work and evaluating the approach that is driving it. If working *for* communities is to be successful, the principles of Primary Health Care need to guide any action that occurs. That is, even when health workers are working for communities, social justice and community participation are guiding principles, ensuring that working *for* communities does not become working *on* communities.

It is not appropriate to expect community development to be the answer to every problem a community faces. There may be times, for example, when this would be unethical because there is an urgent risk to people's health or because people do not feel empowered enough to act. Conversely, people may not be interested in actively participating in an issue and may believe that their taxes provide the wages of health workers so that others do not have to become involved in every health issue that arises. Expecting members of a community to deal with all the things that challenge their health may amount to a form of victim blaming, and be based on an expectation that people — often those with the least resources — should take responsibility for issues over which they have little or no control. At these times, it may be more appropriate to work on behalf of the people concerned to help make the health and social systems more responsive to the needs of the community. Health workers themselves can work — particularly to build healthy public policy and therefore create supportive environments — through the processes of advocacy and mediation, as recommended by the *Ottawa Charter for Health Promotion.*

Finding the balance between working with communities through community development and working for communities is an ongoing challenge for health promotion workers. Finding the appropriate point of balance between these two requires critical reflection by health workers to ensure that the work that is done reflects the principles of Primary Health Care.

Working for healthy public policy

The *Ottawa Charter for Health Promotion,* with its emphasis on building healthy public policy as an integral component of health promotion action, marked the formal recognition of the role that all public policy plays in influencing health and the role of the environment in shaping choices for health. This acknowledgment of the importance of healthy public policy was reflected in the fact that the Second International Conference on Health Promotion, held in Adelaide in 1988, focused on healthy public policy. This acknowledgment is vital because it recognises that people's social and physical environments impact strongly on their health and the health choices they can make, and that all public policies, not just those labelled as health policies, have health consequences.

Healthy public policy is central to the promotion of health because, without the support of healthy public policy, other health promotion actions are likely to be of limited value. As Milio (1990, p. 295) has expressed it:

by definition, even the most effective projects have limits, in time and/or the people who benefit. Projects can demonstrate, but only policies can perpetuate the effects. Projects can create oases of health, but only policies can redistribute and equalize their benefits.

At the same time, healthy public policy 'cannot be developed in a moral vacuum' (WHO 1998, p. 210). The development of such policy requires political will, the support of government, and a commitment to equity and to ensuring that all members of society receive the health benefits of social changes.

Any examination of healthy public policy and action to build healthy public policy must start with a consideration of what policy is, and how it can be influenced.

What is policy?

Defining 'policy' is not easy, because the term is used in a variety of ways. In some instances it is a formal process, in others an informal one. The term 'policy' may be used to refer to a general statement of intention, perhaps resembling a promise; it may refer to a set of actions by government over a period of time in a particular area; or it may refer to a set of standing rules (Palmer & Short 1994, p. 23). In many instances, too, policies may be reflected more by what is not said than what is said.

Public policies are defined as policies that affect the public interest. Many of them are largely the responsibility of governments (Palmer & Short 1994, p. 23). However, they are not determined solely by public interest, as a great many private interests have power in determining the direction of public policy (Gardner & Barraclough 1992, p. 10). For example, the medical profession, guided largely by its interests in private practice and entrepreneurial activity, has a very powerful influence over public policy related to health. Medical insurance companies are in a similar position with regard to health financing.

Until relatively recently health workers have been concerned primarily with health policy, because it was assumed that this was the major policy that impacted on health. It is now recognised, however, that health policy may have very little impact on health by comparison with the impact of social policy and economic policy because it focuses largely on the structure of health care delivery. Social policy, for example, deals with such issues as income distribution, housing and transport provision, while economic policy affects such things as employment rates, inflation and standard of living. Policies that impact on the physical environment include policies on land use, mining and farming. It is clear that all these things do a great deal to structure the environments in which people live. The notion, then, of public policies having a substantial impact on health makes good sense, and the need for economic, social and health policies to be responsive to the requirements of the community is quite apparent. Two recent results of the growing recognition of this fact are the increasing concern for the health of the environment, and concern for the impact of economic rationalism on the quality of life of the community (Pusey 1998).

At the same time, though, Australia has made several significant advances towards making health policy itself more health promoting, through the range of policies that have been developed since our commitment to the Health For All by the year 2000 strategy. These policies, many of which were reviewed in Chapter 1, may place greater emphasis on health promotion, attempt to deal directly with some of the causes of health problems, ensure equitable access to health care for all, or develop services appropriate to the needs of particular groups. However, as some of the policy development in Chapter 1 highlighted, inadequate resources for comprehensive policy implementation may be a barrier to realisation of the vision presented in those policies.

The process of public policy making

Public policy making has been described as a dynamic social and political process (Milio 1988, p. 3). It is also a competitive process, with the competing interests of different groups involved in trying to shape the direction that public policies take (Gardner & Barraclough 1992, p. 11). Public policies result from 'a synthesis of power relationships, demographic trends, institutional agendas, community ideologies [and] economic resources' (Brown 1992, p. 104).

There are three key groups of people involved in the policy-making process — the public (including formal interest groups), political and bureaucratic policy makers, and the mass media (Milio 1988, pp. 3–4). Some interest groups involving themselves in the policy-making process have a great deal more power than others because of their political position and their ability to influence the views represented in the mass media. For example, mainstream medical interest groups are usually listened to by members of parliament and shape the public agenda more strongly than many other groups, and their opinions are reported more often by the mass media.

Public comment on new and developing policies is valuable, and seems to have developed as a result of two quite different phenomena. Firstly, there has been greater recognition of the importance of community participation resulting from recognition of the Primary Health Care approach and the new public health movement, although this has been taken up to different degrees by various governments. Secondly, there has been a growing distrust of politicians to act in the community's best interest and an increasing demand by many community members to influence decisions made by government. Nevertheless, it is the politicians, bureaucrats and powerful interest groups who set the agenda and decide the framework and philosophy of a policy. Members of the public commenting on a document are often in the position of trying to change the policy after the framework has been set.

Several authors have described the public policy-making process using a variety of relatively similar models. Palmer and Short (1994, pp. 33–4) describe it as a five-stage model:

1. *Problem identification and agenda setting.* A public problem is recognised as a political issue, and is placed on the political agenda. This often occurs in response to pressure from an interest group.
2. *Policy formation.* New policies are developed or existing policies are redeveloped. The social and political context in which this occurs is likely to have a significant bearing on the outcome.
3. *Adoption.* A new policy is formally accepted, through either legal enactment in parliament or approval of the appropriate minister.
4. *Policy implementation.* A policy is actually put into practice. The 'product' seen at this point may be quite different from what was imagined when the policy was first formulated. For example, its power may be eroded by the way in which it is implemented, or it may have unforeseen consequences when it is

put into practice. The outcome of policies that are implemented with an in-adequate budget may be quite different from that envisaged when they were originally formulated.

5. *Policy evaluation.* Policies are evaluated for their impact. Clearly, if policy evaluation is to be meaningful, it needs to be an ongoing process. Policy making is a cyclical process, and evaluating policy in action may lead to the policy issue being put back on the policy agenda, and thus to the cycle beginning again.

It is important to note, however, that this model accounts only for policies that are formally developed, not those that develop incrementally and never reach the public agenda.

Community members and groups affected by the policy concerned may be able to influence the policy-making process at any stage in its life, but this is more likely to happen during policy formation and policy evaluation. In addition, because of the cyclical nature of the stages in the public policy-making process, community members and interested groups can be part of the process that puts issues back onto the policy agenda. With regard to issues that have never been formally discussed as policy issues but have developed incrementally, community members may be involved in the important process of getting them onto the public agenda and reviewed critically, perhaps for the first time.

Public policies can be influenced through social advocacy and lobbying. These are discussed in more detail later. It is important to note, however, that affecting public policy in this way is often a slow process, and it may take several years of concerted effort by a number of people to change the major direction of a policy process. Working with people and keeping your sights set on your goal are important. Hancock (1990, p. 29) describes this process of changing public policy as one of 'goal directed muddling through'.

Developing networks for intersectoral health action

If health workers are to influence the direction of policy and action in a way that makes environments healthier, then clearly they need to influence policy and action in a number of sectors. They cannot do this alone, but must work with a range of other people who recognise the health impacts of actions in what are traditionally regarded as non-health areas. These people include workers in

The Victorian Health Promotion Foundation

The Victorian Health Promotion Foundation was established in 1987 following the proclamation of the Tobacco Act, which was supported by all three political parties in Victoria. From its inception it was funded by a 5% levy introduced by the Act on all wholesale tobacco sales, which was estimated to raise $23 million each year. 'VicHealth' was the first health promotion foundation to be established in Australia, and its unique funding arrangement was a source of interest both nationally and internationally. As a result, its work has had an impact beyond the borders of Victoria.

VicHealth was funded for 10 years from revenue raised through tobacco franchise fees, although from 1992 the amount of funding allocated was determined by the Treasurer. However, in 1997 the High Court of Australia ruled that it was unconstitutional for the States to collect such franchise fees. Since that time VicHealth has been supported by annual funding from the Victorian government, as part of funding for the Department of Human Services.

In its early years, VicHealth funded programs in five key areas — tobacco replacement, sport sponsorship, arts and culture sponsorship, health promotion programs, and research. Its tobacco replacement program was the centrepiece of this work until 1992, when most sport sponsorship and other tobacco advertising became illegal.

VicHealth has since continued with a focus on work that improves the environmental supports for healthy choices. In line with both the *Ottawa Charter for Health Promotion* and *The Jakarta Declaration on Leading Health Promotion into the 21st Century*, VicHealth aims to work by developing strategic alliances with government, business and not-for-profit organisations to develop healthy environments in a wide range of settings (VicHealth 1999, p. 1).

VicHealth's current focus is perhaps best reflected in the outcomes it has set for itself in its Strategic Plan for the period 1999–2002 (VicHealth 1999):

1. **Recognised as a leader in health promotion innovation** – VicHealth will be accorded high standing in health promotion agenda-setting and advocacy for policy and practice development locally and globally.

2. **Demonstrable contribution to population health** – Health promotion's contribution to improving health is assessed by the provision of supportive environments for individuals to adopt and sustain healthy behaviours.

3. **Greater investment in population groups most in need** – Population groups that experience social and economic disadvantage have at least twice the risk of serious illness and premature death than more advantaged socioeconomic groups. A critical aim for health promotion is to influence change to support improved health outcomes for these groups.

4. **Shared responsibility for health across setting and sectors** – VicHealth will be an intelligent broker of investments for health promotion across settings and sectors. VicHealth will work with sport, recreation, community, health, the arts, culture, entertainment and business in order to improve the health status of Victorians.

5. **Innovative organisation** - VicHealth seeks to support change processes in other organisations to achieve improved health outcomes. This role is dependent upon VicHealth's own capacity to learn, take risks, communicate and deliver quality responses to complex issues.

VicHealth began as a world leader in innovative funding of health promotion, through its establishment using taxation of tobacco products. Since its development it has developed in response to changing circumstances, to ensure its continuing relevance as a health promotion organisation. As a result of this responsiveness, it continues to contribute to the development of innovative health promotion practice.

Further information about VicHealth can be obtained from:
Victorian Health Promotion Foundation
Suite 2, First Floor
333 Drummond Street
Carlton VIC 3053
Tel: 03 9345 3200
Fax: 03 9345 3222
http://www.vichealth.vic.gov.au

industry, transport, agriculture and education, in addition to members of the community.

It is vital, then, that you plan to make and maintain valuable working relationships with people in other disciplines, other agencies and other sectors in order to maximise the joint actions you can take to promote health. These working relationships can be very powerful, even though there may be times when conflict may arise. More often than not, though, when a working relationship exists between people, it seems much easier to deal with any conflict than when there is no previous working relationship.

Creating supportive environments

The World Health Organization is encouraging the building of healthy public policy because it creates supportive environments in which it is easier for people to make healthy choices. While, as Milio (1990, p. 295) notes, one-off projects do not have the impact that healthy public policy does, one-off projects that impact in a positive way on the environment can support people's healthy choices, and either encourage the establishment of healthy public policy or promote individual

---

Health Action, New Zealand

Health Action is a community-based health project that aims 'to create a social and political environment that supports actions leading to good health' (Langford 1990, p. 14). It has chosen to focus on these aspects of health promotion because they constitute the 'hard edge' of health promotion that tends to be neglected by health workers, who tend to focus on health education (Langford 1990, p. 18). It has done this by working with community groups acting on issues of health concern, supporting them in their endeavours and bringing groups with shared or related concerns together for joint action.

The way in which Health Action addressed the problem of high skin cancer rates gives us some valuable insights into how the *Ottawa Charter for Health Promotion* can be implemented. Rather than focus on sun sense education, Health Action aimed to reduce the emission of ozone-depleting substances in the Nelson region of New Zealand and reduce demand for these products. It formed a coalition of several local groups — the Environment Centre, the Forest and Bird Society, the Cancer Society and a conservation group — and some local health administrators, and worked together to deal with the issue. It informed consumers of the ozone-friendly choices they could make, lobbied the city council to develop a policy on ozone-depleting substances (which has resulted in the local council recycling chlorofluorocarbons [CFCs] and a total of three councils committing themselves to an ozone-friendly policy), contributed at a national level to the development of an Ozone Layer Protection Bill and worked successfully to encourage shop managers to stock only ozone-friendly products. This activity has been very successful and a number of other New Zealand communities have taken similar initiatives.

This is just one example of the work of Health Action. The principles behind its other work are the same and by working with community groups it is achieving healthy change which will be supportive of the community and provide opportunities for health and healthy choices (Langford 1990).

behaviour change. The previous examples of 'Health Action' and 'Tobacco sponsorship replacement at the local level' demonstrate ways in which this can be done.

Social advocacy and lobbying

Social advocacy and lobbying are very much recognised as part of the health worker's role, particularly since the *Ottawa Charter for Health Promotion* acknowledged their importance. They constitute a key strategy with which to work for healthy public policy. Health workers have two key roles to play in social, or health, advocacy: acting as advocates and lobbyists themselves, and encouraging and supporting other community members to take up advocacy and lobbying. Chapter 2, discussing participation, identified the fact that, on the whole, individuals are poorly prepared for participating in the political process and are not encouraged to do so. Developing skills in this area, as well as assisting others to do so, is a vital part of health promotion work if we are to take up our advocacy role effectively.

Joining advocacy groups

People can do advocacy work as individuals, and they can do it as part of an organisation that includes advocacy and lobbying work in its activities. There are a number of key organisations that currently act to advocate for community members and consumers in the health system. Some of them are specifically designed for community and consumer advocacy work, for example, the Consumers' Health Forum and the Health Issues Centre; others are professional organisations which include community and consumer advocacy as part of their role, for example the State-based Community Health Associations and the Public Health Association of Australia. All these organisations are among those you can

---

The Health Issues Centre

The Health Issues Centre is an independent non-government organisation that conducts health policy analysis and social advocacy. It aims to create a more equitable health care system which is more responsive to the needs of its community. It argues for a more balanced system of illness treatment and health promotion, and for more equitable allocation of the health dollar.

As well as lobbying for change to the health system, the Health Issues Centre produces a quarterly journal and regular issues papers. Papers published to date include *What's wrong with the health system?*, *Getting off the sickness-go-round: are we on the right track?*, *Where the health dollar goes*, *Organ transplants: the need for community debate*, and *Our better health: getting it together.*

Membership of the Health Issues Centre and copies of its papers are available by contacting:

Health Issues Centre
Level 11, 300 Flinders Street
Melbourne VIC 3000
Tel: (03) 9614 0500, Fax: (03) 9614 0511

involve yourself in. In addition to adding your weight to the voices behind their advocacy work, you will learn a great deal about effective advocacy work and about work being conducted by others.

Lobbying members of parliament

Appealing to members of parliament to act on issues that impact on the health of the community can be a useful way of having your views represented, and (hopefully) taken account of when decisions are being made at the political level.

There are several possibilities. Firstly, you can approach your own State and federal members of parliament. It is worthwhile when communicating with them to emphasise the impact of your concern on the local people, as parliamentarians are elected by local people in the expectation that they will represent those people's interests. Secondly, you can lobby members of parliament responsible for particular portfolios relevant to the issue at hand. For example, the State and federal ministers of health may be approached regarding your concerns about a health issue. Ministers responsible for other relevant portfolios can also be approached. The transport, agriculture, sport, education and environment ministers are just some of the ministers whom it may be appropriate to approach regarding different health promotion issues. Thirdly, the Prime Minister and the Premier of the State in question can be approached if you believe the issue has more serious or urgent consequences.

Lobbying members of parliament is more likely to be successful if done by a larger number of people, and much of this approach therefore involves working with other people, and educating them about the ways in which lobbying skills can be used to affect the public agenda. Encouraging other people to lobby members of parliament and to keep at it by regularly contacting them until you get the response you want, will increase your chances of success. They are best reached via their electoral offices, as their offices at Parliament House are often unattended (Beauchamp 1986, p. 122). Contacting a member of parliament by letter rather than by telephone is more likely to be successful because a written request is more difficult to ignore (Beauchamp 1986, p. 124).

The mass media is also a very useful tool in lobbying members of parliament and other key decision makers, who are increasingly reliant on the mass media for their understanding of important policy issues. Wallack and Dorfman (1996, pp. 303–7) provide an example of an entire media campaign run with the ultimate aim of influencing just one person — the senior public servant who had the power to implement policy changes in an unsafe public housing estate.

Responding to calls for public comment

Commonwealth and State departments of health, and other government sectors, place advertisements in all the major metropolitan newspapers, usually on a Saturday, when they wish to advise of the availability of a new report for public discussion, canvass public opinion on an issue, invite public involvement in an activity or advertise the availability of funding for health promotion activities or research. Other bodies, for example, the National Health and Medical Research Council, do the same. It is therefore extremely valuable to examine the major newspapers regularly in order to identify these calls for public comment. They provide a valuable opportunity to influence government policy on issues affecting health.

Major Australian newspapers

- The Sydney Morning Herald
- The Courier Mail
- The Age
- The West Australian
- The Advertiser

- The Hobart Mercury
- The NT News
- The Canberra Times
- The Australian
- The Land (rural issues)

Unfortunately, many health workers miss out on opportunities to respond to these calls because they assume that they will gain access to any relevant discussion papers through their workplace. In fact, in many instances these discussion papers do not trickle down through the bureaucracy to health workers. Unless you search for them yourself, in the same way as other members of the public do, you may have no opportunity to influence the direction of public policy and health in your State or region, or Australia-wide.

More often than not, calls for public discussion are responded to by more skilled and articulate members of the community, and many other people do not feel

Some examples of calls for public comment

PARLIAMENT OF THE COMMONWEALTH OF AUSTRALIA

HOUSE OF REPRESENTATIVES STANDING COMMITTEE ON FAMILY AND COMMUNITY AFFAIRS

Indigenous Health

In view of the unacceptably high morbidity and mortality of Aboriginal and Torres Strait Islander people, the Committee has been requested by the Minister for Health and Family Services, with the support of the Minister for Aboriginal and Torres Strait Islander Affairs to inquire into and report on the following matters:

a) ways to achieve effective Commonwealth coordination of the provision of health and related programs to Aboriginal and Torres Strait Islander communities, with particular emphasis on the regulation, planning and delivery of such services;

b) barriers to access to mainstream health services, to explore avenues to improve the capacity and quality of mainstream health service delivery to Aboriginal and Torres Strait Islander people and the development of linkages between Aboriginal and Torres Strait Islander and mainstream services.

c) the need for improved education of medical practitioners, specialists, nurses and health workers, with respect to the health status of Aboriginal and Torres Strait Islander people and its implications for care:

d) the extent to which social and cultural factors and location, influence health, especially maternal and child health, diet, alcohol and tobacco consumption;

e) the extent to which Aboriginal and Torres Strait Islander health status is affected by educational and employment opportunities, access to transport services and proximity to other community supports, particularly in rural and remote communities; and

f) the extent to which past structures for delivery of health care services have contributed to the poor health status of Aboriginal and Torres Strait Islander people.

The Committee Chairman, Mr Peter Slipper, MP, Member for Fisher, invites interested individuals and organisations to make written submissions to the inquiry. An invitation to appear before the Committee at public hearings may be issued on the basis of submissions received.

Further information can be obtained from the Committee Secretary, Mr Bjarne Nordin, on (06) 277 4565. Written submissions should be addressed to:

The Secretary
House of Representatives Standing Committee
on Family and Community Affairs
Parliament House
CANBERRA ACT 2600

Telephone: (06) 277 4566

The closing date for submissions is 1 October 1997.

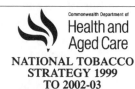

Commonwealth Department of
Health and Aged Care

NATIONAL TOBACCO STRATEGY 1999 TO 2002-03

Release of the draft Strategy document for public comment

The Ministerial Council on Drug Strategy at its November 1998 meeting endorsed the release of the draft National Tobacco Strategy 1999 to 2002-03 for public consultation.

The draft Strategy builds on current national activity in tobacco control and sets strategic directions for future action. Development of the Strategy represents a partnership between the Commonwealth Government, the National Expert Advisory Group on Tobacco, State and Territory governments, the non-government sector and the broader community.

Public comment is invited on this draft Strategy document. These comments, together with invited comment from key stakeholders in tobacco control, will be used to finalise a document that will direct Australia's policy on tobacco and health into the 21st century.

Copies of the draft Strategy accompanied by a background paper and summary document will be available for **PUBLIC COMMENT** from **Monday, 1 March 1999** and may be ordered by:

Fax: (02) 6289 8360
Email: phd.publications@health.gov.au
Phone: **1800 020 103 – ask for extension 8654**

Copies of the documents are also available on the Department of Health and Aged Care web site at: *http://www/pubhlth/strateg/drugs/tobacco/index.htm*

Submissions on the draft Strategy document should be made in writing or on audio tape and sent to:

Tobacco and Alcohol Strategies Section
MDP 103
GPO Box 9848
CANBERRA ACT 2601

Submissions should be received by **Friday, 19 March 1999**. Late submissions cannot be considered.

confident about writing to government departments with their opinion. Regrettably, this may mean that the final reports of government do not accurately reflect a broad range of public opinion, and so it is vital that as many people as possible put forward their views. It is most worthwhile to respond to these calls for submissions, and to encourage as many people as possible around you to do so.

It may be a good idea to arrange for a group of people to get together to discuss these draft documents, and perhaps to put together a group response. This can be very useful if you think the people who may be affected by the proposal are unlikely to respond individually because they do not have enough time, confidence or skills.

Responding to parliamentary inquiries

In situations where a government may need to explore an issue in some depth, a parliamentary committee may be established, to investigate the issue and make recommendations to Parliament. When a parliamentary committee conducts an inquiry, submissions are called for in the press and all members of the public are invited to respond.

Some of the people who make submissions are then invited to appear at a public hearing to answer questions. These hearings are usually open to the public, although it is possible to request to speak to the committee in private if necessary.

Some examples of calls for public comment

Suicide Prevention Task Force
Call for Submissions

The Premier, the Hon. Jeff Kennett and the Minister for Health, the Hon. Rob Knowles h the Suicide Prevention Task Force under the chairmanship of Mr Peter Kirby. The Task conduct an intensive public investigation into the nature and extent of suicide, particul and ways of preventing suicide.

The Task Force will receive individual, community and expert submissions up to 17 Ma will announce a schedule of public consultation meetings commencing 3 March 1997.

The Task Force has been asked to inquire into and, where applicable, make recommer Government on:
1. The nature and extent of suicide, particularly youth suicide, in Victoria and its impa and community in general.
2. The identification of risk factors that contribute to suicide.
3. Strategies to prevent and minimise the incidence of suicide, including the role of th
4. Strategies to enhance the overall capacity of the service system to better meet the who are at risk of suicide.
5. Examples of best practice, locally and internationally, regarding service provision.

The Task Force will also make comment on specific issues as they relate to older Victo rural Victoria.

Individuals or organisations interested in contributing to this important investigation sh submission by 17 March 1997 to:

Executive Officer
Suicide Prevention Task Force Secretariat
Level 1, 555 Collins Street
Melbourne Vic 3000
Telephone: (03) 9616 8310   Fax: (03) 9616 8631

Submissions may be presented in community languages.

🏹ictoria *ON THE MOVE*

LEGAL AID AND FAMILY SERVICES

FAMILY RELATIONSHIPS
SERVICES PROGRAM
Attorney–General's Departmen

FUNDING FOR INNOVATIVE SERVICES TO SUPPORT MEN IN THEIR FAMILY RELATIONSHIPS

The Commonwealth Government, through th Family Relationships Services Program, contrac community-based organisations to help familie achieve and maintain functional relationships ar resolve disputes without the need to resort to th egal system for solutions.

n November 1997 the Prime Minister announce he availability of $6 million over four year or innovative pilot services targeted to better mec he needs of men in their family relationships. Th pilots will aim to achieve more effective outcome or men and their families seeking assistance wit building and maintaining healthy relationship including appropriately managing separation. Th nitiative is part of the Government's "Partnership Against Domestic Violence" strategy.

Applications are sought from community-base not for profit organisations to provide innovativ and effective services which support men i heir relationships with their partner: ex-partners, children, step-children and extende amily members.

To obtain an application package please fa 02) 6250 5962, giving contact name, organisatio address, telephone and fax number. Applicatio packages will be forwarded by mail.

Applications must be postmarked no later tha Friday, 17 July 1998.

Men and Family Relationships Initiative
Family Services Branch
Legal Aid and Family Services
Attorney-General's Department
National Circuit
Barton ACT 2600

Using the mass media

As a key influence in placing issues on the policy agenda, the mass media are powerful tools to use in working for healthy public policy. Using the media in this way is known as media advocacy, which was discussed in Chapter 5. Letters to the editor and media releases can put forward an alternative view and help to reshape the public perception of an issue. In addition, they can widen discussion on draft documents open for public discussion by making other people aware of the documents and their implications.

There is widespread acknowledgment that politicians rely on the mass media for most of their information about public issues, so the value of using the mass media to lobby for change should not be underestimated.

Ensuring community representation on committees

If public committees are to conduct work that reflects a broad view of community opinions, community members or consumers need to be adequately represented on them and have adequate decision-making power. Health workers have an important role to play in lobbying for community representation on, and effective participation in, committees whose work impacts on the life of the community. Working to achieve these two goals is an important way in which you can ensure that the work of these committees remains in touch with community perspectives.

Some people may wonder why community representatives are necessary if health workers are committed to presenting a community perspective. However, there will be times when the perspective of community members may clash with that of health workers, and health workers should not assume that they are always able to represent the community perspective in an unbiased way when representing their professional interests (Consumers' Health Forum 1999, p. 3). Furthermore, accepting community members as partners with health workers means according them partnership status, not simply speaking on their behalf.

However, health workers should take seriously their responsibility to respect and represent the community perspective as much as possible. Even in situations in which community representatives are present, health workers can add support by adding their voice to those presenting the perspective of community members.

Representing consumer interests, whether as the community representative or as a health worker concerned to represent the consumer perspective, is not always a comfortable position to be in. The perspective of community members can be threatening to many professionals if they believe that it is their job to make decisions on behalf of the community and that they know what is best. This is especially so if the consumers or community members do not agree with these professionals' opinions. Recognising that the community perspective may challenge professionals on the committees may help those representing it to deal with any negative feedback they receive from committee members. Supporting members of the community in this position, or finding support for yourself if you are in this position, is vital if the community perspective is to be maintained on the committee for a length of time that enables things to be achieved.

Consumers' Health Forum of Australia

The Consumers' Health Forum is a national peak organisation representing consumers on national health care issues. It provides a balance to the views of government, manufacturers, service providers and other health professionals.

The Consumers' Health Forum aims:
* to contribute towards the improvement of people's health and wellbeing by:
  — ensuring accessibility to the health system and high quality outcomes;
  — improving information available to consumers;
  — addressing inequities in outcomes;
  — strengthening the ability of consumers to participate in, and strategically influence, health policy, planning and service delivery;
* to represent the views and interests of health consumers at a national level by:
  — strengthening relationships with consumer organisations;
  — building strategic alliances;
  — providing advice to the government.

The Consumers' Health Forum establishes policy in consultation with its membership and other consumers. Over the last several years, it has been active in developing consumer oriented policy in many areas including health financing, chronic pain management, mental health policy, rational prescribing of medicines and consumer rights.

In addition to its policy work, Consumers' Health Forum provides an effective mechanism for disseminating information to the community by publishing a journal three times a year, *Australian Health Consumer*.

The Consumers' Health Forum nominates and supports consumer representatives on national government, industry and provider group committees. These representatives put the consumers' perspective.

Consumers' Health Forum activities and policy are coordinated by the governing Committee, which is its governing body. It is elected every 2 years.

The information and resources of the Forum are available directly to consumer groups and individual consumers who wish to avail themselves of this service.

The Consumers' Health Forum has a secretariat based in Canberra and receives funding for its core activities from the Commonwealth Department of Health and Aged Care Services. It has also been successful in attracting funds for specific projects.

For further information on any of the Consumers' Health Forum's activities, please contact:

> Consumers' Health Forum
> PO Box 52
> Lyons ACT 2606
> Tel: (02) 6281 0811; Fax: (02) 6281 0959
> email: info@chf.org.au
> Web site: www.chf.org.au

Tobacco sponsorship replacement at the local level — a success story

In November 1991 the New South Wales State Parliament enacted the Tobacco Prohibition Act, which prohibited community groups from obtaining sponsorship from tobacco companies without specific government approval.

In January 1992 the Mid North Coast Art Society suffered what it saw as a grave financial blow when the Rothmans Foundation withdrew its sponsorship of the society's annual art show. Extensive media coverage, both electronic and print, carried numerous stories of the adverse effects of the Tobacco Prohibition Act on such community events as this. This publicity, we observed, created a backlash against the legislation, and with the loss of their long-term sponsor, small community organisations were left feeling helpless and unsure of which direction to take in fund-raising.

In 1990 the Manning Great Lakes Health Service, in rural New South Wales, had in place a 5-year plan for health promotion in their Health For All program. This plan evolved from the Health for All initiatives of the World Health Organization and the consequent Australian and New South Wales programs. Two major components of this program were the Country Heart-Throb program and the Smoke Free program. The community health centre staff acting as facilitators of these programs proposed to the health service management that, as a one-off demonstration, staff would work to raise money to replace the tobacco sponsorship. The intention of this was to demonstrate to the community that community activities and events could survive and prosper with the new legislation.

Reorienting the health system

As this was a new approach to health promotion, in that fund-raising is not a normal health promotion activity, a proposal was presented to the health service management. It responded enthusiastically and with full support, and a number of guidelines were set:

- all monies raised would be collected by the health service. Donations would be receipted to it and amounts over $2 would be tax deductible;
- the final aggregated donation would be paid to the Mid North Coast Art Society with the following requests:
  - that the Country Heart-Throb and Smoke Free programs be presented on a health promotion display at the art show;
  - that a sponsor board be provided for those donors who wished to be recognised;
  - that publicity by the Art Society acknowledge the health service, in particular its Country Heart-Throb and Smoke Free programs.

When contacted, the president of the art society was sceptical about the ability of the health service to raise sufficient funds to replace tobacco sponsorship.

The announcement that the health service was to take up this challenge received wide media coverage. To facilitate media interest, a direct approach was made to the editor of the local newspaper and to journalists on commercial and ABC radio stations. The local television station was also contacted. As a result, all activities and events received wide media coverage and support, which ensured that the whole issue remained firmly in the community's awareness.

Community involvement

As a result of the media interest, a number of direct donations were quickly made to the fund by members of the public and health service personnel who felt strongly about this issue. These included a donation by a 74-year-old pensioner who had recently stopped smoking after 50 years (this was used to good effect in a press release). It soon became apparent, however, that a more aggressive approach to fund-raising was needed.

As the purpose of the project was to demonstrate to the community that events could be funded by sources other than tobacco sponsorship, it was decided to organise events that involved participation by a wide cross-section of the community. This provided opportunities for health education. The events included:

• a healthy barbecue for health service staff;
• raffling of a T-shirt donated by renowned Australian artist Ken Done;
• a poster design competition in schools;
• a healthy fund-raising breakfast;
• raffling of an original Australian landscape by a local artist.

It is important to emphasise that these activities had more benefits than just fund-raising. Although we maintained the principle of replacement of tobacco sponsorship in fund-raising, a health promotion theme was emphasised during all activities. The first activity was a healthy barbecue for health service staff during their lunch period. As there are a large number of smokers among the staff, the opportunity was taken to highlight the benefits of going smoke free. The barbecue was well attended by both smokers and non-smokers. The Ken Done T-shirt raffle proved popular.

The Manning Base Hospital had already developed its canteen into a public restaurant, called Stitches, which is oriented towards healthy food. A healthy breakfast was offered at Stitches and the general community was invited. To maintain the relationship between fund-raising and art, a local artist and art teacher, Ron Hindmarsh, was the guest speaker. During his talk he began work on an Australian landscape painting, which was then available for us to raffle.

Raising health awareness

Continuing with the art theme, a poster design competition was held throughout the local schools. Children from kindergarten to Year 6 were invited to paint or draw their views on tobacco use and smoking. Teachers were encouraged to include a session on smoking in their health studies. Prizes, in the form of Hot Tuna surfwear and K Mart educational material, made competition keen. The best posters were displayed in the local shopping mall during World No Tobacco Day. This attracted much attention from both school children and adults. Prizes were presented to the winners during school assemblies, which again reinforced the non-smoking message to school-age children. Every entrant in the competition received a certificate of merit.

Each fund-raising event received broad media coverage in which the reason for the fund-raising was emphasised. In addition, as a direct result of its involvement with us, the Art Society lobbied the local council to make the hall they meet in smoke free.

Conclusions

The tobacco sponsorship replacement program was an example of how an adverse event can be turned to advantage and used to create a series of opportunities for health promotion. It has also opened the way for further health promotion activities. Despite criticism by some health professionals that fund-raising is not an accepted health activity, we believe that the principle and the activities clearly demonstrated to previous recipients of tobacco sponsorship that they were not reliant on tobacco sponsorship, and achieved wide-reaching positive results.

The school poster design competition opened up the subject of smoking in the schools and provided a forum for education on tobacco use. Presenting the popular prizes at the school assemblies had beneficial effects. Children whose teachers had not involved them in the competition demanded to know why, and most schools requested that we run the competition annually.

We raised $380 more than our target figure of $1000 and the excess funds were given to the Great Lakes Art Society, which had also lost its tobacco sponsorship. This generated further publicity and extended the benefits of the program to another community. The extensive media coverage throughout the fund-raising ensured that the community was kept constantly aware of the fact that there is art, and sport, and life after tobacco sponsorship.

The art show, which was on for a week, attracted 3000 people. A non-smoking health promotion display and material featured prominently. There was only one thing missing on the opening night — the tobacco company's logo!

After the support provided by the health service in 1992, the Art Society continued to manage very well without tobacco sponsorship. With a strong commitment to a smoke-free environment in the local area, the Arts Show was sponsored first by a local nurse for 2 years, then by a local doctor. This sponsorship has remained until the time of writing, and the Art Society premises continue to be smoke free. A potentially negative community response to tobacco control legislation has been permanently turned into a health-promoting cultural event.

Trish Abbott
(previously) Generalist community nurse, and
Facilitator, Country Heart-Throb program,
Taree Community Health Centre

Bob Berry
(previously) Clinical Nurse Consultant,
Alcohol and Other Drugs Service, and
Facilitator, Smoke Free program,
Taree Community Health Centre

The Consumers' Health Forum has produced a very useful booklet, *Guidelines for Consumer Representatives: Suggestions for Consumer or Community Representatives Working on Committees* (1999), which addresses many issues relevant to community members becoming involved with committees. It is worthwhile ensuring that agencies you work with keep a copy of this booklet and make it available to any community members or budding community representatives, so as to help them increase their effectiveness on committees.

The role of local government in health promotion

Although public policy developed at the State and national levels has a great influence on the way our daily lives are structured, a remarkably large number of policy decisions that shape our environment are taken at the local level, particularly through local government. Responsibility for such issues as land use, placement of industry, housing standards, availability of recreational areas and location of shopping areas is all exercised at the local level. Local government, therefore, is quite a powerful influence on our environments, and the impact of public policy at the local level can be profound. In recognition of this, the 1992 National Review of the Role of Primary Health Care in Health Promotion recommended strengthening the role of local government in health promotion.

Developing healthy public policy at the local level may not be without its challenges. Zabolai-Csekme (1983, p. 3) points out that Primary Health Care may challenge the concept of development quite fundamentally because its focus is on the health of people and the environment. Most local councils operate from a philosophy of development, which usually means expansion of industry and population. These are not necessarily conducive to health, yet they are assumed to be good for the community. Recent acknowledgement of the concept of sustainable development may help to break down this assumption. However, it is unlikely that local councils will embrace the principles of Primary Health Care without considerable encouragement, both from community demand and from legislation at State and federal government levels, because the expansion of industry and population is highly regarded by society generally. Until it is quite clear that other approaches are acceptable, councils may feel compelled to remain with this approach. This may mean that community members have considerable work to do in lobbying local councils to take their concerns about healthy public policy seriously.

Some local Councils, however, are working for healthier communities. The Australian Local Government Association is committed to the idea of the Primary Health Care approach, and several Councils have been engaged in innovative health promotion projects, developed in partnership with the health and other sectors (Smith 1997).

The principles of working to influence local government are much the same as those of working to influence public policy at State and federal levels. How they are put into practice, however, varies slightly and, because local Councils are one step closer to the ground, people often find it easier to involve themselves in working at the local level for change. The issues at stake here arise more often just down the street or in their own backyard and the decisions are taken in a building with which most people are familiar. Because of this, local government does not have quite the same mystique as politics at the State and federal levels, and people may more readily act for change.

As in the case of work for public policy change at State and federal levels, people can work through the media, writing letters to the editor and bringing issues to the attention of local television, radio and newspaper reporters. You can also lobby local councillors, who may feel very committed to representing local councillors seem most open to hearing your views and most concerned about the issues you raise, develop a relationship with them and keep them up to date on the issues you are concerned about to enable them to make more informed decisions when issues come up without notice. They may contact you for information if they recognise you as a trustworthy source of information on issues that impact on health.

Local government is usually dominated by people representative of business and professional groups in an area. Many community groups have put forward candidates to represent the community perspective in local government. You might work to support one of these candidates or you might consider standing for the Local Council yourself and working for change from the inside.

One excellent example of a community health centre working for healthy public policy at the local level is provided by the 'Vote For Health' campaign conducted by the Parks Community Health Service in South Australia. The campaign encouraged people to vote in the local government elections by providing information about how to vote and discussing the central role of local government decisions in promoting the health of the community. The campaign also elicited information from all local government candidates about their attitudes to health issues, and this information was published to provide a basis on which people could make their voting decisions. This information also provided a basis against which local government councillors could be accountable (Phillips-Rees et al. 1992, pp. 54–5).

Health promoting settings

As the discussion in the previous section demonstrates, the idea of implementing the *Ottawa Charter for Health Promotion,* with its focus on healthy public policy, at a societal level is certainly important. At the same time, though, the focus on such a broad target for change is often beyond the scope of most health workers. In addition, society is made up of many smaller institutions, and it is within the context of these settings that people are exposed to healthy or unhealthy environments.

Policies operating at the institutional level can have a big impact on people's lives. The policies of institutions, such as workplaces, schools and hospitals, influence people's lives as they come in contact with these institutions and often influence the lives of community members even when they are not in direct contact with the institution. For example, work-related exposure to hazardous substances results in a great many workers becoming sick or dying (Tesh 1981, p. 382). Moreover, workers who take toxic substances home on their work clothes affect not only their own lives beyond the workplace, but also those of their partners and children, as they too are exposed to the chemicals. It is vital, therefore, to work for healthy institutional policy, in addition to healthy public policy.

A word of warning, however. Working for healthy institutional policy, while valuable, cannot replace working for healthy public policy. In the light of recent attempts by some Australian State health departments to limit the work done in an 'Ottawa Charter' approach to health promotion to work traditionally carried out by health workers, there is a tendency to try to limit public policy work to work for policy change within organisations, rather than addressing broad public policy issues. Health workers need to ensure that they work for public policy change on issues that impact on health at the same time as they work for institutional policy change. Otherwise, we may end up with a sanitised version of health promotion, which may ignore the hard issues that have the biggest impact on people's health and address issues only at the level of the individual or institution.

The ways in which you can work for healthy institutional policy will vary depending on the institution, the ways in which it relates to the public and your relationship with it. Working for change within an organisation for which you work will require you to follow the organisation's normal lines of communication. However, working to change an organisation that sees itself as responsible to the public may require you to follow lines of communication similar to those for working towards change to healthy public policy; that is, in dealing with such an organisation, you can write to its Chief Executive or any people in key positions relevant to the particular issue. Remember that you may need to keep at it and that, if requests for change come from more than one person, they are more likely to be successful. In the case of public services, if you do not have any success you can take your suggestions to others who have influence over the organisation, such as a government minister.

In their search for ways in which to implement the principles and strategies of the *Ottawa Charter for Health Promotion* at a local level, the WHO began exploring opportunities to work for health promotion in particular settings. This process began with the development of the Healthy Cities concept. Other additional settings approaches, such as health promoting hospitals, health promoting schools and health promoting workplaces have since been developed. There is considerable scope to develop this model further, with health promoting prisons, health promoting nursing homes and health promoting universities — just three other settings in which the model is currently being explored.

Health promotion has been identified as including three interrelated processes of personal development, organisational development and political development towards health (Kickbusch 1994, p. 5). Health promoting settings provide an opportunity to strengthen the role of organisational development as a health promotion strategy, while also maintaining the focus on individual and political development.

The aim of the settings approach to health promotion is to do much more than implement health promotion activities within a particular organisation. Rather, its aim is, through organisational development, to create true health promoting settings (Baric 1994, p. 36). To achieve this goal of settings that promote health, at least three approaches are needed:

- *creation of a healthy working and living environment for the participants in that setting;*

- *integration of health promotion into the daily activities of that setting;*

- *creation of conditions for the setting to reach out into the community (social and physical environment) and by means of networking and healthy alliances promote the spread of this concept to other settings.*

(Baric 1994, p. 36.)

Health promoting settings are equally as concerned about the health of people who work within a setting as with those who live, learn or receive care there. It is for this reason that changes that result from health promotion action are developed with employees, not imposed on them, and that organisational development processes are so important to the health promoting settings approaches. The importance of the settings approach to health promotion was reemphasised in the *Jakarta Declaration on Leading Health Promotion into the 21st Century* (see Appendix 3, p. 273).

Healthy Cities

The first area in which the health promoting settings approach was explored was the area of 'Healthy Cities'. The Healthy Cities project is an attempt to establish healthier living conditions in cities through the development of widespread healthy public policy, supported by a broad range of private and public sectors. Developed originally for European cities by the WHO, it was adapted to suit Australian conditions. Following a year-long pilot project in three areas (Illawarra in New South Wales, Canberra in the Australian Capital Territory and Noarlunga in South Australia), it was evaluated quite positively. Other cities or local council areas were then invited to join the Healthy Cities Australia network. The concept has been expanded in recent years to include 'Healthy Communities' and, in the Pacific, 'Healthy Islands'.

When the concept of a health promoting setting was first explored with Healthy Cities, one of the main issues it was attempting to address was how to establish effective intersectoral collaboration at the local level. It was hoped that working in the context of a particular city and its problems would enable practitioners from a variety of sectors to come together for the purposes of solving the particular problems at hand. This aspect of health promoting settings as a rallying point for intersectoral collaboration is a real strength of the settings approach.

Focusing on intersectoral action, the Healthy Cities project espouses the value of the community development process. Many examples of Australian action under the Healthy Cities project are available (see, e.g. Rees 1992; Clarke & MacDougall 1993; Australian Community Health Association 1990a, 1990b; and Healthy Cities Australia 1990). However, the extent to which different cities are using a 'working with communities' approach varies greatly. Some are working to develop a strong community participation base with a focus on community decision making, while others are more directive and have major decisions made by professionals. For example, Short (1990) has described the way in which professionals are more 'on top' than 'on tap' in the Illawarra Healthy Cities project.

Regrettably, the Federal Government decided against refunding the Healthy Cities project at a national level when funding for the project ran dry in June 1992. This decision was taken before the evaluation of Healthy Cities was completed. It decided instead to 'target fewer and more specific areas of strategic importance' (Department of Health, Housing and Community Services, cited by Lennie 1992). Unfortunately, this hardly explains the removal of funding from the program. Loss of national funding for Healthy Cities is a great shame, since it is one of the few health promotion activities that could have been funded to enable Australia to take a broad structural approach to health. The National Review of the Role of Primary Health Care in Health Promotion has recommended the continued funding of the Healthy Cities project in Australia (National Centre for Epidemiology and Population Health 1992). In the meantime, many of the cities and localities already involved in the Healthy Cities movement will continue with the processes set in train. However, without ongoing support and network building, its future impact as a national program is unclear. However, some local-level work is continuing. Queensland, in particular, appears to have an ongoing commitment to the concept through its Healthy Cities and Shires project (Chapman & Davey 1997). The concept of Healthy Cities continues to have considerable potential in the Australian context.

Health promoting hospitals

By far the largest amount of health promotion work conducted by the health system in Australia is done within the community health sector, a sector that receives, with public health, just 4.4% of the health budget. Clearly, greater funding for that sector is an important part of effectively implementing Primary Health Care. However, if we are to effectively reorient the current health system towards a greater emphasis on Primary Health Care and health promotion, we need to do more than shift the spending priorities within the health system. Primary Health Care and health promotion cannot work effectively if they are established in opposition to the hospital-based system. The hospital system itself needs to become an integral part of the Primary Health Care system, working in direct response to community needs and promoting the health of the community as a whole. This will require hospitals to work much more closely with community health centres, Aboriginal Medical Services and medical practices and on many more activities than discharge planning. This is clearly quite a different approach from the one currently prevailing in most hospitals, although there are some important exceptions, particularly in some rural areas of Australia. We need to ensure that we maximise the role of health promotion within the present health system by increasing the role that hospitals play in health promotion, and increasing their commitment to the Primary Health Care philosophy. This approach has been urged by WHO (WHO 1987; Ebrahim & Ranken 1988, p. 85).

Hospitals clearly present several major opportunities for health promotion. Firstly, they come into contact with a large number of people who are sick and those close to them. Secondly, they are one of the largest public sector employers in the country and so have a large workforce whose skills are a major resource. Thirdly, they utilise some potentially dangerous and environmentally damaging methods and practices. Fourthly, they are effectively 'total institutions' and have their own often peculiar and pervasive culture, particularly in the area of human relationships. And finally, they draw to them a large proportion of the health dollar.

It is a major challenge for hospitals to adopt the health promoting settings approach in a meaningful way, rather than merely 'add on' health promotion activities. The extent to which they can do this will depend on the barriers that exist in each hospital and the level of commitment that health workers and health administrators have towards this reorientation. What can be achieved in large teaching hospitals, for example, may differ greatly from what can be achieved by smaller rural hospitals who may already have close contacts with their community. However, many hospitals are now experimenting with the health promoting hospitals concept and many are moving beyond 'health promotion in a setting' to a true health promoting settings approach.

The Vienna Recommendations on Health Promoting Hospitals

Fundamental principles

Within the framework of the health for all strategy, the Ottawa Charter for Health Promotion, the Ljubljana Charter for Reforming Health Care and the Budapest Declaration on Health Promoting Hospitals, a health promoting hospital should:

- promote human dignity, equity and solidarity, and professional ethics, acknowledging differences in the needs, values and cultures of different population groups;
- be oriented towards quality improvement, the wellbeing of patients, relatives and staff, protection of the environment and realization of the potential to become learning organizations;
- focus on health with a holistic approach and not only on curative services;
- be centred on people providing health services in the best way possible to patients and their relatives, to facilitate the healing process and contribute to the empowerment of patients;
- use resources efficiently and cost-effectively, and allocate resources on the basis of contribution to health improvement; and
- form as close links as possible with other levels of the health care system and the community.

Strategies for Implementation

The HPH project provides opportunities throughout the hospital to develop health-oriented perspectives, objectives and structures. This means in particular:

Fostering participation and creating commitment by:

- encouraging participatory, health-gain-oriented procedures throughout the hospital, including the active involvement of all professional groups and building alliances with other professionals outside the hospital;
- encouraging an active and participatory role for patients according to their specific health potential, fostering patients' rights, improving patients' wellbeing and creating health promoting hospital environments for patients and relatives;
- creating healthy working conditions for all hospital staff, including the reduction of hospital hazards, as well as psychosocial risk factors;
- enhancing the commitment of hospital management to health gain, including the principles of health in the daily decision-making processes;

Improving communication, information and education by:

- improving communication within and the culture of the hospital so that they contribute to the quality of life for hospital staff (communication styles used by hospital staff should encourage interprofessional cooperation and mutual acceptance);
- improving the communication between the hospital staff and the patients so that it is guided by respect and humane values;
- enhancing the provision and quality of information, communication and educational programmes and skill training for patients and their relatives;
- integrating the principles of the health promoting hospital into the hospital's routine through developing a common corporate identity within the hospital;
- improving the hospital's communication and cooperation with social and health services in the community, community-based health promotion initiatives and volunteer groups and organizations, and thus helping to optimize the links between different providers and actors in the health care sector;
- developing information systems that measure outcomes as well as serving administrative purposes;

Using methods and techniques from organizational development and project management:

- to change and reorient existing hospital routines to make the hospital a learning organization;
- to train and educate personnel in areas relevant for health promotion, such as education, communication, psychosocial skills and management;
- to train project leaders in project management and communication skills;

> **Learning from experience:**
> - exchange of experience with implementing health promoting hospitals projects at the national and international level should be promoted so that participating hospitals can learn from different approaches to problem solving;
> - health promoting hospitals should commit themselves to regional, national and international exchange and communication.

In 1991, the WHO established the International Network of Health Promoting Hospitals and, in the *Budapest Declaration of Health Promoting Hospitals,* set down the minimum requirements of a health promoting hospital. Regular international Health Promoting Hospitals conferences have been held, and there is a growing wealth of experience in the area. As a result of these developments, the Vienna Recommendations on Health Promoting Hospitals were produced in 1997. These provide a more comprehensive set of principles and strategies towards which hospitals should aspire (see opposite).

Needless to say, though, many challenges remain and, as pressure increases on hospitals to contain their costs or become more profitable, there is the danger that longer term approaches reflected in health promoting hospitals will be neglected as they focus on addressing immediate and short-term problems.

One important development that has been occurring parallel with health promoting hospitals and is very complementary to it, is the development of more environmentally friendly hospitals. There have been some major success stories of hospitals reducing their waste, not just by recycling but also by reducing unnecessary use of disposable items. This has required major changes in practice, including reductions in the number of paper towels and dressing packs used, recycling of suction tubing and a return to non-disposables to give just some examples. It has also involved a major reduction in chemical use within hospitals.

At a 1993 conference on health and ecology, hospitals from around Australia described how they had made substantial reductions in their waste and chemical use, and the cost savings that have stemmed from these. These initiatives have been strongly supported by staff of the hospitals, with action driven by enthusiastic multidisciplinary committees (Newman 1993). There are three important points to be made here. Firstly, this kind of change cannot be imposed upon people. Secondly, there is a ground swell of health workers keen to change their practice to reduce their impact on the environment. Thirdly, many of the barriers to changing practice that have been described as infection control are not insurmountable, and often have more to do with ritual than infection control (McPherson 1993).

Hospital-based health workers do not have to wait for major policy changes within hospitals to occur before increasing their individual health promotion action. In particular, they can lobby their employing organisations to take a greater role in health promotion. They can also choose to increase their commitment to health education in the hospital setting; they can use their rights as community members to write to their Members of Parliament and lobby for changes to unhealthy public policy; and they can join community groups and work for a healthier community. Such actions recognise that health workers are part of their community

From health promotion in a hospital to developing a health-promoting hospital — the experience of Flinders Medical Centre

Flinders Medical Centre, a 440-bed teaching hospital in the southern metropolitan region of Adelaide, was the first Australian hospital to become an affiliated member of the World Health Organization (European region) Health Promoting Hospitals network. The process of achieving international recognition in health promotion can be traced back to 1984 when Flinders Medical Centre became the first hospital in the country to establish a Health Information Centre. From humble beginnings, the Health Information Centre eventually became a Health Promotion Unit, employing five staff members.

In its early years, the Health Promotion Unit focused on the provision of health education and lifestyle information through counselling, group programs and participation in statewide health promotion campaigns. The quality displays and pamphlets developed by the Health Promotion Unit gained recognition throughout South Australia. Staff initiated the first 'smoke-free' policy for an Australian hospital and supported the development of a hospital food policy. Although the Health Promotion Unit had undertaken policy initiatives, the role and function of the Unit was primarily that of providing health promotion in a hospital, rather than that of developing the hospital as a health-promoting setting.

As practitioners around the world gained experience in implementing health promotion as laid down in the *Ottawa Charter for Health Promotion* (1986), a broader range of strategies and actions were recommended for health protection, maintenance and improvement. In addition, the *Budapest Declaration on Health Promoting Hospitals* (1991) established a set of aims, based on the Ottawa Charter, to reorient hospitals towards health and challenged them to become more than centres of quality health treatment and care. Organisational development strategies were required to incorporate concepts, values and standards of health promotion into the structure and organisational culture of the hospital. The Budapest Declaration aimed to enable health promotion to become an integral part of the hospital system.

Following several years of successfully providing health promotion, and breaking down negative attitudes towards health promotion in the hospital culture, the Health Promotion Unit underwent a change in management in 1994. In line with international developments, the Unit embarked on a process of change to build the organisational capacity of the hospital to promote health. This process began by building capacity among staff in the Health Promotion Unit to enable them to reconceptualise their roles as change agents, adopting Primary Health Care principles and approaches to health promotion. Staff seized opportunities to demonstrate this changed approach and began to advocate for access and equity issues and to work for system change. Examples of this include addressing previously ignored multicultural and indigenous health issues. The success of addressing these issues with multi-strategy processes is evident. Statistics reveal a significant increase in the hospital's use of interpreters. An Aboriginal Health Unit has been established with an indigenous manager and staff working in both primary prevention and in developing the organisation to provide a more culturally supportive environment.

Organisational development requires support from senior management. Flinders Medical Centre has this support and leadership. This has resulted in health advancement being reflected throughout the hospital's strategic plan (1998) and in its mission, which states that 'Flinders Medical Centre is an international leader in integrated patient care, teaching, research and health promotion' (FMC Mission statement, 1996).

This has given legitimacy and recognition to health promotion, and has enabled staff of the Unit to take the organisational development approach further. For example, a Health Enhancement Research Grant enabled collaborative processes to be modelled in establishing cardiac rehabilitation in community rather than hospital settings. Participants in the study became co-researchers who found that the impact of social isolation and anxiety contributed to readmission to hospital. A self-help group providing social support and exercise at appropriate intensity reduced hospital readmission for people in the study. This project became a catalyst for a further project involving three hospitals and community health services, who developed a comprehensive plan for more coordinated cardiac rehabilitation in the region. The collaborative process modelled by Health Promotion staff and the comprehensive plan produced attracted considerable attention and respect from senior administrators and medical specialists.

The three key elements of a health-promoting setting identified by Baric (1994 — see p. 185) have been used to structure the work of the Unit, and are evident in the following examples:
- integrating health promotion into all activities of the setting:
  - developing capacity among ward staff to be health promoting in their practice to create health promoting wards;
  - enabling staff to improve the quality of written health information;
  - ensuring that people from non-English-speaking backgrounds are offered interpreters and treated in culturally appropriate ways. This is supported by a Language Services Policy and Multicultural Health Plan;
- creating a healthy environment for staff and consumers:
  - recognising the impact of the physical environment of the hospital on health; for example, by enhancing healing through participatory Arts in Health projects developed initially by Health Promotion staff;
- Creating alliances with other settings, consumers and the community:
  - inviting hospitalised people to become co-researchers in a project aimed at meeting consumers' needs in developing sustainable cardiac rehabilitation in community settings;
  - improving the health care provided to country people attending city hospitals was begun through a project titled 'Building Bridges for Country–City Health'.

Examples of initiatives undertaken by other staff that demonstrate organisation wide commitment to the development of a health-promoting hospital include:
- reducing the hospital's contribution to environmental degradation through developing comprehensive strategies for energy and waste reduction practices. This project saved the hospital $300 000 in its first year and has won many awards. It has become the benchmark for other hospitals;
- reducing accidents and injuries among staff through developing comprehensive strategies for Occupational Health, Safety and Welfare;
- involving staff groups in identifying and implementing strategies to improve and develop the organisation in a project called 'Making it Better for Patients and Staff';
- participating in the national process of reconciliation between Aboriginal and other Australians through recognition of prior ownership of the land on which the hospital is built. The employment of an Aboriginal Health Team is creating a more supportive environment within the hospital for Aboriginal people and

operating service) addresses many issues, such as organising home care, equipment and resources more appropriately for older people rather than placing them unnecessarily in the hospital system.

Many challenges and barriers were encountered in the process of moving from 'doing' health promotion to becoming a health promoting setting. As work practices moved away from dealing with immediate problems by offering instant solutions, staff felt frustrated by the time required to bring about change in a large and complex hospital. With their focus on organisational change and supporting other frontline staff to implement health promotion in their work practices, Health Promotion staff no longer sold books, took blood pressures or ran stress management groups. As their work became less visible, frustrations were expressed regarding the amount of time spent in processes involving organising and running meetings, communicating and networking. Without immediate outcomes, staff at first felt that they were not really doing their work. There was a need to communicate and justify their new role and function to other hospital colleagues, who had expectations for Health Promotion Unit staff to fulfil earlier roles. Clear communication of the limitations of the previous roles and the health benefits from comprehensive approaches were generally well accepted and the credibility of health promotion was enhanced.

A further difficulty experienced has been that of territorialism. Health Promotion Unit staff were not recognised as having either a legitimate role or expertise in some of the areas in which they were becoming involved in order to advance health and reduce readmissions to hospitals. This was an initial reaction from some staff to the entry of Health Promotion staff into cardiac rehabilitation. However, as discussed above, the outcomes demonstrated and validated the involvement of Health Promotion staff.

Health promotion is no longer a marginalised activity at Flinders Medical Centre but is part of the hospital's core business and strategic plan. Dedicated Health Promotion staff understand their broadened roles as agents of change, developing capacity across the hospital for the system and all stakeholders to move beyond clinical and curative care, towards providing services that aim to enhance and improve the health of the community. Health Promotion staff are continually challenged to look critically at their strategic directions to fine tune the systems and structures to ensure they support health enhancement.

Developing health promoting hospitals represents a considerable challenge, particularly during these times of budget restraint, ageing populations, technological advances and a political climate withdrawing from public sector service provision. Advocating for health, particularly for the disadvantaged, negotiating and mediating between conflicting interests, is perhaps more important than ever, to protect, maintain and improve the health of our communities. By developing into a responsive health promoting setting, Flinders Medical Centre plans to have a central role in this process.

Cynthia Spurr
Manager, Health Promotion Unit
Flinders Medical Centre
Bedford Park, South Australia

and that they have a right and responsibility to protect their health and that of their community.

The health promoting settings approach can be expanded further to be applied to all health care settings, such as health and medical centres. Certainly the AHCSS review process was designed to encourage just that (see pp. 122–124). Fawkes (1997, p. 392) has identified several elements required of any health setting if it is to be health promoting:

- *principles that inform the policies and strategies for health care service delivery, such as equity, empowerment, participation and access;*
- *organisational capacity to implement these principles through activities such as leadership, professional technical and political skills, culture, resources, and networks and partnerships;*
- *programs and services (core business for health care organisations) geared to promoting health; and*
- *facilities whose design, location and function contribute to the health and wellbeing of service users and employees, and the amenity of the local community.*

Health promoting schools

The third major area in which the health promoting settings concept has been well developed is that of health promoting schools. Schools play a central role in the lives of children all around the globe, and their potential as health promoting settings is enormous. Schools have long been the site for much health education, with the development of healthy behaviours during childhood having positive flow-on effects in adulthood (Smith et al. 1992, p. 171).

At the same time, though, school environments have not always made the most of their potential as supportive environments. School health education may be either reinforced or undermined by aspects of the school environment (Smith et al. 1992, p. 171). Also, schools are not always positive experiences for students, and negative experiences within the social environment of the school, such as bullying, may have far-reaching effects.

For these reasons, there has been considerable enthusiasm for the development of schools as health promoting settings, with the WHO supporting and encouraging this development since the mid-1980s.

A health promoting school has been defined as a school:

> ... *which systematically and deliberately sets out to promote and encourage a healthy lifestyle for its students, staff and wider community, by developing school community policies, curriculum, programs, resources and a physical environment which emphasises a shared concern for community health issues.*

> (Dommers et al. 1996, p. 17.)

To achieve this, action needs to involve all three elements of the school as an organisation — the school curriculum, the school environment (or hidden curriculum), and the interaction between school and community (or school outreach) (Nutbeam 1992, p. 152). That is, health promoting schools may begin with better incorporation of health into the school curriculum. However, as they develop the

Working for healthy institutions — the problem of asbestos

It could be assumed that knowing about an environmental health hazard and taking appropriate action to minimise the hazard would go hand in hand. Not so — at least not in the case of one higher education institution.

When the problem of very substantial amounts of friable and powdery asbestos lagging around heating pipes was raised in the institution, there was general nonchalance by the management. Finally, under sustained pressure from a small group of employees, aided by the Workcover Authority, removal of the asbestos was initiated. Then the problems really began.

The initial problem was to get the contractors to carry out the removal in accordance with the Asbestos Removal Code of Practice, and to get the institution's management to enforce the contractor's compliance.

Subsequent problems arose in the institution's own maintenance staff, who, although some of the supervisors had been trained in asbestos work, had what could only be described as a cavalier attitude to asbestos. This attitude was demonstrated by repeated breaches of the Code of Practice for working with asbestos. Many of the maintenance staff seemed to treat the issue of asbestos exposure as insignificant and amusing, despite the wealth of evidence to the contrary. Again the institution's management seemed either unwilling or unable to deal with the situation. Every attempt was made to stifle discussion of the issue and suppress knowledge of the problems.

Change in the institution's attitude to asbestos did not come easily. It took concerted and sustained action to reach even a minimal level of acceptance of the need for safe work practice in relation to asbestos. The change was brought about by appropriate use of union industrial muscle, in conjunction with the provisions of the NSW Occupational Health and Safety Act (1983), although this alone would not have achieved the desired result.

It was necessary for unions to work closely with the site Occupational Health and Safety Committee and the Workcover Authority. It was also necessary to make full and judicious use of the media, both print and electronic. The media made the real difference to the initial campaign. Before media involvement the institution was loathe to take any rectifying action. When the media became involved and the general public became aware of the situation, it was suddenly an acute embarrassment for an institution of higher learning to be shown to have serious defects in environmental safety.

The results of this intensive and multifront campaign were heightened awareness of asbestos hazards in some of the staff and a change in management attitude. The most senior managers began to take the issue of asbestos seriously and this filtered down to most of the supervisors. However, in the end it took a Workcover prosecution to really force the issue.

It would be nice to be able to end this story on a positive note, but it's the old story: winning the battle doesn't necessarily mean winning the war. Breaches of the Asbestos Removal Code of Practice still occur. The institution has to be closely scrutinised and constant vigilance is essential to ensure that safe work practices are maintained.

> The important role of unions in working within institutions and with statutory authorities in promoting health on difficult issues such as that described above cannot be overestimated.
>
> *Jenny McParlane*
> *Senior Lecturer, School of Health*
> *University of New England, Armidale*

settings approach further, leading schools are broadening their focus to include such things as the physical environment of the school and its contribution to the wider community, and the culture and social milieu of the school, including relationships between children and between children and teachers.

To ensure that mental health as well as physical health is high on the agenda of health promoting schools, MindMatters, a National Mental Health in Schools Project, is being developed. Its aim is to develop a whole school approach to promoting mental health, based on the health promoting school model. As a result, it works to create school enivronments that are supportive of individual students and supportive of mental health, by creating positive school culture in which inclusiveness, diversity and participation are encouraged and caring relationships enable the development of resilience in students (Cahill 1999, pp. 2–3.)

MindMatters provides a valuable opportunity to strengthen the mental health components of the health promoting school concept, enabling the development of a positive social environment and positive coping skills, central to the promotion of mental health.

With considerable support at both national and international levels, health promoting schools provide a valuable opportunity to integrate health promotion into a key setting in the lives of children.

Health promoting workplaces

Workplaces illustrate extremely well the importance of establishing healthy institutional policy as the basis of institutional health promotion. In recent years, despite the framework for action provided by the *Ottawa Charter for Health Promotion,* a great deal of the focus of workplace health promotion has remained on individual behaviour change for healthy lifestyles. Workplace health promotion must accord priority to the issues that arise in the workplace, particularly those that require changes to policy. Within workplaces, this may need to be done in close partnership with occupational health and safety workers and with unions.

Conclusion

This chapter has reviewed some of the ways in which we can work for healthier communities. It is in this area more than in any other area of health promotion that change and development are occurring, as practitioners develop more innovative ways to work for communities. It is in working for communities that we are most working to change the environment, rather than the individual.

Doing this in a manner that enhances rather than constrains people's choices is perhaps the biggest challenge facing health workers in this area of health promotion. You are encouraged to keep developing your skills in this area and to keep critically evaluating your practice, so that your ability to work for communities continues to be enhanced.

References and further reading

Aiello, J., Barry, L., Lienert, L. and Byrnes, T. 1990, 'Health Promotion: a Focus for Hospitals', *Australian Health Review,* 13 (2), 90–4.

Ashton, J. (ed.) 1992, *Healthy Cities,* Open University Press, Milton Keynes.

Australian Community Health Association (eds) 1990a, *Healthy Environments in the 90's: the Community Health Approach: Papers from the 3rd National Conference of the Australian Community Health Association,* Australian Community Health Association, Sydney.

Australian Community Health Association (eds) 1990b, *Making the Connections: People, Communities and the Environment: Papers from the First National Conference of Healthy Cities Australia,* Australian Community Health Association, Sydney.

Baldry, E. and Vinson, T. (eds) 1991, *Actions Speak: Strategies and Lessons from Australian Social and Community Action,* Longman Cheshire, Melbourne.

Baric, L 1992, 'Promoting Health – New Approaches and Developments', *Journal of the Institute of Health Education,* 30 (1), 6–16.

Baric, L. 1994, 'Implication for Policy and Strategy', in *The Settings-Based Approach to Health Promotion: an International Working Conference in Collaboration with the World Health Organization Regional Office for Europe.* Conference report, Hertfordshire Health Promotion, Welwyn Garden City, Hertfordshire.

Barraclough, S. 1992, 'Policy Through Legislation: Victoria's Tobacco Act', in Gardner, H. (ed.), *Health Policy: Development, Implementation, and Evaluation in Australia,* Churchill Livingstone, Melbourne.

Beauchamp, K. 1986, *Fixing the Government: Everyone's Guide to Lobbying in Australia,* Penguin, Ringwood, Victoria.

Booth, M. L. and Samdal, O. 1997, 'Health Promoting Schools in Australia: Models and Measurement', *Australian and New Zealand Journal of Public Health,* 21 (4), 365–70.

Brown, V. 1992, 'Health Care Policies, Health Policies, or Policies for Health?', in Gardner, H. (ed.), *Health Policy: Development, Implementation, and Evaluation in Australia,* Churchill Livingstone, Melbourne.

Cahill, H. 1999, 'Why a "Whole School" Approach to Enhancing Resilience?", *MindMatters Newsletter,* March, 2-3.

Catford, J. 1991, 'Primary Environmental Care: an Ecological Strategy for Health', *Health Promotion International,* 6 (4), 239–40.

Chapman, P. and Davey, P. 1997, 'Working "With" Communities, not "On" Them: a Changing Focus for Local Government Health Planning in Queensland', *Australian Journal of Primary Health – Interchange,* 3 (1), 82-91.

Chu, C. and Simpson, R. (eds), *Ecological Public Health: From Vision To Practice,* Centre for Health Promotion, University of Toronto and Griffith University, Brisbane.

Chu, C., Driscoll, T. and Dwyer, S. 1997, 'The Health-Promoting Workplace: an Integrative Perspective', *Australian and New Zealand Journal of Public Health,* 21 (4), 377–85.

Clark, B. and MacDougall, C. (eds) 1993, *The 1993 Community Health Conference:*

Vol 1: Papers and Workshops, Australian Community Health Association, Sydney.

Colquhoun, D., Goltz, K. and Sheehan, M. 1997, *The Health Promoting School: Policy, Programmes and Practice in Australia,* Harcourt Brace and Company, Sydney.

Consumers' Health Forum 1999, *Guidelines for Consumer Representatives: Suggestions for Consumer or Community Representatives Working on Committees,* Consumers' Health Forum of Australia, Curtin, ACT.

Corti, B., Holman, C. D. J., Donovan, R., Frizzell, S. K. and Carroll, A. M. 1995, 'Using Sponsorship to Create Healthy Environments for Sport, Racing and Arts Venues in Western Australia', *Health Promotion International,* 10 (3), 185–97.

Corti, B., Holman, C. D. J., Donovan, R., Frizzell, S. K. and Carroll, A. M. 1997, 'Warning: Attending a Sport, Racing or Arts Venue May be Beneficial to Your Health', *Australian and New Zealand Journal of Public Health,* 21 (4), 371–6.

Davies, J. K. and Kelly, M. P. (eds) 1993, *Healthy Cities: Research and Practice,* Routledge, London and New York.

Dommers, E., Ingoldby, M. and Heart Foundation (Victorian Branch) 1996, *The Health Promotion Handbook: Action Strategies for Healthy Schools,* Harper Schools, North Blackburn.

Ebrahim, G. J. and Ranken, J. G. 1988, *Primary Health Care: Reorienting Organisational Support,* Macmillan, London.

Elder, J. and McBride, T. 1989, 'Local Government Embraces Health Promotion', *Health Issues,* 19, 6–8.

Everingham, R. and Woodward, S. 1991, *Tobacco Litigation: the Case Against Passive Smoking: AFCO V TIA,* Legal Books, Sydney.

Evers, A., Farrant, W. and Trojan, A. (eds) 1990, *Healthy Public Policy at the Local Level,* Campus Verlag, Frankfurt am Main, Germany.

Fawkes, S. 1997, 'Aren't Health Services Already Promoting Health?', *Australian and New Zealand Journal of Public Health,* 21 (4), 391–7.

Gardner, H. (ed.) 1992, *Health Policy: Development, Implementation, and Evaluation in Australia,* Churchill Livingstone, Melbourne.

Gardner, H. (ed.) 1989, *The Politics of Health: the Australian Experience,* Churchill Livingstone, Melbourne.

Gardner, H. and Barraclough, S. 1992, 'The Policy Process', in Gardner, H. (ed.), *Health Policy: Development, Implementation, and Evaluation in Australia,* Churchill Livingstone, Melbourne.

Gillies, P. 1998, 'Effectiveness of Alliances and Partnerships for Health Promotion', *Health Promotion International,* 13 (2), 99–120.

Goldstein, G. and Kickbusch, I. 1996, 'A Healthy City is a Better City', *World Health,* 49th year, (1), January–February, 4–6.

Goumans, M. and Springett, J. 1997, 'From Projects To Policy: "Healthy Cities" as a Mechanism for Policy Change for Health?' *Health Promotion International,* 12 (4), 311–22.

Hancock, T. 1985, 'Beyond Health Care: From Public Health Policy To Healthy Public Policy', *Canadian Journal of Public Health,* 76 (Suppl.), May/June, 9–11.

Hancock, T. 1990, 'From "Public Health in the 1980s" to "Healthy Toronto 2000": the Evolution of Healthy Public Policy in Toronto', in Evers, A., Farrant, W. and Trojan, A. (eds), *Healthy Public Policy at the Local Level,* Campus Verlag, Frankfurt am Main, Germany.

Harris, E. and Wills, J. 1997, 'Developing Healthy Local Communities at Local

Government Level: Lessons from the Past Decade', *Australian and New Zealand Journal of Public Health,* 21 (4), 403–12.

Harris, E., Wise, M., Hawe, P., Finlay, P. and Nutbeam, D. 1995, *Working Together: Intersectoral Action for Health,* Australian Government Publishing Service, Canberra.

Health Promotion Unit 1991, *Health Promotion in the Workplace,* NSW Department of Health, Health Promotion Unit, Sydney.

Healthy Cities Australia 1990, *Making the Connections: People, Communities and the Environment: Papers from the First National Conference of Healthy Cities Australia,* Australian Community Health Association, Sydney.

Howat, P., O'Connor, J. and Slinger, S. 1992, 'Community Action Groups and Health Policy', *Health Promotion Journal of Australia,* 2 (3), 16–22.

Kickbusch, I. 1994, 'An Overview to the Settings-Based Approach to Health Promotion', in *The Settings-Based Approach to Health Promotion: an International Working Conference in Collaboration with the World Health Organization Regional Office for Europe,* Conference report, Hertfordshire Health Promotion, Welwyn Garden City, Hertfordshire.

Kickbusch, I. and Jones, J. 1996, 'A Health-Promoting School Starts with Imagination', *World Health,* 49th year, (4), July–August, 4.

Kickbusch, I. and O'Byrne, D. 1997, 'Promoting Health Where the People Are', *World Health,* 50th year, (3), May–June, 4–5.

Labonte, R. 1993, 'A Holosphere of Healthy and Sustainable Communities', *Australian Journal of Public Health,* 17 (1), 4–12.

Langford, B. 1990, 'Community Action in Health Promotion', in Australian Community Health Association, *Healthy Environments in the 90's: the Community Health Approach: Papers from the 3rd National Conference of the Australian Community Health Association,* Australian Community Health Association, Sydney.

Legge, D. and Sylvan, L. 1990, 'Community Participation in Health: the Consumers' Health Forum and the Victorian District Health Council Programme', in Evers, A., Farrant, W. and Trojan, A. (eds), *Healthy Public Policy at the Local Level,* Campus Verlag, Frankfurt am Main, Germany.

Lennie, I. (Executive Officer, Healthy Cities Australia) 1992, *Letter To Healthy Cities Supporters, 26 August,* Australian Community Health Association, Sydney.

McPherson, M. 1993, 'Greening a Hospital', in *Health and Ecology: a Nursing Perspective,* proceedings of a national conference, Australian Nursing Federation, Melbourne.

Mason, C. 1990. 'Healthy Public Policy for Women and Workers: an Australian Case Study of Employment Discrimination, Occupational Health and Safety Legislation', in Evers, A., Farrant, W. and Trojan, A. (eds) 1990, *Healthy Public Policy at the Local Level,* Campus Verlag, Frankfurt am Main, Germany.

Mason, C. 1992, *Opportunities for an Ecological Strategy for Health in NSW: Possibilities for The Health Sector: an Issues Paper,* Health Promotion Unit, NSW Health Department.

McMichael, A. J. 1993, *Planetary Overload: Global Environmental Change and the Health of the Human Species,* Cambridge University Press, Oakleigh, Victoria.

Milio, N. 1986, *Promoting Health through Public Policy.* Canadian Public Health Association, Ottawa.

Milio, N. 1988, *Making Policy: a Mosaic of Community Health Policy Development,* Department of Community Services and Health, Canberra.

Milio, N. 1990, 'Healthy Cities: the New Public Health and Supportive Research',

Health Promotion International, 5 (3), 291–7.

Municipal Association of Victoria and Victorian Health Promotion Foundation 1990, *Healthy Localities Project: Second Progress Report, October 1989–June 1990,* Melbourne.

National Centre for Epidemiology and Population Health 1992, *Improving Australia's Health: the Role of Primary Health Care: Final Report of the Review of the Role of Primary Health Care in Health Promotion in Australia,* The Australian National University, Canberra.

National Health and Medical Research Council 1989, *Health Effects of Ozone Layer Depletion,* Australian Government Publishing Service, Canberra.

National Health and Medical Research Council 1996, *Effective School Health Promotion: Towards Health Promoting Schools,* Australian Government Publishing Service, Canberra.

National Health and Medical Research Council 1996, *Health Promoting Sport, Arts and Racing Settings: New Challenges for the Health Sector.* Australian Government Publishing Service, Canberra.

Newman, N. 1993, *Health and Ecology: a Nursing Perspective,* proceedings of the First National Nursing the Environment conference, Australian Nursing Federation, Melbourne.

Nutbeam, D. 1992, 'The Health Promoting School: Closing the Gao Between Theory and Practice', *Health Promotion International,* 7 (3), 151–3.

O'Byrne, D., Jones, J., Sen-Hai, Y. and Macdonald, H. 1996, 'WHO's Global School Health Initiative', *World Health,* 49th year, (4), July–August, 5–6.

Palmer, G. and Short, S. 1994, *Health Care and Public Policy,* Macmillan, Melbourne.

Pelikan, J., Lobnig, H. and Krajic, K. 1997, 'Health-Promoting Hospitals', *World Health,* 50th year, (3), May–June, 24–5.

Phillips-Rees, S., Sanderson, C., Herriot, M. and May, A. 1992, *The Changing Face of Health: a Primary Health Care Casebook,* South Australian Health Commission and South Australian Community Health Association, Adelaide.

Playdon, M. 1997, 'Promoting Health in Hospitals', *Australian Nursing Journal,* February, 4 (7), 18–19.

Pratt, R. 1992, 'The Health of Planet Earth: the Greening of Nurses', in Gray, G. and Pratt, R. (eds), *Issues in Australian Nursing 3,* Churchill Livingstone, Melbourne.

Pusey, M. 1998, 'Incomes, Standards of Living and Quality of Life: Preliminary Findings from the Middle Australia Project', in Eckersley, R. (ed.), *Measuring Progress: Is Life Getting Better?,* CSIRO Publishing, Collingwood.

Rees, A. (ed) 1992, *Healthy Cities: Reshaping the Urban Environment: Proceedings of the Second National Conference of Healthy Cities Australia: 13–15 May,* Australian Community Health Association, Sydney.

Ryan, P. 1992, *Cases for Change: CHASP in Practice,* Australian Community Health Association, Sydney.

Salmon, J. W. 1993, 'Whose Health? Re-Examining Public Health Policy', in Lafaille, R. and Fulder, S. (eds), *Towards a New Science of Health,* Routledge, London and New York.

Shields, K. 1991, *In the Tiger's Mouth: an Empowerment Guide for Social Action,* Millennium, Sydney.

Short, S. 1990, 'Professionals On Tap or On Top in the Illawarra Healthy Cities

Project?', in Australian Community Health Association (ed), *Healthy Environments in the 90's: the Community Health Approach: Papers from the 3rd National Conference of the Australian Community Health Association,* Australian Community Health Association, Sydney.

Smith, C., Roberts, C., Nutbeam, D. and Macdonald, G. 1992, The Health promoting School: Progress and Future Challenges in Welsh Secondary Schools, *Health Promotion International,* 7 (3), 171–9.

Smith, S. 1997, *Primary Health Care Policy Design and Implementation in Local Communities – What Local Government Contributes,* paper presented at the Designing the Future: Strategic Directions for Primary Health Care in Economically Advanced Countries' conference, Brisbane, March 12–14.

Summers, D. (ed.), 1987, *The Longman Dictionary of Contemporary English,* Longman, Harlow, Essex.

Tassie, J. 1992, *Protecting the Environment and Health: Working Together for Clean Air on the Le Fevre Peninsula,* Le Fevre Peninsula Health Management Plan Steering Committee, Port Adelaide.

Tesh, S. 1981, 'Disease Causality and Politics', *Journal of Health Politics, Policy and Law,* 6 (3), 369–90.

Tsouros, A. D. 1995, 'The WHO Healthy Cities Project: State of the Art and Future Plans', *Health Promotion International,* 10 (2), 133–41.

Tsouros, A. D. 1996, 'A Nine Year Investment', *World Health,* 49th year, (1), January–February, 7–9.

VicHealth 1999, *Strategic Directions 1999–2002,* Victorian Health Promotion Foundation, Melbourne.

Wallack, L. and Dorfman, L. 1996, 'Media Advocacy: a Strategy for Advancing Policy and Promoting Health', *Health Education Quarterly,* 23 (3), 293–317.

Went, S. (ed) 1991, *A Healthy Start: Holistic Approaches to Health Promotion in School Communities,* Faculty of Education, Monash University, Melbourne.

Whelan, A., Mohr, R. and Short, S. 1992, *Waving or Drowning? Evaluation of the National Secretariat: Healthy Cities Australia Final Report,* Australian Community Health Association, Sydney.

WHO Regional Office for Europe 1997, Vienna Recommendations on Health Promotiing Hospitals, WHO Regional Office for Europe, Copenhagen.

World Health Organization 1987, *Hospitals and Health For All: Report of a WHO Expert Committee on the Role of Hospitals at the First Referral Level,* Technical Report Series 744, World Health Organization, Geneva.

World Health Organization 1991, *The Budapest Declaration on Health Promoting Hospitals,* adopted at an International Conference on Health Promotion, Budapest, Hungary, 31 May to June 1991, World Health Organization, Geneva.

World Health Organization 1997, *Promoting Health Through Schools: Report of a WHO Expert Committee on Comprehensive School Health Education and Promotion,*World Health Organization, Geneva.

World Health Organization 1998, *The World Health Report 1998: Life in the 21st Century. A Vision For All,* World Health Organization, Geneva.

Zabolai-Csekme, E. 1983, *Adult Education: an Agent of Primary Health Care,* Adult Education and Development, 20 March, 1–10.

CHAPTER 8

Working with groups

*M*uch health promotion, whether it is lobbying for political change, community development work or more formal health education, involves working with groups of people, both community members and work colleagues. These groups often have dynamics that are so much more than the sum of the individuals in them. It is possible to develop an understanding of group dynamics and skills in working with a group, so that the group works effectively for what it is trying to achieve, rather than allowing its dynamics to work against what it is trying to achieve. This chapter will examine some of the important components of the group process and some practical strategies for working with groups.

Group theory

Group theory has been developing since the turn of the century, with several social psychologists researching the dynamics of group behaviour. After World War II, as concern for the future of democracy grew, there was a further increase in interest in group dynamics and the ways in which groups could be encouraged to operate democratically and collaboratively (Johnson & Johnson 1997, p. 40). It is from this base that group theory has developed, and so belief in the principles of democracy and collaboration underpins group theory and its application. This focus means that the principles of group work are compatible with the Primary Health Care approach, and have much to contribute to the practice of health promotion.

Group theory has not been developed with any collection of individuals in mind. Rather, for the purposes of theory, Johnson and Johnson (1997, p. 12) define a small group as 'two or more individuals in face-to-face interaction, each aware of their positive interdependence as they strive to achieve mutual goals, each aware of his or her membership in the group, and each aware of the others who belong to the group'. Clearly many groups that meet do not fit this definition. However, by recognising and working with the principles of group dynamics, health workers can help groups move toward this definition, enabling people to gain as much as possible from group membership.

The typical life of a group

Several theorists have proposed that groups typically go through a series of stages as they establish themselves, develop and ultimately wind down. Probably the most commonly used model is Tuckman's model of group development. It has been further developed by others and is known now as a five-stage model, suggesting that a group typically goes through a series of stages in its life — forming, storming, norming, performing and ending (or mourning). These stages describe the way in which the group goes about its activities (that is, the *process* of its behaviour). Groups will be attempting to get on with the business that brought them together at the same time as these processes are developing. The development of group process may, however, structure the way in which a group tries to do its business, and the effectiveness of the group may depend to a large extent on how it develops through the five stages. It is worthwhile, therefore, examining Tuckman's model, as it provides a useful framework for understanding behaviours that can commonly occur at different times in a group's life.

Despite the impression that Tuckman's model may give, it is important to acknowledge that the stages of a group's life do not necessarily occur in a neat straight line. Moreover, groups may not go through all these stages; for example, some groups may get stuck in the storming process, not resolve the power and control issues, and so not perform effectively. On another level, however, this series of stages may be experienced to some extent every time a group gets together (Brown 1992, p. 111). Tuckman's model provides a useful guide to what we might normally expect in the life of a group. However, it is not definitive, and other models also have merit and are worthy of examination (see, e.g. Sampson & Marthas 1990 or Bundey et al. 1989). Also, as you examine groups with which you are involved, you will see the extent to which the life of individual groups varies in relation to those models, and you may like to add important points of your own. The following explanation of Tuckman's model is based on the summary given by Brown (1992, pp. 101–10).

Forming

When the group first comes together, and for some time afterwards, it may be little more than a collection of individuals, rather than a group with its own identity. People may be feeling apprehensive about joining and anxious about their role in the group and how they should perform. At this point, if the group has a designated leader, that person usually plays a significant role, the members of the group being reluctant to take responsibility for decision making. Members rely on the leader to make decisions and control the direction of the activity at hand. At this time, they may be examining the group and their role in it to decide if it has something to offer them. Formal group leaders therefore have an important role to play in making clear what the aims of the group are, and in negotiating with the group regarding what it will set out to do and how it will do it. In those cases where there is no designated leader, the group may be tentative at this stage as a leader begins to emerge or as various people take up leadership positions.

Storming

In the storming stage of the group's life, people look for the role or roles they can play. Issues of power and control are often most prominent at this stage as group members jockey for position. At the same time, people may be afraid of losing their individuality and being absorbed into the group. Both these factors may cause the group to be quite fragile at this stage. The leader may need to ensure that dominant people are not permitted to take over and that all members have an opportunity to establish an equal role. This may take some skill and this stage may be the most difficult for the leader to deal with.

Norming

Once most of the issues of power and control have been sorted out, the group is in a position to develop a sense of cohesion and trust between members. Norms of appropriate behaviour are set so that people have a sense of where they stand and what is acceptable behaviour. As a result, group members may start to settle into the group. At this point its leader may need to harness the cohesion developed and use it to get the group working effectively on its tasks.

Performing

When members start taking responsibility for the group and its tasks, they are in the performing stage of its life. At this stage, there is a high level of cohesion and trust between members and the group is largely self-sufficient in relation to the leader. In many respects this stage is similar to the previous one: they differ only in the degree to which the group is performing its tasks and the level of self-sufficiency with which it is doing this.

Mourning

When the time comes for a group to come to an end, this will have an impact on it, even if it was convened to work for change and the ending of the group signifies success (as, for example, in the case of a community action group working to resist the development of a highway through their town). In this final stage of the group, it is important for it to evaluate its achievements and deal with any unfinished business. Some members may want to postpone the end of the group because they may have benefited a great deal from being a group member and may want to continue enjoying the company of other members and the sense of achievement that the group may have been experiencing. Having some form of ritual ending, such as having a meal together or carrying out a 'group closure' activity (see Pfeiffer & Jones, 1974–1985) may help the group to finalise its activities and members to acknowledge its ending.

Elements of successful group work

Johnson and Johnson (1997, p. 31) suggest that an effective group is one that accomplishes its goals, maintains good working relationships and develops in response to changing circumstances. Groups are more likely to be effective when:

- Goals are clear and relevant to all group members;
- Communication is accurate and clear, and two-way;
- Participation and leadership are shared among members;
- Decision-making procedures suit the issue being dealt with;
- Power and influence are shared, based on expertise not power;
- Controversy is encouraged, and creativity and problem-solving promoted;
- Conflicts are resolved constructively (Johnson & Johnson 1997, pp. 32–4).

In observing a group, therefore, and deciding which aspects of its operations are effective and which may need improving, several issues are worth examining.

The task, maintenance and individual activities of the group

The activities that a group performs can be roughly divided into three types: those that get the group's task done; those that maintain the life of the group and therefore may help it to get its tasks done; and those that individuals perform to look after their own needs. It is important that groups address these sets of activities.

If members try to push through to accomplish their tasks while ignoring the needs of individuals, the group may soon become ineffective. If, on the other hand, a group concentrates on maintaining itself, people may communicate effectively and enjoy meetings for a while, but may leave the group without having addressed the issue that brought them to it in the first place. They may leave feeling frustrated at the group's lack of achievement.

Of course, not all activities fit neatly into task functions or maintenance functions. Some activities may have components of both, and whether an activity is a task or maintenance function of a group may vary depending on the context and the particular group. For example, a support group's task activities may be the development of friendship and support networks, an activity that may be regarded in another type of group as having a maintenance function. To succeed, all groups need to address both their task functions and their maintenance functions, although there is no set proportion of activities that should be assigned to either category. What is important is for each group to strike a balance between the two types of activities. This balance will depend on the reason each group is meeting and, to some extent, on the individual needs of people in each group.

You could ask yourself the following questions when observing task, maintenance and individual activities in a group:

• Who keeps the group from getting too far away from its task?
• Who asks the group for suggestions about how to deal with a problem?
• Does anyone summarise group discussion?
• Does anyone try to involve people who do not seem to be participating (Bundey et al. 1989, pp. 101–2)?
• Does the group take time out to talk socially and find out how everyone is doing?
• Do the needs of any individuals in the group dominate?

Leadership

The pattern of leadership within a group is well worth examining, as it will tell us a great deal about how the group operates and how involved members are. Many people assume that the originator of the group is the only person who should exhibit leadership behaviours, but this is not so. Even in a group where a worker has some responsibility for it, if the group is to be effective, its leadership should be shared.

You could ask yourself the following questions when observing the leadership patterns in a group:

• What leadership behaviours are exhibited in the group?
• Is leadership shared by members of the group, or does one person maintain control?
• Who exhibits leadership behaviours and who does not?

Power and influence

Power and influence are very much linked to leadership in a group. Indeed, if the people with the power and influence in a group are not its leaders, conflict may result. However, people with power and influence may not be those who talk the most or are the most active in the group. Bundey et al. (1989, p. 100) point out that some people may have a great deal of influence, but say little; however, when they do speak, others take notice.

You could ask yourself the following questions when observing power and influence in a group:

- Are there any people in the group whose opinions are listened to very carefully?
- Are there any people whose opinions are ignored?
- Are people with influence helping the group to achieve its goals?
- Are there conflicts between people with influence?

Decision making

There are several aspects of decision making that need to be considered when observing group process. They are:

> *when* decisions are made (timing);
> *how* decisions are reached (process);
> *who* is responsible (who monitors the decision making process);
> *what* issues are to be decided.

(Bundey et al. 1989, p. 40.)

When decisions are made reflects a number of important elements of the group process. In a formal health education group, for example, this might include examining what decisions the group leader makes before the group actually starts, thus preventing the whole group from being involved in those decisions. In community action groups it might include consideration of whether important decisions are left until the end of long and arduous meetings, when people may not be as fresh and capable of good decision making as they could be, or when people with other commitments have had to leave. Conversely, decisions taken early in meetings may leave people feeling there was inadequate discussion.

How decisions are made may determine what degree of ownership is felt by group members over these decisions and help determine their level of satisfaction with the group's performance.

You could ask yourself the following questions when observing decision making in a group:

- How are decisions made in this group:
  - by one person?
  - by a small dominant group?
  - by simple majority?
  - by consensus?
- Who controls the decision-making procedures in a group?
- Are there issues that feature prominently in the group over which it has no decision-making power?

Group goals

A key issue in determining whether people feel involved in a group is the extent to which they share the group's goals. If the goals of an individual do not match the goals of the group, it is unlikely that he or she will be committed to it. Once again, this is just as relevant for community groups as for groups participating in health education activities. In either case, if someone or a small group of people dominate the goal-setting process, others can be left out of the group or drop out because of lack of commitment. In formal health education groups, this can happen when the group leader alone establishes the goals of the group without involving members in the process. The goals of the group might then suit no one in the group, and might reflect only the group leader's ideas of what people want. What a waste of energy when simply determining or clarifying group goals together could prevent this!

You could ask yourself the following questions when observing goal setting in a group:
- Does the group have clear goals?
- Who was involved in establishing them?
- Who 'owns' goals that are set?
- Are there members of the group who do not seem to share the group goals?

Communication

Patterns of communication in a group are extremely important. Distribution of leadership, participation, power and control, and conflicts of interest, will all be reflected in observable patterns of communication. Communication is both verbal and non-verbal and occurs between individuals and between an individual and the group. It has a key role in facilitating the group's achievement of its tasks and group members' comfort and sense of belonging.

You could ask yourself the following questions when observing communication in a group:
- Who talks and to whom?
- Who keeps the interaction going in the group?
- Are people silent, and if so, how does the group respond (Bundey et al. 1989, p. 46)?
- Do people address the whole group when they talk or just some people?
- What non-verbal communication is happening?
- How powerful are the non-verbal messages?
- Is anyone giving mixed messages?
- Is more being not said than said?

Rules and norms

Many groups will establish appropriate rules of behaviour or ground rules to guide their activities. For example, it might be decided that only one person will speak at any one time, that only the spokesperson will speak publicly for the group or that discussions at group meetings are confidential. In addition to the rules themselves, what is important is how they were developed. Did the group as a whole decide on them and agree with them, or were they imposed on the group by a leader?

In addition to these explicit rules by which the group operates, there may be a number of norms guiding the group, of which group members may or may not be aware (Bundey et al. 1989, p. 103). Norms are implicit rules that guide the activities of the group, often more strongly than the explicit rules. They influence the group powerfully, and can either support its activities or hinder its progress, depending on the norms themselves and what the group is trying to achieve. Some examples of group norms are that it is acceptable to turn up to group meetings 15 minutes late because they will not begin on time; that it is acceptable to talk about each other when no one else is around; that it is acceptable to interrupt each other during discussions and dominate discussion; or that it is unacceptable to disagree with someone else in the group.

In deciding whether a norm is unhelpful, it is important to look carefully at what is happening and what role it plays in the group's behaviour overall. For example, what may at first glance seem like an unhelpful norm may actually act as a valuable means of releasing tension. Laughter and games interrupting meeting procedure may be one example of this. It is vital that cultural norms also be considered. For instance, what may seem like an unhelpful norm of people consistently being late for group meetings may stem from particular cultural views of time in which being ruled by the clock is not as strong as it is in Anglo culture. In these cases, it is more likely to be the group leader, not the group, that will need to do the adapting.

However, in instances when unhelpful norms are minimising the group's ability to function, it will be necessary for the group leader to deal with the issue. This will mean making the group aware of what is happening, since it may not be conscious of the norm operating. Sometimes this will be enough: individuals will recognise how they are contributing to the norm and will agree to change their behaviour. If this does not happen, the group as a whole will need to decide how best to deal with it. Perhaps they will decide to leave things as they are and accept the consequences, or they may establish new ground rules and agree to stick to them. Alternatively, the norm may have arisen because a particular aspect of the group did not suit some group members, and the group may therefore decide to make the appropriate changes. For example, if people are consistently arriving late, it may be that the starting time for meetings needs to be altered to fit in with other commitments that people have.

You could ask yourself the following questions when observing rules and norms in a group:
- What are the rules guiding behaviour in the group?
- Which of these are 'written' (rules) and which are 'unwritten' (norms)?
- Which seem to be supporting the group's activities and which seem to be hindering its progress?
- Are there any that are hindering the group's progress and that group members do not seem to be aware of?

Controversy and creativity

Controversy can be extremely important to the life of a group. From it come new ideas and challenges to people's thinking. Unfortunately, people sometimes think that controversy is bad and to be avoided at all costs, and so do not allow it to be explored. Not only does this deprive the group of the opportunity to develop new and innovative solutions to the problems they are addressing, it can also run the risk of damaging the group. Irving Janis has highlighted the great danger posed by 'groupthink' if controversy is not allowed to exist in a group.

Groupthink is described as a process that can occur when disagreement and creativity are stifled, and it results in extremely poor decisions, often out of touch with reality. It has been highlighted as the cause of some of the disastrous decisions made in political history. It typically occurs when the group has a strong directive leader, when criticism within the group is stifled and when opportunities for criticism from outside the group are removed. As a result, uncritical acceptance of the leader's opinions leads to extremely poor, even dangerous, decisions.

Janis (1982, cited by Johnson & Johnson 1997, pp. 256–8) has outlined eight symptoms of groupthink:

1. *Self-censorship.* Group members censor themselves by not voicing any concerns about the issue being discussed.
2. *Illusion of unanimity.* Because of the lack of discussion, group members assume that everyone else is in agreement about the issue.
3. *Direct pressure on dissenters.* If anyone does speak out, pressure is brought to bear on that person to conform.
4. *'Mind guards'.* Some particular group members take on the role of discouraging objections.
5. *Illusion of invulnerability.* Members assume that the group is in a powerful position and cannot be criticised by outsiders. This results in very risky decisions.
6. *Rationalisation.* Group members rationalise the decision taken, in order to justify to themselves the position adopted by the group.
7. *Illusion of morality.* The group does not consider the ethical issues involved, and assumes that it is morally above reproach.
8. *Stereotyping.* Group members stereotype critics or competitors ('they are all stupid') in order to rationalise any outside opposition.

Groupthink provides an extreme example of what can happen to a group and its decision making when creativity and controversy are discouraged. Many people have experienced at least mild forms of groupthink and been concerned about its impact.

You could ask yourself the following questions when observing controversy and creativity in a group:

• How do the others respond when a group member makes an unusual suggestion or disagrees with the group leader?
• Does the group use processes to encourage creative thinking among its members (e.g. brainstorming)?

Conflicts of interest

If controversy in a group is extreme, it may be that real conflicts of interest are present. Perhaps members of a community action group are there for very different reasons, so that the group cannot agree on an action plan. Perhaps a worker acting as group leader is in a group because of his or her agency's expectations, and not because of a personal commitment to helping people facing the particular issue being addressed. In any case, when conflicts of interest are not handled well, they can damage a group and hurt individuals involved in it. It is therefore vital for group leaders to be able to recognise conflicts of interest and, where possible, structure activities to minimise the damage caused by those conflicts. The possibility of conflicts of interest is one reason why clarifying the group's

Rules for fighting fair

Do I want to resolve the conflict?
• BE WILLING TO FIX THE PROBLEM.

Can I see the whole picture, not just my point of view?
• BROADEN YOUR OUTLOOK.

What are the needs and anxieties of everyone involved?
• WRITE THEM DOWN.

How can we make this fair?
• NEGOTIATE.

What are the possibilities?
• THINK UP AS MANY SOLUTIONS AS YOU CAN. PICK THE ONE THAT
  GIVES EVERYONE MORE OF WHAT THEY WANT.

Can we work it out together?
• TREAT EACH OTHER AS EQUALS.

What am I feeling?
• AM I TOO EMOTIONAL NOW? COULD I GET MORE FACTS? TELL THEM
  HOW I FEEL?

What do I want to change?
• BE CLEAR. ATTACK THE PROBLEM, NOT THE PERSON.

What opportunity can this bring?
• WORK ON THE POSITIVES, NOT THE NEGATIVES.

What is it like to be in their shoes?
• DO THEY KNOW I UNDERSTAND THEM?

Do we need a neutral third person?
• COULD THIS HELP US TO UNDERSTAND EACH OTHER AND CREATE
  OUR OWN SOLUTIONS?

How can we both win?
• WORK TOWARDS SOLUTIONS WHERE EVERYONE'S NEEDS ARE
  RESPECTED.

©*The Conflict Resolution Network*
PO Box 1016 Chatswood NSW 2057

goals and involving everybody in their establishment are so important. These may not be enough to prevent conflicts of interest but they are an important start.

You could ask yourself the following questions when observing conflict in a group:
• Are there issues that always bring out anger?
• Is the group working through conflicts that arise or are these a barrier to action?
• Are there any people who seem to be always disagreeing and unable to allow others' viewpoints?
• How does the rest of the group respond to this?

Working with experiential groups

Experiential groups are groups run with the emphasis on the process of group involvement and what people can learn about themselves and relating to others through the experiences of the group. They can play an important role in mental health promotion. However, working effectively with groups in this way requires skills that cannot be developed through reading alone. If you wish to work effectively in this manner, you need to complete a training course in working with group process. There are many reputable counselling, relationship and group training courses available for this purpose.

This brief overview of the various elements of group dynamics should provide you with a standpoint from which to observe these elements at work. Being able to observe these dynamics in operation will enable you in many cases to steer the group away from unproductive patterns towards those that better enable the group to achieve its goals.

Hints for working with groups

There are several practical points that may make working with groups a more positive process for both facilitator and group members. These have been developed on the basis of the experience of people working with groups over a number of years. The following hints for working with groups have been developed from Ewles and Simnett (1985, pp. 122–6).

Numbers

In considering the optimal size of a group, the first consideration will be the purpose for which the group is meeting. If it is a public meeting designed to canvass opinion on an issue, the actual size of the group may not influence effectiveness. If it is a structured meeting where members of several interested parties need representation, the size of the group may be determined by the number of such parties.

If, on the other hand, the group is a health education group built on the principle of maximum participation by its members, it will be important to keep it to a manageable size. In such cases, the optimal size of a group is regarded as being between 8 and 12 people. If there are fewer than 8 people in a group, people may feel exposed and be unwilling to participate. Moreover, an insufficient number of ideas may be generated in a problem-solving group. However, if there are more than 12 people in a group, it is difficult for everyone to get involved, and often the louder members will dominate.

If you need to have more than 12 people in a group, consider whether you can split it up into smaller groups for discussion and activities. Alternatively, it may be worthwhile running two separate groups alongside each other. Which solution to choose will depend on the reason the group is meeting (can the topic 'cope' with a large group?) and the amount of resources you have (can you afford to run the same group twice?). If, however, you are dealing with a sensitive topic, it may be appropriate to have a group of fewer than eight people in order to enable people to speak comfortably about the topic. In these cases, you may also consider whether it is more appropriate to discuss the topic on a one-to-one basis.

Timing

The length of time that a group meets for is very important in determining whether members feel it is valuable or not. Groups need to be together long enough to break the ice, settle down and achieve something, but not so long that people begin to get bored or feel they are wasting their time. Generally, between an hour and an hour and a half is a reasonable amount of time. Breaks or changes in the group's activity will enable it to stay fresh for that length of time, or even longer if necessary. However, meetings lasting more than one and a half hours would need to be well planned, and you would need a good reason to justify them. Planning the length of meetings with the participants will increase the likelihood that the duration planned is realistic and fits in with the other needs of group members.

The day and time that the group meets will have a considerable bearing on who will attend. There are some commonsense rules you can follow to ensure that the timing does not prevent people from attending. For example, after school in the afternoon may not be a good time to run a single parents' support group unless child care is available. Meetings between 5.30 p.m. and 7 p.m. may be unpopular, as this tends to be meal time for many people.

All the planning in the world, however, will not enable you to prevent clashes with the other commitments that members of each particular group may have. It therefore makes good sense to check at the group's first meeting whether the day and time suit members and, if they do not, to negotiate a day and time that suit most of them. Not only does this increase the likelihood that people can attend the group, it also makes it quite clear that the group belongs to everyone, not just the group leader. Furthermore, you may want to experiment with different meeting times to maximise attendance and ensure that people who want to attend the groups are not consistently missing out because of poor timing.

Location

Location can also be negotiated. It is important that group members feel comfortable in the venue. Obviously, if people feel threatened, they are unlikely to continue going to the group. For example, many Aboriginal people have had negative experiences in hospitals, and may not feel comfortable in a hospital or community health centre. If there is no local Aboriginal Medical Service, the local Aboriginal Land Council offices may be a comfortable place to meet.

Remember that hospitals and, to a lesser extent, community health centres, have a history of being authoritarian and of being places where people lose control over themselves. It may be difficult for these associations to be broken and so, in the meantime, if there is any doubt, find a more neutral place. Church halls, Country Women's Association halls, youth clubs, senior citizens' centres, Aboriginal Land Council offices and people's homes are just some examples of possible meeting places. Which venue is most appropriate will depend very much on the members of the group.

Another important point about location is that it needs to be accessible to group members. Organising a group to meet in a venue that is not accessible by public transport is likely to prevent some people from being able to attend.

Seating

If a group is to work successfully, all members need to feel that they have an equal right to participate. Obviously, seating such as that in a typical classroom is not likely to make people feel equal members of the group. For this reason, comfortable seating, arranged so that everyone can see each other is most likely to be effective. Ewles and Simnett (1985, p. 122) suggest that it is important to remove desks and other furniture that is likely to create a barrier between people. However, until group members get to know one another, such barriers are sometimes useful because they stop people feeling exposed or threatened.

Green and Kreuter (1991, p. 77) point out, however, that even when seated in a circle people may not have equal opportunity to participate because sitting directly in front of the facilitator makes it easier to speak owing to the additional eye contact likely to be received. The facilitator might therefore sit opposite shy people in order to encourage them to speak, or next to someone who is talkative in order to minimise eye contact with that person, enabling others in the group to participate.

Getting the group started

How the group is established and the atmosphere that is created when it first meets will help determine whether or not people will go to future meetings. It is therefore important to start the group in a way that breaks the ice and enables people to feel comfortable in their surroundings and with each other. If you are organising a group meeting for community development or action work, this may be done fairly informally through introductions and discussion of the particular issues involved. However, for an educational or support group, it might be done more formally.

Icebreakers

Several things can be done at the beginning of a group's life, and at other times when necessary, to break the ice and help relax people into the group. These icebreakers may provide an opportunity for people to introduce themselves to one another in a fun way or discuss their reasons for being involved with the group and what they want to accomplish. There are several resources containing examples of icebreaker activities that can be useful in various groups (e.g. West 1997). Some icebreaker activities can also serve as goal-setting activities, when they provide people with an opportunity to discuss why they have joined the group.

Introducing the group

Once the ice is broken and people are settled in you can introduce the group and its goals. If you have asked people during the icebreaker to tell you what they want to achieve from the group, you can now all use this information to plan together the group goals. You may find at this time that your own goals for the group go out the window to some extent, and the group together plans its goals.

By the time you have finished the introduction, members should have an understanding of the group and what it will achieve, and should have had an opportunity to change the group plan so that it more accurately meets their needs.

Experiential activity

Having met one another and determined which issues will be covered during the group's life, group members should leave the first meeting also having had a taste of what the group will be doing. You might therefore involve the group in an activity that begins its formal life or demonstrates just what you will achieve. For example, a stress management group might discuss the particular stressors of its members and do a relaxation exercise. In this way, members are able to leave the first meeting with some sense of whether the group is likely to be beneficial for them or not, and whether or not they plan to return.

Facilitating group discussion

So very often people plan to have a discussion in a group, but they do not plan how it will actually happen. They assume that if they say, 'Let's discuss … ' a discussion will just begin. Unfortunately, the times when that will happen are more the exception than the rule. Most times, it is necessary to structure activities that will enable a discussion to develop (Ewles & Simnett 1999, p. 253). You may not need them, but more often than not you will. It will be necessary to have an idea of group members' attitudes to the topic before launching into discussion, so that you have a sense of the best approach to take. Can you be provocative in order to encourage a vigorous debate, or do you need to begin gently and lead the group into the controversial areas? You will need to bear this in mind when planning discussion. Ewles and Simnett (1999, pp. 253–5) suggest that the activities discussed below may be useful in encouraging discussion.

Using trigger materials

Show a film or play a game that touches on the issues you hope to cover. If it is slightly controversial, it will motivate people to discuss the issues. Then ask specific questions to draw out the pertinent issues. Make sure that you plan a set of questions before the event and that these are open-ended, so that you do not simply receive only 'yes' or 'no' answers.

Debate

Break the group into two, provide both sides with information if necessary, give them time to prepare and then have them debate the issue. Of course, if you want to encourage participation you may be better to keep the debate informal. Having group members argue the position they disagree with is one way of enabling them to clarify their views and hear the views of their 'opponents'.

Brainstorming

Brainstorming is a good way to pool everyone's ideas and come up with innovative ones, especially if you are trying to find solutions to a problem. It could be used, for example, to come up with ways to change the attitudes of local government councillors towards child care facilities, convince businesses to become envir-

Northcote Hydrotherapy and Massage Group

We are a group of older women who had been attending hydrotherapy classes organised by the Northcote Community Health Centre's physiotherapist. We had a range of physical problems, with many of us experiencing great difficulty in getting about.

Because of increasing demands on her work, the physiotherapist suggested that we organise ourselves. One member with swimming qualifications became the group leader for the exercises, following advice from the physiotherapist. The group members work their own way through the hydrotherapy exercises now if the leader is not there, and we all contribute new exercises as we hear of useful ones. The group lobbied for two years to have the Melbourne City Council adjust the water temperature in the swimming pool, and were successful.

In 1987 massage was introduced into the group. We applied to the Women's Trust Fund and received funds for a masseur to teach us how to massage each other and to assist when specialist treatment was required. Everyone who is massaged has to massage one of the others. The health centre made a room available. Five men joined the group for massage, but left when their health improved.

We began more formal meetings when we had to put together a submission to apply for funding for the masseur. We recognised that the company and support we provided one another was a big plus, and so we decided to organise some bus trips we could go on together. We applied for more funds, this time to the Department of Sport and Recreation, for a bus driver (we were able to borrow the Council bus). The physiotherapist helped with the submission writing and the health centre assisted by offering its treasury and auditing services. Much to our delight we received $4000 of the $5000 we had applied for. Since then we have organised a variety of outings, which have been wonderful events for all.

The group holds a committee meeting once a month. Decisions are made democratically and several people have taken on specific roles as a result of their expertise. We have had some frail older people referred to us, as professionals have heard about the value of the group's activities. We also have been involved in writing a book, entitled *Put Your Whole Self In* (McDonald 1992). Stories about the exercises we do in the water are included in it.

We think that our success is due much to the support and positive attitude of the Northcote Community Health Centre staff, who have given assistance when necessary, without taking over. We are encouraged to make our own decisions, and enjoy the independence. Remaining independent is very important to us.

Many of our lives changed dramatically as a result of the group. As we have said before, 'Our group will continue going probably until we drop dead, or as long as we can get onto a bus or tram. Our ambition is to spread this message of self-help, dignity and independence to senior citizens groups, health centres and such places around the country. Our work should help do that' (Community Development in Health Project 1988, p. 42).

We have been through several changes since we first started getting together, but we continue to enjoy the group and sharing its benefits with new members, other groups and students.

Members of the Northcote Hydrotherapy and Massage Group

onmentally responsible, devise effective overeating avoidance tactics or plan stress release activities into a normal working day.

The typical strategy for brainstorming is as follows: put the problem or issue to the group; ask participants to think up as many ideas as possible, without judging their own or other people's ideas; accept all suggestions and write them down; keep going until all ideas are exhausted and people cannot think of anything else.

What you do next depends on the reason for the brainstorming. If the group was trying to find the most appropriate solution to a problem, the next step would be to prioritise the suggestions made. This may require group members simply to vote, or there may be lengthy discussion, depending on the issue and the philosophy of the group. If the brainstorming was designed to answer a question, you may want simply to group the answers into similar categories.

Rounds

Rounds are good because they ensure that everyone has an equal opportunity to participate. They can therefore be used both to encourage shy group members to speak and to prevent dominant group members from monopolising conversation. Ewles and Simnett (1999, p. 254) suggest four rules that are necessary if rounds are to be successful:

- *no interruptions until each person has finished his statement;*

- *no comments on anybody's contribution until the full round is complete (i.e. no discussion, praise, interpretation, criticism or I-think-that-too type of remark);*

- *anyone can choose not to participate. Give permission, clearly and emphatically, that anyone who does not want to make a statement can just say 'pass'. This is very important for reinforcing the principle of voluntary participation.*

- *it does not matter if two or more people in the round say the same thing. People should stick to what they wanted to say even if someone has said it already; they do not have to think of something different.*

Rounds can be valuable for beginning and ending sessions and getting feedback, or as a measurement of the entire group's opinion.

Buzz groups

Breaking the group into smaller groups to discuss a key issue may enable everyone to participate more fully in the group. As a rule, these small groups need occur for relatively short periods of time, after which they can report back to the main group.

Self-help groups

Self-help groups have been growing in popularity over the last few years and can offer a great deal to people who join them. They may work for social change or for personal change in their members, or a combination of both. The challenge for such groups is to find the appropriate balance between these two approaches (Biklen 1983, pp. 206–7). 'Self-help refers to groups developed and controlled

The rise and fall of Club 2430

In 1982 the first case of the human immunodeficiency virus (HIV) was diagnosed in Australia. Most Australians took very little notice. By 1989, with the release of the *National HIV/AIDS Strategy,* Australia began to sit up and take notice. As a result of this strategy, Australia has been relatively successful at stemming the spread of HIV/AIDS, compared with many other countries. Despite this, around 16 550 individuals (as of September 1998) in Australia — male, female, old, young, black, white, heterosexual, bisexual, homosexual — have been infected with the HIV virus. This virus does not discriminate.

However, conservative rural communities of Australia continue to see HIV/AIDS as a metropolitan disease and to believe they are not at risk. The challenge of addressing the needs of those who are at risk in a rural area is a difficult one. Accessing those at risk seemed to me, a high-profile middle-aged female community health worker, an impossible task. Could someone in my position contact those at risk and, more importantly, would I be accepted and trusted? Had I adequately addressed and dealt with my own prejudices?

By 1991, the AIDS Council of New South Wales (ACON) in Sydney had appointed a rural outreach worker who was touring rural New South Wales trying to contact those men who have sex with men, so as to provide peer support programs. His visit inspired me to make a concerted effort to address the needs of gay men and women. An advertisement was placed in the local newspapers (four in all) asking anyone interested in forming a gay support group to meet at the local community health centre on the third Tuesday in November 1991. A total of 19 people, both male and female, came along.

At this inaugural meeting a steering committee was formed. Members came and went and within 2 months membership remained steady at five. In 1992, the group decided to call itself Club 2430.

To stimulate public interest, to present a positive image of the gay community and to show that HIV/AIDS was indeed a virus to be reckoned with, the club's first venture was to host a visit of the AIDS Memorial Quilt. Over 1400 people viewed the display, and three new quilts were handed over to join the existing 400. The success of this promotion prompted the quilt project representatives to ask the club to write a booklet on how to host a rural quilt display.

Twelve months passed and the first annual general meeting was held on 3 November 1992. Chairperson, secretary, treasurer and social secretary were the elected positions. Meetings were held monthly. Membership was $20 a year. In December 1992 there were 19 financial members.

The first 12 months of the group were not all plain sailing. Personalities, financial conflicts and differences of opinion caused concern both for me and for members of the group. However, the group's achievements far outweighed any difficulties:

- six club members attended ACON's peer support workshop;
- one volunteer member regularly accessed the local beats, offering support, HIV/AIDS and safer sex information, condoms and lubricant;
- contact was made with the local police to provide support services for gay members of the community who have been assaulted or bashed, and to provide positive networking between gay people and police;
- members represented the club at national and state HIV/AIDS conferences, with some presenting papers and workshops;

- support, counselling and respite services were made available to HIV-positive persons and theirng families;
- two gay and lesbian fund-raising dances were held, with new members making contact on both these occasions;
- a monthly newsletter, distributed to over 40 contacts, was published. It contained updated information on HIV/AIDS, treatments, future social activities, workshops, conferences and contacts from other gay groups;
- a brochure, providing contact numbers and listing the aims and objectives of the club, was distributed to health and support services in the local area.

Club 2430 provided an identity for an otherwise unidentified group within our small rural community. It provided educative and supportive services, networked with government departments and allowed members to socialise and interact with their community at large. Members reported that their self-esteem, confidence and pride in their sexuality had all increased since joining the club. Comments from members included the following:

- 'I now feel that I belong';
- 'For the first time in over 50 years I now feel that I am part of a group that truly understands me and where I can be myself';
- 'I am no longer afraid to go to clubs. We have strength in numbers';
- 'My self-esteem has greatly increased and I now feel I can talk openly about the death of my lover'.

Club 2430 was an attempt to provide an avenue to stimulate a positive image of the gay community within a rural setting and as a consequence normalise HIV infection. Club 2430 members' positive focus on support, socialisation and education, not homosexuality, enabled them to be accepted and respected by the local community. Their enthusiasm, support and networking were maintained for about 3 years. Over this period membership numbers varied, never exceeding 40, but there was an overall feeling of unity and shared vision.

By the end of 1994, however, the group dynamics had altered and friction and discontent among the ranks became commonplace. Personality clashes, disagreement over group incorporation and over whether the group should engage in high-profile or low-profile events created conflict. The lack of a definite direction or 'mission' saw the group flounder, with no consensus from the membership as to whether they were a social or a support group. Some members felt strongly about providing support to members who were HIV positive, while others were adamantly opposed to this suggestion.

The membership of the group had changed. Gay men who had previously lived in Sydney and experienced the 'hectic out lifestyle' challenged gay members who had lived closeted lives within a small rural community. They were threatened with exposure and realistically concerned about the possible loss of their jobs. In addition, there was a strong move from lesbian women to join the group. Having female membership changed the overall vision and many of the gay male members felt that the women were too dominant in what they believed was a male-oriented group.

The request from some members to incorporate the group created havoc. Some members saw this as a 'control situation' with bureaucratic overtones.

Membership began to wane. Attempts to provide exciting, stimulating and in some cases unusual group activities resulted in small attendances. The need for education and resourcing was no longer seen as a priority and as a consequence the morale of the small number of group members who were keen to continue, waned.

Unfortunately, word of the group's difficulties had reached the ears of the general public. As the HIV/AIDS educator I found it increasingly difficult to encourage new arrivals, who were seeking gay contact, to join Club 2430. The situation needed reassessing.

To the north there existed a very large active gay group (around 350 members). This group had been established for many years, and had clear group direction and well established meeting procedures. Membership participation and open forums for discussion were the norm. The last of the Club 2430 members decided to approach the northern group to see if they would consider providing an outreach service to our area. Responsibility for the organisation of local events would rest with local members, but the philosophy of this larger group would be adopted, providing a multitude of avenues that catered to all members.

This amalgamation provided an acceptable solution and today many of the original members of Club 2430, plus new arrivals to town, have the opportunity to continue to seek support and networking from a larger, well established gay group.

The experience of Club 2430 highlighted for me some of the difficulties of working with groups and enabling them to function effectively. The group had a successful start, had seemed to be functioning well and was always intended as a self-help group, so I had backed away, remaining only as a sounding board. However, after 3 years of apparently successful activity, during which Club 2430 had achieved a great deal, the group still remained relatively fragile.

Membership of the group was changing regularly. This had the effect that the dynamics of the group were changing constantly, preventing a stable set of roles and relationships from developing. As a result, the group was heavily reliant on its leadership, and this too changed frequently. When the leadership was good, the group fired on all cylinders. When leadership was fragile, though, the group lost its direction.

Also, despite group members having the shared experience of their sexuality, the differences between people were often very great. Their sexuality often seemed to be the only thing they had in common. Finding enough common ground between people for the group to function well was often very difficult.

Despite these difficulties, and the apparent demise of the group as an independent body, Club 2430 played an important role, both in the lives of the individuals, for whom it provided a sense of belonging, and through the provision of some practical services that helped to break down attitudinal and structural barriers.

Liz Meadley
(previously) Health Education Officer — HIV/AIDS
Mid North Coast Area Health Service (Southern Sector)

by affected people themselves, by consumers and by victims. They are, by their nature, committed to self-determination' (Biklen 1983, p. 185). Their roles include 'mutual support ... education, advocacy, lobbying, research and information and service provision to both their members and other consumers of the health system' (Markos 1991, p. 4).

Self-help groups often develop as a challenge to the mainstream health system, or find themselves challenging the system once they are established. This is because they often form in response to inadequate services for their needs. Whether they actively challenge the system or not, professionals may feel threatened by people addressing their own needs because they are unhappy with the way in which the system addresses them. Self-help groups demand information from professionals when many are still unwilling to share it, and in so doing challenge the status and power differences between professional and client. They may even question the limits of professional knowledge and the basis on which it is developed (Biklen 1983, pp. 201–4). There have been instances where health workers have been unhappy with consumers having control over their own health care and have felt threatened by consumers suggesting that they have knowledge and competence not possessed by the health worker (see, e.g. Hunt 1990, p. 181).

Consciousness raising plays an important role in the development of many self-help groups. Through talking together and sharing their experiences, members of these groups discover their shared ground and the common sources of oppression or indifference (Biklen 1983, pp. 193–4). Self-help groups may work to create their own alternative services or to change those already in operation (Biklen 1983, p. 195). In either case, they often demand greater control over services so that they may better meet their needs.

Unless they are appropriately funded, self-help groups may be encouraged by government in a way that exploits the community members who join them, particularly those who put considerable energy into organising and running them on a day-to-day basis. That is, governments may support self-help groups because they are a cheap option and because they assume the burden of responsibility for action in what are often difficult or previously ignored areas. Health workers need to reflect critically on suggestions to encourage the development of self-help groups, so as to ensure that these groups do not develop more for the benefit of the health system than the community itself.

In deciding whether a self-help group should be established, health workers must consider whether the people concerned actually want such a group — that is, whether felt need is present. As obvious as this may sound, on many occasions health workers establish self-help groups and then wonder why people do not participate. Clearly, community members will not participate in a group if they do not feel they need to do so. Attempts to impose self-help groups are likely to be unsuccessful, and may well set similar groups up to fail, once a community perception of a self-help group as failing has been established.

Another problem with some health workers' approaches to self-help groups is that professionals may sometimes support the idea of these groups being support groups, but are less supportive of, and even discourage, self-help groups that take on action group activities. However, supporting these groups for their support work only, while discouraging social action, amounts to a form of social control in which group members are expected to put all their energy into achieving tasks that could perhaps be achieved legitimately by the health system, and are not supported in their work for the necessary changes.

Health workers have an important role to play with self-help groups in supporting them and acting as consultants, when groups request this. They should act as resources, and not take over the decision-making process (Kearney 1991,

p. 31). Developing a partnership between self-help groups and health workers may enable them to continue their work effectively. Like any good partnership, the relationship between health workers and self-help groups should be one of mutual respect.

Self-help groups contribute a great deal to the health of members of the community. The examples of the 'Northcote Hydrotherapy and Massage Group' and 'Club 2430' provide some insight into the development and activities of two locality-based self-help groups. Both these groups were developed with the support and assistance of health workers and both went on to be largely self-sufficient for a period of time. As these examples demonstrate, though, the paths of their existences have differed somewhat. Together they reflect some of the range of experience possible in the life of self-help groups, and the ways in which group dynamics can be reflected in the fortunes and progress of a self-help group.

Conclusion

Awareness of group process is an extremely useful component of working effectively with groups, whether they are work teams, social action groups, participants in a health education group or members of a family. Working with groups in a supportive, enabling way, rather than a limiting or controlling way, is an important part of work to promote health using a Primary Health Care approach.

Group theory provides a valuable foundation for developing skills in working with group process. Working to encourage the self-sufficiency of groups, whether they be self-help groups or other forms of group activity, can be an important contribution to the development of individual and community capacity and to the relevance and sustainability of health promotion action.

References and further reading

Benson, J. F. 1993, *Working More Creatively with Groups,* Routledge, London.

Biklen, D. P. 1983, *Community Organizing: Theory and Practice,* Prentice Hall, Englewood Cliffs, New Jersey.

Brown, A. 1992, *Groupwork,* Ashgate, Aldershot, UK.

Bundey, C., Cullen, J., Denshire, L., Grant, J., Norfor, J. and Nove, T. 1989, *Group Leadership: a Manual About Group Leadership and a Resource for Group Leaders,* Western Sydney Area Health Promotion Unit, Westmead.

Commonwealth Department of Human Services and Health 1994, *Talking Better Health: a Resource for Community Action,* Department of Human Services and Health, Canberra.

Community Development in Health Project 1988, *Community Development in Health: a Resource Collection,* Community Development in Health Project, District Health Council, Preston/Northcote, Vic.

Corey, M. S. and Corey, G. 1997, *Groups: Process and Practice,* Brooks/Cole, Pacific Grove, CA.

Douglas, T. 1983, *Groups: Understanding People Gathered Together,* Tavistock, London.

Douglas, T. 1991, *A Handbook of Common Groupwork Problems,* Routledge, London and New York.

Douglas, T. 1995, *Survival in Groups: the Basics of Group Membership,* Open University Press, Buckingham and Philadelphia.

Ewles, L. and Simnett, I. 1985, *Promoting Health: a Practical Guide to Health Education,* John Wiley and Sons, Chichester, UK.

Ewles, L. and Simnett, I. 1999, *Promoting Health: a Practical Guide,* Bailliere Tindall in association with the Royal College of Nursing, Edinburgh.

Green, L. W. and Kreuter, M. W. 1991, *Health Promotion Planning: an Educational and Environmental Approach,* Mayfield, Mountain View, California.

Hart, L. B. 1981, *Learning from Conflict: a Handbook for Trainers and Group Leaders,* Addison-Wesley, Reading, Massachusetts.

Hunt, S. 1990, 'Building Alliances: Professional and Political Issues in Community Participation: Examples from a Health and Community Development Project', *Health Promotion International,* 5 (3), 179–85.

Johnson, D. W. and Johnson, F. P. 1997, *Joining Together: Group Theory and Group Skills,* Allyn and Bacon, Boston.

Kearney, J. 1991, 'The Role of Self Help Groups: Challenging the System and Complementing Professionals', *Health Issues,* 28, 29–31.

Lawson, J. and Callaghan, A. 1991, 'Recreating the Village: Groups for New Mothers', *Australian Journal of Public Health,* (15) 1, 64–6.

Markos, S. 1991, *Self Help Groups and the Role they Play in the Health Care System,* Health Issues Centre, Melbourne.

McDonald, M. 1992, *Put Your Whole Self In,* Penguin, Ringwood, Victoria.

Nelson-Jones, R. 1991, *Leading Training Groups: a Manual of Practical Skills for Trainers,* Harcourt Brace Jovanovich, Sydney.

Pfeiffer, J. W. (ed) 1983, *The Encyclopedia of Icebreakers: Structured Activities that Warm-Up, Motivate, Challenge, Acquaint, and Energize,* Pfeiffer and Company, San Diego, California.

Pfeiffer, J. W. (ed) 1989, *The Encyclopedia of Group Activities: 150 Practical Designs for Successful Facilitating,* University Associates, San Diego, California.

Pfeiffer, J. W. (ed) 1991, *The Encyclopedia of Team-Building Activities,* Pfeiffer and Company, San Diego, California.

Pfeiffer, J. W. (ed) 1991, *The Encyclopedia of Team-Development Activities,* Pfeiffer and Company, San Diego, California.

Pfeiffer, J. W. and Jones, J. E. (1974–1985), *A Handbook of Structured Experiences for Human Relations Training, Volumes 1–10,* University Associates, San Diego, California.

Richards, C. and Walsh, F. 1990, *Negotiating,* Australian Government Publishing Service, Canberra.

Roe, M. 1995, *Working Together to Improve Health: a Team Handbook,* Queensland Primary Health Care Reference Centre, University of Queensland, Brisbane.

Sampson, E. E. and Marthas, M. 1990, *Group Process for the Health Professions,* Delmar, New York.

Scott, D. 1981, *Don't Mourn for Me – Organise,* Allen and Unwin, Sydney.

Scott, S. 1988, *Positive peer groups,* Human Resource Development Press, Amherst, Massachusetts.

Shields, K. 1991, *In the Tiger's Mouth: an Empowerment Guide for Social Action,* Millennium, Sydney.

Tyson, T. 1998, *Working with Groups,* Macmillan, Melbourne.

West, E. 1997, *Icebreakers: Group Mixers, Warm-Ups, Energizers and Playful Activities,* McGraw-Hill, New York.

Women and Addiction Support Group 1991, 'Self Help is Expert Help', *Health Issues,* 28, 22–4.

CHAPTER 9

Education for health

Education plays a central role in health promotion. Not only is education itself a common health promotion strategy, it is also involved to some extent in just about every other health promotion strategy used. Working for public policy change, community development, using the mass media, and working with individuals and groups, all involve education in some form or another — whether it be education of policy makers, health workers or community members. Education is therefore inextricably linked with all other forms of health promotion. This chapter reviews some of the principles of health education, or education for health, and considers the particular approaches to education that sit most comfortably with the Primary Health Care approach.

Values in health education

Chapter 2 reviewed several key values in health promotion, many of which have particular relevance to health education. In particular, the attitudes of health workers towards community members, the presence or absence of victim blaming or labelling, and whether health workers see education as an opportunity for encouraging compliance or empowerment, all have a major impact on both the way in which education occurs and the likely outcome of that education.

Health workers using a Primary Health Care approach work in partnership with community members, recognising the expertise that community members bring to the learning process. They are also careful to avoid victim blaming, working with people to help change the environment as well as individual behaviours when people determine they need assistance to change these. Health workers using the Primary Health Care approach also recognise education as an enabling strategy rather than one to encourage compliance with others' wishes. For this to occur the focus is on participation in which community members have decision-making power, not merely token involvement. Because of the central role of these values in health education, you are encouraged to review Chapter 2 if you are not familiar with these issues.

The changing focus of health education

Until relatively recently, education of individuals to change their behaviours, out of the context of changes to the environment in which they live, was regarded as the only goal of health education. With the development of the new public health movement, however, this focus on health education fell from favour, as health workers recognised that imploring individuals to change their behaviour would not address problems created by an unhealthy environment or the actions of other people. With this recognition has emerged a focus on health promotion in its broadest sense, and a shift of emphasis away from health education.

It would be a mistake, however, to believe that health education is no longer important. Rather, health education remains central to health promotion, both because health education is the basis from which the current approach to health promotion has developed, and because health education plays a vital role in attempts to promote health using other strategies (Green & Kreuter 1991, p. 14). Moreover, education that focuses on helping individuals acquire new skills and knowledge still has an important place if we are to help people further develop their skills for dealing with the variety of situations they encounter.

Nonetheless, the change in philosophy that is marked by the new public health movement has resulted in a shift in emphasis within health education. Education has been recognised as having an important role to play in work for social change (Freudenberg 1984, p. 40), and emphasis has moved away solely from educating individuals to change their behaviour towards recognising the power of education to help create a healthy environment. Tones and Tilford (1994, pp. 33–4) describe the two key ways in which education is used to help create and support healthy public policy as 'agenda setting' and 'conscientisation'.

Agenda setting is the use of education at the community level to explain and convince people why public policy changes are important. Recent Australian examples of the use of agenda setting include the education campaigns that preceded the reduction of legal blood alcohol levels from 0.08 to 0.05 mg/L, education about the benefits of car seat belt wearing before legislation making car seat belts compulsory, and education about the importance of cycling helmets before legislation making them compulsory. In agenda setting, education can occur through formal education campaigns, and through public discussion and debate within the mass media. While working at the social rather than the individual level, agenda setting uses an approach to education that is fairly traditional. That is, agenda setting is predominantly a one-way process, with the aim of creating a more compliant population.

Conscientisation, or critical consciousness raising, may be regarded as the more radical approach to education for social change (Tones & Tilford 1994, p. 34). This is very much a two way educational process, with the specific intention of empowering community members. Critical consciousness raising is discussed in further detail below because of its central importance in Primary Health Care.

Defining health education

Health education is typically defined as: 'any combination of learning experiences designed to facilitate voluntary actions conducive to health' (Green & Kreuter 1991, p. 17). This definition is important for its recognition that any changes must be made on the voluntary decisions of the person or people concerned and that health education often involves a variety of strategies or interactions. It also includes scope for a variety of health promoting actions, rather than limiting health education to individual behaviour change, although this point is perhaps less obvious. Freudenberg (1984, p. 40) has attempted to make this final point more explicit and account for the broader range of activities that form part of education for social change by defining health education as 'those efforts that educate and mobilize people to create more healthful environments, institutions and policies (as well as lifestyles)'. The scope of health education is therefore quite broad, as is reflected in Ewles and Simnett's seven dimensions of health education (1985, p. 28):

- *Health, and therefore health education, is concerned with the whole person, and encompasses physical, mental, social, emotional, spiritual and societal aspects;*
- *Health education is a life-long process from birth to death, helping people to change and adapt at all stages;*
- *Health education is concerned with people at all points of health and illness, from the completely healthy to the chronically sick and handicapped, to maximize each person's potential for healthy living;*
- *Health education is directed towards individuals, families, groups and whole communities;*
- *Health education is concerned with helping people to help themselves and with helping people to work towards creating healthier conditions for everybody, 'making healthy choices easier choices';*
- *Health education involves formal and informal teaching and learning using a range of methods;*
- *Health education is concerned with a range of goals, including giving information, attitude change, behaviour change and social change.*

Within a Primary Health Care approach, then, health education is used across a broad spectrum of activities, from patient education, through individual education for healthy choices, to education for social change. However, the philosophical positions from which these kinds of education have traditionally occurred is quite different (Tones, Tilford & Robinson 1990, p. 6). Both patient education and health education for individual behaviour change had their roots in the medical model, and much education of this nature remains within the medical model. However, this does not mean that all education of this kind occurs from a medical model perspective. Nor does it mean that all education that can be described as education for social change is necessarily built on a social model of health. The difference between agenda setting and conscientisation provides a clear demonstration of this. Remaining focused on the principles of Primary Health Care and applying these principles to the conduct of education, no matter what the setting or the impetus for education, is therefore a major challenge for the health worker.

Education for critical consciousness

The concept of education for critical consciousness, critical consciousness-raising, or conscientisation was developed in its original form by Paulo Freire, although similar ways of working have also been developed by others. For example, the consciousness-raising techniques of the women's movement have much in common with Freire's education process. This approach to education offers a great deal to Primary Health Care because of the focus on working *with* people and because it provides a framework for action in dealing with the root causes of problems as recognised by people themselves. It provides an important link between the lives and experiences of individuals and change at a structural level.

Freire (1973, p. 13) criticised traditional notions of education and agricultural extension (closely related to community development) for amounting to cultural invasion, as representatives of powerful groups impose their view of the 'facts' on less powerful members of society. He argued that education is never neutral because it in some way either confirms or challenges the status quo. On the basis of this premise, he argues for education that challenges the status quo and thus enables the empowerment of oppressed members of society and the development of a more just social system. Education for critical consciousness focuses on changing the environment rather than the individual alone, by working with people to examine the underlying issues behind their problems and to change the structures around them.

Freire (1968, cited by Minkler and Cox 1980, p. 312) argues that social change can be achieved only by the active participation of the people as a whole — it cannot be achieved by strong leaders alone. Therefore, action for change must be built on critical reflection and action by everyone concerned. This process of critical reflection and action is described by Freire as 'dialogue', a two-way process occurring between 'teachers' and 'learners', in which both are teacher–learners.

Education for critical consciousness is a process of problem posing that leads people through analysis of their personal situation and then of the underlying social issues to making a plan for action to address the issues they have discovered. The four steps involved in the process are:

- *reflecting upon aspects of their reality (e.g. problems of poor health, housing, etc.);*

- *looking behind these immediate problems to their root causes;*

- *examining the implications and consequences of these issues; and finally,*

- *developing a plan of action to deal with the problems collectively identified.*

(Minkler & Cox 1980, p. 312).

Before such a process can occur, however, facilitators need to listen carefully to the needs articulated by community members and take the time to understand their problems as they see them (Wallerstein & Bernstein 1988, p. 382). They also need to observe the dynamics of the groups and individuals concerned to determine what sense of belonging or community exists. Some sense of community or group belonging seems to be important for the conscientisation process to work effectively (Minkler & Cox 1980, p. 320). It is for this reason that education for critical consciousness often goes hand in hand with community development.

Education for critical consciousness as described by Freire may not fit every learning situation that arises. However, the principles of problem posing, two-way communication and sensitivity to people can be used in any learning situation, so that it becomes an enabling process for the people involved. The following general guidelines for more traditional health education give some indication of how this can occur.

The teaching–learning process

Leddy and Pepper describe three key assumptions that should underpin effective teaching–learning (1989, pp. 317–33):
- Teaching–learning is a process, not a product — that is, new information and skills are not the only goals. How that learning occurs is equally important and may contribute greatly to the learning process.

Talking better health

Talking Better Health is a training program for health workers and community members, based on the conscientisation process described above. Developed from the Healthwise programs prepared for Victoria, South Australia and Tasmania, Talking Better Health provides a framework for exploration, understanding and action on health issues.

Talking Better Health is a five-step process based on storytelling and group discussion. It provides an opportunity for people to examine their own and each other's experiences in the health system, look for common issues in those experiences, explore the underlying causes of those experiences, and together plan action to address the issues identified. Talking Better Health enables people to move beyond commonly held beliefs to a more complex examination of health problems and solutions.

The Talking Better Health process provides a vivid demonstration of the importance of skills in facilitating group process in health education. The health worker's ability to facilitate discussion and enable group members to contribute to the discussion and planning process will be a large determinant of the success of the process. Health workers who attempt to impose their views or be too directive are unlikely to effectively implement the process.

Talking Better Health is offered as a training course in several Australian States and as a written manual (Commonwealth Department of Human Services and Health 1994). There are two supplementary manuals addressing the particular issues involved in using the Talking Better Health process with indigenous Australians (1996) and people from non-English speaking backgrounds (1998).

The Talking Better Health manuals and information about Talking Better Health workshops are available from the Centre for Development and Innovation in Health, Level 5, Health Sciences Building 2, La Trobe University, Bundoora VIC 3083. Tel: 03 9479 3700, Fax: (03) 9479 5977. email: cdih@vicnet.net.au   Web site: http://www.cdih.org.au

- The teaching–learning process occurs between people who all bring their own expertise to the situation, whether it be the expertise of personal and collective experiences or the more theoretical expertise carried by health workers.
- The teaching–learning process needs to be built on effective communication and mutual respect.

These principles demonstrate the importance of a partnership approach to working with community members. Both the community member (or members), and the health worker contribute to the discovery of potential solutions in a supportive atmosphere in which learners are allowed the dignity of risk and assume responsibility for decisions they make (Ewles & Simnett 1999, pp. 174–6). In such an approach, education is a guided problem-solving process in which both 'teacher' and 'learner' are open to learning from each other.

Facilitating the teaching–learning process

Several principles guide effective teaching–learning and build on the philosophical base of the teaching–learning process described above. They provide some general

The Murri Mums' Birthing Classes

In 1991, a group of older Aboriginal women living in Moree, New South Wales, approached me as the Coordinator of Community Health with their concern about the lack of pre-natal classes for Aboriginal women in the area. Only a very small number of Aboriginal women were using the pre-natal classes provided, although these classes were well attended by non-Aboriginal women.

The Aboriginal women who approached me were concerned about the quality of life and health of the young Aboriginal mothers and babies, who they recognised were not taking advantage of the service available. As mothers themselves, though, they felt they understood why Aboriginal women were staying away, and wanted to improve the situation. At the same time, the Moree Plains Health Service had identified the need for culturally appropriate health services if they were to have an impact on the poor health status of the local population, one third of whom are Aboriginal.

From the outset, it was recognised that the Aboriginal women themselves needed to be involved in the planning process to ensure that any action taken would be relevant to their needs and be owned by the women. Phone calls were made to several Aboriginal women working in service agencies around the town and to a local Aboriginal woman who was known to be particularly interested in the classes. We met to discuss the issues. As reasons why they felt Aboriginal women did not attend the available classes, the women cited the lack of specific Aboriginal teaching materials, the fact that Aboriginal women felt uncomfortable being the minority, and their embarrassment at the presence of non-Aboriginal supporting men in what was to them 'women's business'.

The women present agreed to be involved in the process of finding out if Aboriginal women in the town would support Aboriginal birthing classes. A questionnaire was devised and given to the women. As they worked in areas where they came into contact with young Aboriginal women, they arranged to assist these women to complete the questionnaires.

Analysis of the questionnaires indicated support for the idea of the classes and gave us some useful information about their existing knowledge and about areas in which they felt they needed to know more. A final meeting was held with the Aboriginal service providers at which their commitment to the idea, a plan of proposed sessions (day, time and venue for the classes), the key people who should be involved in the classes, and the questionnaire results were discussed. There was unanimous support for the classes, which they decided to call the 'Murri Mums' Birthing Classes'. A midwife with whom the women felt comfortable and who was already a successful childbirth educator was approached and agreed to lead the classes.

The first 6-week program began in February 1992 and was well attended, the plan was to break for 2 weeks and recommence classes. However, the second program was not attended and it was clear that there was a problem. Discussions with the key Aboriginal women indicated that class-free weeks led to confusion about when the classes were on, so it was decided to offer the classes continually. It also became apparent that transport to the classes was difficult, so several Aboriginal workers undertook to provide transport to the classes.

Evaluation of the classes by the Aboriginal women was very positive. Nonetheless, it would have been a mistake to think that we had 'arrived' and that the classes would roll smoothly on. We needed to continually listen to the women who attended the classes and adapt what we did according to their needs. This process was as central to the Murri Mums' Birthing Classes as the actual skills and knowledge that we aimed to help the women develop.

Programs such as this may remain fragile, dependent on changing needs and circumstances and on the ongoing relationships between health workers and community members. The early 1990s was a time of change and, after health service restructuring and a number of staff changes, the Murri Mums' Birthing Classes were unable to continue. Nonetheless, the process used in the establishment of these classes remains a useful example of how to work with community members to develop relevant meaningful health education.

Jennifer Brett
(previously) Coordinator, Community Health
Moree Plains Health Service

guidelines that can be applied to any teaching–learning situation:
• allow people to direct the learning process;
• get to know people's perspective;
• be aware of the context of people's lives;
• build on what people already know;
• be realistic in what you set out to achieve;
• take account of all levels of learning;
• present information in logical steps.

Allow people to direct the learning process

The active participation of community members in the education process is paramount to successful education. Client-controlled education is much more likely to address the issues of concern to people, when they are ready, and in the order that will help them to learn most effectively.

Participation to the point of control over the education process fits comfortably with the Primary Health Care approach. It is also supported by the principles of adult learning, which recognise the need for learners to direct the learning process and for learning to address the problems that learners themselves want to address. This principle was originally thought to apply only to adult learners, but there is growing recognition that it is just as relevant to child learners (Kalnins et al. 1992).

Client-controlled learning is most likely to occur if people themselves set the goals of learning. Chapter 8 discussed how this can be incorporated into group work, and the same approach can be taken with individuals. Helping people clarify just what it is they want to learn is therefore an important part of the education process.

Active participation can also be encouraged by maximising interactive teaching techniques and activities, rather than taking an 'empty vessel' approach and 'filling' passive recipients with information. People need to be able to have their say, use their initiative, experiment and find out what works for them. Structuring education so that these things are possible is therefore another priority for health workers who are eager to facilitate learning. Which interactive techniques and activities are appropriate will vary depending on the situation, the people involved and on whether you are involved in education for individual change or education for social change. Commonly used interactive activities include debating contentious issues, using structured group activities, planning action to address a problem, and practising the action required (whether that be drafting a letter to a local councillor, role-playing the negotiation between work colleagues about smoking in the workplace, or preparing a low-fat meal).

It is important to point out, though, that interactive techniques do not by themselves ensure interactive learning, nor is interactive learning precluded by the use of what are traditionally regarded as non-interactive techniques, such as lectures. Rather, it is how teaching techniques are used that ultimately determines the extent and success of interactive learning. Once again, emphasis should focus on how the health worker and learners use the teaching techniques, rather than solely on which techniques are used.

Get to know the people's perspective

Teaching–learning is effectively a communication process and as such is built on an understanding of the background and ideas of the other person or people. This is often a long slow process and not necessarily one that can be completed before the teaching–learning begins. Rather, you need to be open to learning about the other person's perspective throughout the teaching–learning process, and to adapt your approach accordingly. A person's attitudes towards relevant issues, their cultural background, their life experience and topics currently of priority for them may all influence their approach to learning and their ability to act. To ensure that communication is effective, pay particular attention to the needs of people who have impaired sight or hearing, low literacy skills or any other communication problem.

Be aware of the context of people's lives

The active participation of people in directing the learning process will help to ensure that education does not occur out of the context of their lives. This will again enable learning to be directed to the specific needs of the learners, taking account of such things as the particular barriers to action that they need to address and any other issues that may be more important to them than those identified by health workers.

Being aware of the whole situation with which people are dealing will also help to identify other strategies that may be needed to address the issue at hand. Using conscientisation, this would then mean that these other strategies would become part of the education process. For example, letters may be written to members of parliament regarding the re-routing of a main road, while road safety education may be conducted to deal with the problem in the short term.

Build on what people already know

The active participation of community members in the learning process will help to ensure that you start from the point where it is easiest for people to begin to learn. This will enable you to build on what people already know, providing new material in a format and at a pace that is appropriate to the learner or learners. Finding out what people know in a way that does not leave them feeling vulnerable is an important skill here. For example, 'can you tell me what you have heard about osteoporosis?' provides people with more scope to express ideas they are unsure of than asking people what they 'know' about the topic.

Be realistic in what you set out to achieve

Education is much more likely to be effective if you set realistic, achievable goals rather than expecting to achieve too much all at once. It will be useful, therefore, to spend some time with the people you are working with, finding out what they want to achieve and assisting them to adapt their plans if they seem unrealistically high or low. Helping people to plan what they want to achieve so that it is divided into a number of manageable pieces can also help them to keep track of their progress.

Take account of all levels of learning

Learning has traditionally been regarded as occurring on three levels — knowledge, attitudes and behaviour. While this schema has been criticised in recent years, it provides a useful guide. Consideration of whether knowledge development, attitudes and values clarification, or behaviour change and skill development are needed will help determine on what level or levels learning needs to occur.

Several health education books describe teaching strategies and the level or levels of learning to which they are suited. However, these descriptions are, on the whole, of limited use because it is the way in which strategies are used, rather than the actual strategies, that determines on which levels learning occurs. Also, in reality it is often impossible to separate knowledge, attitudes and behaviour, so attempting to separate them during the learning process is not always realistic.

Present information in logical steps

If people are to learn effectively, new ideas need to be provided in a logical sequence in which more complex ideas are built on simpler ones. Some planning is therefore needed to structure ideas so that they are presented in an ordered fashion. Of course these plans may be let go, to some extent, as learners direct the process through their questions and other activities, but the plan remains a useful framework.

The notion of learning having to start with simple ideas before moving on to more complex ones has been questioned in recent years. As with the notion of starting with achievable issues in community development, there is growing recognition that people may be quite able to deal with complex ideas when they relate to their own experiences or the problem to be solved, without needing to discuss the more simple ideas first. In these instances, people are likely to be motivated to learn about the complex issues, since they relate to the problem at hand.

Teaching–learning strategies

By now it is probably quite apparent to you that all the health promotion strategies described in this book so far are useful health education strategies. Mass media campaigns, community development, lobbying and advocacy, and group work often result in education of more than one group of people, and often at several different stages in the process.

In addition, we discussed conscientisation above, and several other common health education strategies are discussed below. Which strategies are most appropriate depends on the issue at hand, the needs of the people with whom you are working, the context in which the learning is taking place and the particular skills that you and the people you are working with have. In addition, strategies can be adapted and new ones developed to better suit each situation. The following brief descriptions provide an introduction to some common education strategies.

Talks and lectures

Talks and lectures tend to be regarded as a relatively efficient way to pass on a lot of information to a group of people. They allow an audience to participate passively and learn in a relatively unthreatening way. However, their effectiveness can be limited in a number of ways. Firstly, people may attempt to provide too much information in a talk, swamping the audience in a way that tends to inhibit rather than foster learning. Secondly, unless combined with other strategies, talks tend to be one-way communication in which little interaction (and therefore little participative learning), occurs. While this may not always be a bad thing, it is also possible to combine talks and lectures with other interactive strategies, using a variety of approaches to get the message across.

Icebreakers may be used during long presentations to help energise the group and keep the presentation interesting (West 1997). In these situations, though, it is worth confirming whether such a long presentation is necessary.

Discussions and debates

Discussions and debates provide an opportunity for people to examine an issue by comparing a variety of views. They are a much more participative approach to learning than talks and lectures, although care still needs to be taken to ensure that they are effective. Firstly, discussion may need to be guided (perhaps through a series of questions) or provoked (such as through a challenging video or opinion). Secondly, if group discussion is to be a participative process for everyone, it may need to be facilitated so that everyone has a chance to participate.

Demonstration and practice of skills

Observing and then practising behaviour can be a valuable way to learn and may be vital when people are attempting to learn a new skill. If demonstration is to be effective, planning the demonstration as a series of logical steps, reserving explanation to the necessary key points, will help simplify the process for learners.

Role-play

Role-playing often provides a useful opportunity for people to practise new or unfamiliar behaviour with others. It can also be used to provide an opportunity to explore values and feelings within a group. A word of warning about role-plays, though: they should be used to explore emotional or challenging issues only by health workers with the knowledge and skills to assist participants to debrief and de-role at the end of the process. Otherwise, role-playing may do more harm than good.

Games

There is a great variety of educational games or activities available to trigger learning. One example of these is the series of structured activities for group learning (Pfeiffer & Jones 1974–1985). However, if games and activities are to be effective learning tools, they need to be relevant to the issue at hand and well facilitated. Like other teaching–learning strategies, games and activities are not ends in themselves and need to be integrated with other learning processes to be used to full effect. For example, a series of open-ended questions to guide discussion after a game may help draw out the key learning points and link the message of the game to real life experience.

Self-contracting

Self-contracting provides a mechanism whereby people can contract with themselves to change their behaviour in some way and then support the behaviour change through rewarding the behaviour they wish to encourage. Despite the discomfort some people feel with its behaviour modification origins, self-contracting has often been found to be a useful tool in helping people change their behaviour. Very important in this process is that people themselves determine what they should change and how they should support their new behaviour.

Action

Enabling people to act on an issue of concern to them can provide an excellent opportunity for them to learn and make a difference at the same time. Writing a letter about an issue of concern, planning and conducting a health survey or media campaign, or developing educational materials for use with peers are just some examples of action for change that in itself may teach the protagonists a great deal. In these situations, educators may play an important role as resource people, but otherwise allow people to act independently.

Community level education

Education at the level of the community or population is a more complex process than education at the individual or group level — even more planning and teamwork is needed if it is to be successful. Nonetheless, the same general principles apply. The World Health Organization (1988, p. 175) suggests three points to keep in mind if you need to develop successful education at the community level:

- *You should get the support of influential people in the community — those who are called 'opinion leaders' or 'key people';*

- *You should be sure that all the people of the community are informed about the problem and are kept up to date on plans and progress. All available channels of communication should be used for this purpose;*

- *You should get the maximum number of people involved so that the community will really strengthen its capacity to do things for its health. This can be done through community health committees, advisory or planning boards, etc.*

'The Rural Access and Self Esteem Program: a learn to drive program for rural women'

The Learn to Drive and Self Esteem Program for isolated rural women was developed in 1989 by a clinical nurse consultant in women's health and the coordinator of a neighbourhood centre based in a small rural township. The need for the program was identified as a result of consultation with women living in isolated rural communities and personnel from the Community Health Centre, Community Youth Support Scheme, Area Transport Association, and the Women's Refuge and Accommodation Service.

The aim of the program was to extend the independence of rural women who didn't hold a driver's licence. The self-esteem component of the program was developed by the group facilitators in response to recognition by the group participants that lack of self-confidence had hampered their previous attempts to acquire a driver's licence.

The Southern Sector of the Mid North Coast District in New South Wales comprises the two large rural centres of Taree and Forster and is dotted with small, isolated poorly-serviced communities. Public transport is limited to school bus routes to and from rural villages and commercial centres. These factors contribute to personal and family isolation as well as stress in women of all age groups. Single parents in these areas are often disapproved of and domestic violence is tolerated as a way of life (Office of the Status of Women, 1989, p. 21).

The original target group of the program consisted of women with young children living in small villages, who were unable to drive and therefore unable to access medical services, employment opportunities and further education, and who had to negotiate with partners, friends or relatives for shopping opportunities. Retired women were later identified as another target group. They had come to the area with an ageing partner from cities with adequate public transport, to idyllic beach resorts with no transport or support services and very limited and expensive food outlets.

The pilot program was financed with a grant from the North Coast Department of Adult Education. The program was developed from modules originally used for Skill Share programs involved with adult literacy. The modules have been completely replaced by a redeveloped Roads and Traffic Authority handbook, developed in a user-friendly format. Audio tapes in different languages are available from the Roads and Traffic Authority to support people with low literacy levels and from non-English speaking backgrounds. Women's health education is blended through the program, depending on the needs of each group of women. The program is conducted over six sessions, each of 4 hours, with up to 16 participants. Group facilitators need to be skilled in assertiveness training and conversant with the *Road Traffic Handbook*. The support of group members for each other is essential, so facilitators also need a well rounded knowledge of group leadership and group dynamics.

The participants are encouraged to apply for their learner's permit at any time during the program. Practice using the computer questionnaire is an essential component of the course. Driving instructors are invited to meet the participants and describe their service. This component allows participants to select the instructor who best suits their needs. Course participants pay for their own driving instruction and licence test.

The course participants and group leaders meet 3 months after the completion of the course to assess their progress. The comments of the participants allow the group leaders to evaluate the program's outcome. Also at this time, suggestions for future programs are encouraged from the women.

The program outcome has been very exciting, with women not only gaining their driver's licences but also making positive lifestyle changes. Women have demonstrated repeatedly that they are able to overcome most obstacles, such as lack of financial resources, support in practice driving and access to a car if they are empowered by the program and the group. Many have gained employment, accessed services and undertaken further education. Some women have subsequently left abusive relationships. A few women have decided not to gain their driver's licences, for various reasons. Some of these women have been refused access to the family car and have been coerced by their partner to discontinue. Indeed, the program has challenged several relationships and this is evident in some of the comments made by the women's partners. These comments included that the car wouldn't be available for him when he needed it, 'you can imagine what women get up to if you let them drive', 'she gets smart enough now', and 'I'll take her when she needs to go somewhere'.

One woman recruited for the program cancelled her place because her husband informed her that 'he would give her a good beating if she continued'. This woman has since left the relationship and has gained her driver's licence.

Some of the reasons which women have given for not acquiring a driver's licence before the driving course have been:
- they might hurt someone;
- they would fail both the computer and practical tests;
- they didn't have the skills, ability or temperament to drive;
- they believed they were too old to drive;
- they were told they were too stupid to drive.

Over 200 women within the Southern Sector of the Mid North Coast have undertaken the course between its inception and the end of 1998. Women's refuge clients and Aboriginal women have specifically requested courses. Participants have ranged in age from 18 years to 70 years old. Each group conducted attracts at least one woman from a non-English speaking background. The program's evaluation reveals a 98% success rate of gaining a driver's licence as well as increases in self-esteem. Other gains identified by the women include employment, further education and involvement in community activities. Some comments that indicate the breadth of this impact include:
- 'It's wonderful — my children are so proud of me since I've gained my licence. I'm able to buy groceries as I need them for the first time in my life';
- 'I take a friend to church every Sunday. I feel marvellous,' a woman who is over 70 years of age stated;
- 'My daughter couldn't have taken the job if I hadn't got my licence,' said a woman living on a farm who was able to transport her 16-year-old daughter to a Saturday job;
- 'I'm going to enter my name on the electoral roll now. I've never felt I was important enough before,' a 40-year-old woman said at the completion of a course;
- 'Slowly I have come to learn that I am important person';

- 'I was able to negotiate a wage increase because of the confidence I have experienced since attending the course';
- 'I now face problems realising my opinion is important';
- 'I think I have a clearer view of how to achieve more independence for myself'.

When asked to name one or more components of the course that were valuable, some of the responses were:

- 'companionship';
- 'accepting the reason why I was not reaching my goals';
- 'learning not to be negative';
- 'I am the same person but facing a problem openly';
- 'I have a quiet time for me';
- 'losing weight';
- 'eating a healthier diet';
- 'I am able to make choices I didn't have before'.

Courses continue to be run regularly, with results similar to those described above, both in terms of success in gaining driver's licences and the other positive results related to confidence and self-esteem.

In 1997 the program was identified as an example of best practice in women's health by the evaluation of the NSW National Women's Health Program (NSW Health Department 1997). It is important to note, though, that after its original pilot funding in 1989, this program had not received any specific funding and was simply developed and funded as a part of ongoing community health work in the area. However, in 1996 a successful grant application resulted in funds from the NSW National Women's Health Program to develop a formal package of the program. The 'Rural Access and Self Esteem Program: a learn to drive program for rural women' is now available as a program plan for other centres to implement. In addition, the program has been sold to all area health services throughout New South Wales, sponsored by the NSW Cervical Screening Program.

The 'Rural Access and Self Esteem Program: a learn to drive program for rural women' provides rural women without a driver's licence with the opportunity to access the basic services most of us take for granted, in an environment that is supportive and positive. As a result, this program has greatly increased the choices available to the women who have participated and has gone quite some way to promoting the health of these women within the context of their lives.

Lorna Neal
Area Coordinator (Women's Health)
Mid North Coast Area Health Service

Community-level education draws particularly on mass media and community development strategies. If it is to be effective, it needs to be built on the recognition of the nature of communities as being composed of a variety of groups, often with competing interests. This is likely to mean that a variety of different approaches are needed to work effectively with each of these different groups.

Minkler's 10 commitments for community health education

Start where the people are
Respecting community members' own perspectives and priorities and working with them on the issues they identify is the basis for effective meaningful health education.

Recognize and build on community strengths
Paying as much attention to the strengths of communities as their needs acknowledges the resources of the community and itself strengthens the community.

Honor thy community — but do not make it holy
While this focus on the community is vital, we need to ensure that we maintain our focus on social justice, or we run the risk of blindly committing ourselves to divisive community attitudes.

Foster high level community participation
True power sharing and control by the community should be the aim if people are to participate meaningfully in health education.

Laughter is good medicine — and good health education
Humor and light heartedness itself have health benefits, as well as improving the quality of good health education.

Health education is educational — but it is also political
Health education should not ignore the political aspects of health issues, but should instead recognize the social and political context in which health issues arise.

Thou shalt not tolerate the bad 'isms'
Health educators should ensure that they do not work in ways which encourage or ignore racism, sexism, ageism, homophobia or other attitudes which act to exclude people.

'Think globally, act locally'
Work at both the macro level and the micro level to address the immediate problem and the broader causal issues.

Foster individual and community empowerment
'If we do start where people are; if we work with, rather than on, communities; if we believe in and work for high level community participation; and if we see our work in terms of its political and economic contexts, we will be doing empowering health education.'

Work for social justice
Work to advocate for social justice and improvements in public health, to help create an environment which is more 'conducive to individual and community empowerment'.

(Minkler 1994, pp. 527–34)

Minkler (1994) has developed a set of 10 principles or 'commitments' for community health education (see box). In examining these it is apparent that they draw together the wide range of principles examined throughout this book, demonstrating the way in which these points all come together in community health education. This also serves to highlight the linkages and similarities between community health education and other strategies identified here.

Conclusion

This chapter has briefly reviewed the role of health education in health promotion and discussed some of the key principles to be considered in education for health from a Primary Health Care approach. Two-way communication and respect, learning based around needs identified by people themselves and active learning form a foundation for effective education for health. On the whole, health workers already have much scope within their traditional roles to incorporate health education readily into their work, to do so in a way that enables people to take greater control over their lives, and to use education as a springboard to other health promotion strategies when these are of value.

References and further reading

Brookfield, S. 1983, *Adult Learners, Adult Education and the Community,* Open University Press, Milton Keynes, UK.

Carr, M., Kuo, H., Fong, A., Jones, L. and Taylor, P. 1991, *Healthwise Tasmania: a Handbook for Facilitators,* Tasmanian Department of Health, Hobart, Tasmania.

Colquhoun, D. 1992, 'Dominant Discourses In Health Education', in *Health Education: Politics And Practice,* Deakin University, Geelong, Victoria.

Commonwealth Department of Human Services and Health 1994, *Talking Better Health: a Resource for Community Action,* Department of Human Services and Health, Canberra.

Cox, K. R. and Ewan, C. E. (eds) 1988, *The Medical Teacher,* 2nd edn, Churchill Livingstone, Edinburgh, UK.

Draper, P., Griffiths, J., Dennis, J. and Popay, J. 1980, 'Three Types of Health Education', *British Medical Journal,* 16 August 493–5.

Ewles, L. and Simnett, I. 1985, *Promoting Health: a Practical Guide to Health Education,* John Wiley and Sons, Chichester, UK.

Ewles, L. and Simnett, I. 1999, *Promoting Health: a Practical Guide,* Bailliere Tindall in association with the Royal College of Nursing, Edinburgh.

Freire, P. 1973, *Education for Critical Consciousness,* Sheed and Ward, London.

Freudenberg, N. 1984, 'Training Health Educators for Social Change', *International Quarterly of Community Health Education,* 5 (1), 37–52.

Glanz, K., Lewis, F. M. and Rimer, B. K. (eds) 1991, *Health Behavior and Health Education: Theory, Research and Practice,* Jossey-Bass, San Francisco.

Green, L. W. and Kreuter, M. W. 1991, *Health Promotion Planning: an Educational and Environmental Approach,* Mayfield, Mountain View, California.

Hill, P. S. and Murphy, G. J. 1992, 'Cultural Identification in Aboriginal and Torres Strait Islander AIDS Education', *Australian Journal of Public Health,* 16 (2), 150–7.

Johnson, S. (1992), 'Aboriginal Health through Primary Health Care', in Gray, G. and Pratt, R. (eds), *Issues in Australian Nursing 3,* Churchill Livingstone, Melbourne, Vic.

Kalnins, I., McQueen, D. V., Backett, K. C., Curtice, L. and Currie, C. E. 1992, 'Children, Empowerment and Health Promotion: Some New Directions in Research and Practice', *Health Promotion International,* 7 (1), 53–9.

Kiger, A. M. 1995, *Teaching for Health,* Churchill Livingstone, Edinburgh.

Laura, R. and Heaney, S. 1990, *Philosophical Foundations of Health Education,* Routledge, London.

Leddy, S. and Pepper, J. M. 1989, *Conceptual Bases of Professional Nursing,* J. B. Lippincott, Philadelphia.

Lorig, K. 1991, *Common Sense Patient Education,* Fraser Publications, Ivanhoe, Vic.

Mather, P. L. 1988, 'Educating Preschoolers About Health Care', *Childhood Education,* Winter, 94–100.

Minkler, M. 1989, 'Health Education, Health Promotion and the Open Society: an Historical Perspective', *Health Education Quarterly,* 16 (1), 17–30.

Minkler, M. 1994, 'Ten Commitments for Community Health Education', *Health Education Research,* 9 (4), 527–34.

Minkler, M. and Cox, K. 1980, 'Creating Critical Consciousness in Health: Application of Freire's Philosophy and Methods to the Health Care Setting', *International Journal of Health Services,* 10 (2), 311–22.

NSW Health Department 1997, *Evaluation of the New South Wales National Women's Health Program,* NSW Health Department, Sydney.

Office of the Status of Women 1989, *National Agenda for Women Implementation Report,* Australian Government Publishing Service, Canberra.

Priest, J. and Schott, J. 1991, *Leading Antenatal Classes: a Practical Guide,* Butterworth Heinemann, Oxford.

Pfeiffer, J. W. and Jones, J. E. (1974–1985), *A Handbook of Structured Experiences for Human Relations Training, Volumes 1–10,* University Associates, San Diego, California.

Redman, B. 1988, *The Process of Patient Education,* C. V. Mosby, St Louis, Missouri.

Reid, J. and Trompf, P. (eds) 1990, *The Health of Immigrant Australia,* Harcourt Brace Jovanovich, Sydney.

Tones, K. 1992, 'Health Promotion, Self-Empowerment and the Concept of Control', in *Health Education: Politics and Practice,* Deakin University, Geelong, Victoria.

Tones, K. and Tilford, S. 1994, *Health Education: Effectiveness, Efficiency and Equity,* Chapman and Hall, London.

Tones, K., Tilford, S. and Robinson, Y. 1990, *Health Education: Effectiveness and Efficiency,* Chapman and Hall, London.

Wallerstein, N. 1992, 'Powerlessness, Empowerment, and Health: Implications for Health Promotion Programs', *American Journal of Public Health,* January/February, 6 (3), 197–205.

Wallerstein, N. and Bernstein, E. 1988, 'Empowerment Education: Freire's Ideas Adapted to Health Education', *Health Education Quarterly,* 15 (4), 379–94.

Wallerstein, N. and Sanchez-Merki, V. 1994, 'Freirian Praxis in Health Education: Research Results from an Adolescent Prevention Program', *Health Education Research,* 9 (1), 105–18.

Werner, D. and Bower, B. 1982, *Helping Health Workers Learn,* The Hesperian Foundation, Palo Alto, California.

West, E. 1997, *Icebreakers: Group Mixers, Warm-Ups, Energizers and Playful Activities,* McGraw-Hill, New York.

World Health Organization 1988, *Education for Health: a Manual on Health Education in Primary Health Care,* World Health Organization, Geneva.

Zabolai-Csekme, E. 1983, 'Adult Education: an Agent of Primary Health Care', *Adult Education and Development,* 20 March, 1–10.

CHAPTER 10

Putting it all together

*I*t is now time to consider how you can put all the approaches and strategies *discussed in this book into practice. There are two ways in which to 'put it all together'. Firstly, the principles and skills of health promotion and Primary Health Care can be incorporated into the way in which health workers approach their everyday work. Secondly, the principles and skills of health promotion can be put together to create specific health promotion programs that health workers may implement as individuals or as part of a team.*

Applying Primary Health Care principles in practice

No matter where health workers are placed, opportunities exist to further apply the principles of Primary Health Care and make work with community members, clients or patients more health promoting. Community health centres, workplaces, hospitals and residential institutions such as group homes, hostels and nursing homes all require work on both the structural level and the individual level to make action and interaction more health promoting. Within these organisations, then, you can be guided by the principles of Primary Health Care in your daily work with community members, clients or patients and staff, and work for change at an organisational level so that the organisation is more responsive to the needs of the people it is designed to serve and more supportive of health through the policies it implements.

On a structural level, services that operate with a Primary Health Care approach:
• respond to the needs of the population;
• are operated with an openness to community members;
• are structured in a way that enables community members to make informed choices;
• are developed in a way that maintains or increases people's control over their own health;
• place emphasis on promoting health.

Such services make maximum use of appropriate low technology and are guided by an agency philosophy of promoting the health of the community or population whose needs they are designed to address.

Individual interactions within such services should be built on recognition of the expertise that community members have with regard to their own lives and their experiences of living with the issues that have brought them in contact with the service. They need to be driven by the right and ability of community members to make informed decisions about their own lives, and so provide what is necessary to enable them to do this.

It is important to reiterate here the importance of the principles of Primary Health Care guiding any work to promote health. This is because, while the skills of use in health promotion are valuable, they do not by themselves ensure the implementation of Primary Health Care principles. Any health promotion strategy can be used in a way that is more controlling than enabling. It is the implementation of Primary Health Care principles that ensures that the strategies are used in a way that is supportive of people and therefore enables them to take greater control over their lives.

Focusing in this way on the principles of Primary Health Care rather than on which particular strategy to use is valuable, because you are then able to respond to the situation and the particular needs of people with whom you are working in the way that is most appropriate. From this perspective, a whole range of variations and combinations of strategies may become apparent and be appropriate for the particular situation with which you are working. Focusing on the known strategies alone, rather than on the principles of Primary Health Care, may limit your possible responses and result in your action being driven more by the strategies themselves than the needs of the people and the situation.

As health workers become more experienced in implementing the principles of Primary Health Care, this is exactly what we are seeing occur. Responses to problems and situations are becoming more individualised and more sophisticated because of the focus on the individual needs of the situation. Effective Primary Health Care practice requires health workers to draw on, rather than rely on, skills and strategies. You are encouraged to examine the publications reviewed in Appendix 4 for some excellent examples of how health promotion skills and strategies have been tailored to fit local need. Some of the important issues have also been reflected in the practice examples provided throughout this book.

Planning health promotion

Planning health promotion will require you to draw on all the information in this book as well as many other skills you have developed as a health worker. That is, planning health promotion requires that you clarify your values, assess the needs of the people for whom the program is being developed and work collaboratively with them to determine the best way to respond to their needs. And because of the involvement of these people themselves and the fact that needs are dynamic, you will need to remain flexible and responsive to changing needs and circumstances.

Health promotion activity is planned on a range of different levels and at different levels of formality and informality. Planning for one activity may take just a few minutes and may be simply thought through by a health worker or community member, while planning for another activity may take considerable time and the involvement of many people. This planning may simply occur and the plan be implemented, or time may be spent documenting the whole planning process. Whichever description best fits the planning you do will depend very much on the situation. Whichever of these approaches is used, the points raised here will be relevant.

The way in which you plan and implement a health promotion program may also differ, according to the particular ways in which things are organised in each State, region and agency. For example, some States and regions allow a more developmental or 'bottom up' approach to health promotion activity in which action is developed with local people, while others expect a more 'top down'

Midwifery care for pregnant teenagers — Primary Health Care in action

At 'The Warehouse', an outreach centre of the Family Planning Association in Penrith, New South Wales, a service is being run to meet the antenatal care needs of pregnant teenagers, managed by midwives from the Nepean hospital and staff from 'The Warehouse'.

'The Warehouse' clinic aims to provide effective, high-quality midwifery and Primary Health Care that meets the needs of its clients. The midwives believe that it is essential to foster a therapeutic relationship so that there can be effective antenatal care (that is, care that has a positive effect on the teenage woman herself, as well as on her pregnancy and parenting). By providing a more appropriate service the clinic is attempting to address the major issue of pregnant adolescents not relating to (and therefore not using) the traditional medical model of care and services. Clark (1984, p. 16) outlines the common problems described by adolescents attending public hospital clinics as:

> *seeing a different health worker each time … losing confidence in the quality of the service … inadequate transport and access … perceived moralising attitudes of staff … [feeling] that their control and responsibility [are] threatened.*

'The Warehouse' clinic attempts to address these issues and demonstrates a Primary Health Care model in several ways, as described below.

Being socially acceptable and accessible

The clinic is socially acceptable and accessible to the clients, who have the choice of attending clinics at either the hospital or The Warehouse, a community based Youth Health Centre, easily accessible and located in a central shopping district within easy reach of public transport. There is an open friendly atmosphere, with partners and friends welcome.

Focus on illness prevention and health promotion

The focus of care is on illness prevention and health promotion. As a group, teenagers tend to have poor nutritional habits and in pregnancy this may result in low haemoglobin levels. There is consensus among the teenagers themselves that calcium and protein intakes are often inadequate. Added to this are the high levels of psychosocial stressors, including smoking, that may further contribute to a less than optimal foetal environment. In addition, pregnancy for the teenager may contribute to increased feelings of powerlessness, low self-esteem and/or psychological and social difficulties. Prenatal visits are a time for assessment and reassurance regarding foetal wellbeing and provide an opportunity to give positive feedback to women about their achievements and progress. Each prenatal clinic session is preceded by an education/discussion group. Topics are broad and include nutrition, exercise, smoking, lifestyle changes and emotional health. Partners and friends are included in these informal classes, and participants are eager to learn.

Multidisciplinary approach

Assistance with finance, housing and education is available through the Youth Centre staff and hospital social worker. This ensures that all available resources that all available resources are utilised to provide an optimal service. The collaboration of all disciplines and service groups is essential to facilitate an effective service. There is a strong vital belief in a social view of health, recognising that for many young women and their partners, the psychosocial stressors and disadvantages of being young parents will far outweigh the physical and practical demands. For this reason, the service aims for a well coordinated holistic approach, with efforts made to minimise the number of health workers with whom each client has to come in contact.

Shared health assessment

The approach to antenatal care is one of shared health assessment, with midwife and client engaging in a relationship that aims to be empowering for the client, maximising her involvement, and endeavouring to promote an atmosphere of mutual trust and respect. The essence of providing effective care to the young pregnant woman is to first examine one's own beliefs and attitudes to teenagers and teenage pregnancy. It is crucial that the midwife likes teenagers and is willing to be their strongest advocate. She or he must be free from the historical beliefs and myths regarding teenage pregnancy and avoid becoming involved in patronising or stigmatising dialogue. Such dialogue serves only to alienate the woman, and once this occurs, it will be virtually impossible to retrace one's steps in order to develop a relationship of mutual trust and respect.

Individualised care provides an excellent opportunity to build effective relationships based on open communication. An atmosphere of mutual trust and respect should be the goal, so that care is effective, productive and rewarding. When the teenage woman has developed a strong sense of this occurring, she is perhaps more likely to listen to advice, change some aspects of her lifestyle or make serious attempts to do so. Gillian Checkley (1990, p. 26) makes a valuable point when she states: 'Teenagers respond well to sincerity, they don't expect you to be always right but they do expect honesty'.

At 'The Warehouse', antenatal care is provided predominantly by two midwives. This allows for greater continuity of care and is crucial if we are to succeed in building a therapeutic trusting relationship that promotes the teenagers' personal growth, self-esteem and knowledge.

Low technology

Minimal appropriate technology is available on site; routine ultrasound, for example, is not provided. Clients are referred to a visiting obstetrician for any assessment or intervention if it is required. The first antenatal visit takes place, together with the maternity booking-in procedure, at Nepean Hospital with the primary midwife involved in the 'The Warehouse' program and a medical officer.

Psychosocial support

One midwife has a full-time commitment for psychosocial support of the women throughout their pregnancies and the early months of parenting. By making early and regular contact as problems arise, admission rates and length of stay for this previously high-risk group are kept to a minimum.

Midwives in 'The Warehouse' program are aware that they must provide care that meets each person's individual needs, including support, information, encouragement, advocacy and empowerment, through working in partnership with each woman. Through this approach to midwifery services for pregnant teenagers, the health of the women and their babies is promoted.

For further information, contact 'The Warehouse', 20 Belmore Street, Penrith NSW 2750. Tel: (02) 4721 8330

Pat Brodie
Midwife

approach to health promotion in which action is planned separately from the community and implemented as an intervention. While both approaches may have important roles to play in promoting health, the imposition of centrally planned health promotion at the expense of local responses to local need can present real problems for health workers attempting to work from a Primary Health Care approach. Similarly, the particular approach taken by local managers will influence the ways in which you can work for health promotion. You will need to work with the realities of your own particular working environment, although you may also be working to change that reality if it does not sit comfortably with a Primary Health Care approach or the needs of your community.

The term 'health promotion program' is used to describe a combination of health promotion activities designed to address a particular need. You may decide that the need you are addressing can be dealt with appropriately by one local health promotion activity or a program consisting of a series of local activities, or that it will require a major national or international campaign. Alternatively, you may plan to design a local program to tie in with a national or State campaign if it is relevant to your area.

When you are planning health promotion, there are several key issues you will need to address. These will be useful for you and your partners in the process enabling you to effectively prepare and implement your ideas. In addition, your own administrators or funding bodies may want to have much of this information to judge the merits of your activity or decide if they will support your plans.

Some of the detail of what will need to be planned will vary depending on the issue you are addressing and the strategy you decide to be most appropriate. For example, if you decide that health education is the most appropriate response, there will be some issues specific to health education that may need consideration. This section, however, will consider the issues common to any health promotion action. Also, the specific details required by the organisation to whom you are accountable may vary, but the sets of issues below should be generally applicable.

To plan health promotion effectively, you will need to:
• assess the needs of the population or community to whom you are responsible;
• prioritise the needs or issues you find;
• examine in some detail the particular issue you are going to act on;
• identify your critical reference group;
• set aims and objectives;
• decide the most appropriate response to the problem;
• calculate what resources you will need in order to act effectively;
• plan how you will evaluate your activity.

Of course, planning is not a simple linear process, and the order in which the above steps occur will vary according to the particular situation. Moreover, it is worthwhile to note once again the fine line between all stages of assessment, planning, implementation and evaluation. Indeed, the steps described above may themselves be part of the action of health promotion in some situations, and are not limited to the planning process.

Examine in detail the issue you are planning to act on

In Chapter 3 we examined needs assessment and discussed the need to set priorities on the issues identified to determine which issue or issues you will address first. When priorities have been set, you will need to examine in more detail each issue you are going to address. This will require you to draw together as much relevant information as possible. It will also require critical discussion of the issue by the people involved (that is, community members, other health workers and anyone else who has concerns about the issue) so that you can review the issue and determine just what the problem is. This is necessary to ensure that the strategies you then choose for addressing the problem are the most appropriate. This examining of a problem in order to move beyond immediate perceptions to a more complete analysis was also discussed in Chapter 3.

Conducting a literature review may enable you to find out more about the problem or issues you are dealing with. It may also enable you to find out how other people have dealt with similar issues if others have already developed a program to meet a similar need. You can then learn from their experiences and mistakes so as to build on their program, or adapt it to meet your needs. Of particular value here is the Health Education and Promotion System (HEAPS), a database containing details of previously developed health promotion programs from around Australia.

Determine your critical reference, host or target group

To ensure that you are addressing an issue in the most appropriate way, you will need to clarify just whose needs the particular program is designed to address. For example, an approach that is relevant to a group of teenagers is unlikely to be relevant to a group of older people living in a nursing home. Even if you are addressing a health need that is relevant to an entire community, you may need to take a slightly different approach to work appropriately with different groups within the community. Most commonly, the group that a particular health promotion program is designed for is known as the target group.

Unfortunately, however, the term 'target group' gives the impression that people are passive and waiting to be 'hit' by the program being implemented. As Yoland Wadsworth (1997, p. 16) has described, this approach regards people as 'sitting ducks'. Such an approach to people does not sit comfortably with Primary Health Care. For this reason, and to encapsulate the importance of the collaboration of people themselves in the planning and implementation of health promotion activity, the term 'critical reference group' has been coined to refer to the group of people for whom a project is designed (Wadsworth 1997, pp. 15–17).

Another term, 'host community', has been coined to refer to the community with whom you are working in community development. This term reflects the fact that you are involved with the community at their request — the community

HEAPS

HEAPS, the National Health Promotion Database, is an easy-to-use computer-based library of information about health promotion resources, projects and programs developed by agencies in the primary health care field. It is an excellent way for health promoters to tap into the growing field of health promotion and avoid reinventing the wheel by learning from others' experience.

The HEAPS project was established in response to the recommendations of the Australian Health Ministers' Conference in April 1985, which identified the lack of well organised and easily accessible information as one of the major obstacles to the growth of health promotion in Australia.

The HEAPS database has developed from the contributions of primary health care practitioners. When an agency has developed a health education or health promotion program, they can complete a summary report of the project, and this information is included in the database. In this way, the database has steadily increased to the size it is today, with over 6000 entries. In this way, HEAPS provides an opportunity for health promotion practitioners to share ideas, resources, program planning and evaluation instruments or protocols. This has been particularly useful with the shift from health education to a more comprehensive approach to sustainable health promotion programs, and the increased expectation that health workers have good planning, evaluation and research skills.

The HEAPS database aims to capture the breadth and diversity of current activities in the Australian health promotion field. HEAPS aims to improve health promotion by:
- building a network of people involved in health promotion;
- documenting their projects and activities;
- enabling the sharing of health promotion ideas and information;
- enhancing health workers' planning skills through training, networking and highlighting examples of good practice;
- improving the coordination of programs across the health promotion field.

HEAPS is supported by health promotion training workshops designed to enhance participants' understanding of key health promotion concepts and to develop their skills in applying these concepts to their work. The action learning workshops focus on how to plan, document, implement and evaluate health promotion activity and how to use the HEAPS for Windows database. Goals and activities of the workshops can be tailored to meet local needs and conditions.

By participating in the HEAPS network, individuals and organisations can:
- share the benefits of what has been learnt by others working in health promotion;
- add to the body of knowledge on good practice in health promotion;
- raise the profile of organisations involved in health promotion;
- be recognised by peers for contribution to the field of health promotion.

Health promoters can benefit by accessing HEAPS during conceptual thinking, planning and evaluation. It is at these times that reviewing others' work can challenge practitioners to think more creatively about possible approaches.

HEAPS is dependent on individuals and organisations subscribing to the database and contributing information. For the past 4 years, considerable effort has been invested in expanded content for HEAPS. This includes specific indicators covering rationale, literature reviews, achieved or anticipated outcomes, what has or hasn't worked and evaluation status of the project.

Contribution to HEAPS is best during the different phases of implementation and evaluation; that is, firstly, when program planning is documented, secondly, throughout the various stages of the implementation, and thirdly, during evaluation. Participating in this ongoing way enables others to see the living development of health promotion, and contributing to the HEAPS network in this way provides a sense of contributing to the national effort of developing health promotion as a discipline.

As of December 1997, the Commonwealth Health Department stopped funding the HEAPS project. Contributions from the health promotion field, however, continue to be collected and annual updates to the existing HEAPS database disseminated.

At the same time, Prometheus Information, the coordinators of the project, are committed to maintaining and further developing HEAPS, in collaboration with the health promotion sector across Australia, in response to the growing requirements of health promotion practice. The HEAPS project is unique nationally and globally. Every effort will be invested into ensuring the intent behind its establishment will be maintained and facilitated by Prometheus Information.

Further information about HEAPS can be obtained from the national coordinator at:

> Prometheus Information
> PO Box 160
> Dickson ACT 2602.
> Tel: 02 6257 7356, Fax: 02 6241 5284
> email: heaps@prometheus.com.au
> Web site: http://www.prometheus.com.au

Alison Miles
Promotion Coordinator
Prometheus Information

is 'hosting' you. This is one more attempt to break free of the disempowering connotations of the term 'target group'. Unfortunately, the term 'host community' is not relevant to all situations and the term 'critical reference group' is somewhat cumbersome and perhaps more directly relevant to evaluation alone, for which it was originally coined. Nonetheless, these two suggested terms constitute important attempts to replace the term 'target group' and the approach it represents.

Clarifying for whom your project or activity is being developed needs to go hand in hand with determining what the problem is. Indeed, these two steps are inextricably linked, as the people for whom the project is developing need to be involved in its development. How this actually occurs, however, will depend very much on the situation. You will need to determine how it can most appropriately occur in each particular instance.

It is important to note that there will be times when the individual or group for whom the action is designed may not be the individual or group with whom you need to work, although they will in these circumstances remain the people for whom you will work. For example, educating local councillors about the dangers of certain environmental toxins used in local industries may be of benefit to members of the community living near those industries if changes occur as a result. In this case, the critical reference group is the community members, not the local councillors. This distinction between who will benefit from the action and whom the action is directed towards is an important one.

Decide how you will respond

Once you feel you have a good understanding of the problem, you will be able to decide on the most appropriate way to respond. Doing this is not a simple task and there are no tricks of the trade to make it easy. As Egger, Spark & Lawson (1990, p. 120) have stated, 'it all depends'. This is the point at which you will have to rely on your assessment skills and judgment, and those of the people with whom you are working. However, the more thoroughly you have examined the issue itself, the more likely you are to be able to respond appropriately. This does not mean that the assessment process must go on interminably, but rather that you must aim to be comprehensive.

As a general rule, addressing an issue on several different levels will increase the likelihood that you will be successful. In deciding on what level or levels you need to work, the *Ottawa Charter for Health Promotion* can be a useful guide. Can you act to work for healthy public policy to address the need? Is there some other way in which you can work for more supportive environments? Will you need to encourage and support community action? Can you help people further develop their own skills in dealing with the issue? Do you need to work for a reorientation of the system so that more emphasis is put on the prevention of this problem?

Take some time to consider (perhaps through brainstorming with the community members involved or some of your colleagues) which strategies you could implement to address the problem on each of these levels. This is a good way of ensuring that you do not assume that the most appropriate strategy is education alone, an assumption that health workers often make.

Set aims and objectives

You can make clear for yourself and any funding or management bodies what you want to achieve from the program or activity by setting aims and objectives. This may occur relatively informally, with community members taking the time to decide exactly what it is they want to achieve and how they want to achieve it. It may also occur more formally, with health workers documenting aims and objectives against which the program may be evaluated.

This is one area where a great deal of apparently contradictory information has appeared in recent years. Many books on health promotion and guidelines for the development of health promotion programs outline varying combinations of goals, aims, targets and objectives, often defined differently. The following use of 'aims' and 'objectives' has been chosen for its simplicity, though it is not meant to be definitive. The key element here, which is likely to be found in any good combination of categories used, is that one is a broad statement of what you wish to achieve and the other is a more detailed explanation of the steps required to achieve it. In larger programs, other categories may need to be used to break the program activities down into manageable pieces.

An aim is a clear statement of what you wish to achieve through your program or activity. There is some disagreement among authors as to whether an aim should be a very general statement of intent or a specific measurable goal against which the program is evaluated. However that may be, it is probably valuable to establish both a general statement of intent, towards which your activity will contribute, and a more specific aim against which your action can be evaluated.

Objectives describe the steps that you will need to take in order to achieve your aim. As far as is realistically possible, they should be written in a manner that enables them to be evaluated: that is, they are specific and measurable. Objectives may describe what action will occur (e.g. an environmental action group may set objectives of writing letters to their local member of parliament, the minister for the environment and the chief executive officers of relevant companies in their local areas to express concern at pollution levels) or they may describe what changes will occur as a result of the action (e.g. the same group may set objectives of putting environmental health issues firmly on the local and State government agendas). These two types of objectives are referred to as process objectives and outcome objectives, respectively. Generally, evaluating against objectives that describe the outcomes will more readily enable you to determine if your program or activity has been effective than evaluating against objectives that simply describe the action of the protagonists, or process. While the action that occurs may be very valuable, you may want to know whether it has actually made the difference you hoped it would. Outcome objectives are extremely valuable because they enable you to do that.

Within health education, these two types of objectives are described as learner-centred and teacher-centred objectives. Teacher-centred objectives describe what the teacher will have accomplished as a result of his or her activity (e.g. the teacher will have explained the principles of effective writing), while learner-centred objectives describe the change which you hope will result (e.g. the learner will be able to write a letter for publication in the local paper). Once again you can see how the implementation of the teacher-centred objective may be important, but its value may be reduced if it does not result in the changes described by the learner-centred objective.

Objectives, then, make clear statements about what you want to achieve and how you want to achieve it. It is worth noting that the more clearly you have defined the need you are addressing, the easier it will be to set objectives for the program. This is one example of how each of the steps in planning a health promotion program or activity described here is inextricably linked to the others.

Calculate what resources you will need

You will also have to calculate just which resources you will need, to implement your ideas and what resources you already have. A key component of this is examining which skills are needed and whether staff members or community members have these skills or whether others will need to be involved to pass them on or to participate directly in the program.

It is important that you make maximum use of the skills of people who are available to work with you. Doing that makes good sense because it means effective use of resources. It may also be a positive process for community members themselves because recognition of and respect for their abilities is something most people appreciate. Also, working with community members so that they develop the skills to continue the activity will enable them to keep working for their health and will result in increasing the resources of the community.

Other health workers can also be regarded as valuable resources. For example, workplace health promotion programs implemented from outside the organisation need to actively involve any occupational health and safety workers in the organisation, as these people also have a health promotion responsibility and work in the organisation on a daily basis. Similarly, involvement of teachers in school health promotion programs, Aboriginal health workers in Aboriginal health promotion programs and local midwives or women's health nurses in women's health promotion programs will increase the chances that local people will have access to local resources and that the program will continue in the community in one form or another. Indeed, you will need to seriously consider whether these people should be leaders in health promotion activity in these areas, with other health workers acting as resources.

You will have to estimate how much time, in terms of preparation, implementation and evaluation, the program will take, so that you can make an informed decision about what it will cost the agency and decide whether it is worth the effort that will go into it. You will then be in a better position to decide whether the agency can run the program using existing resources or whether you will need to apply for additional funds. Alternatively, if the program appears too costly, it may be able to be adapted to reduce its cost. Maintaining the spirit of the program then becomes an important issue.

You will also need to consider just which physical resources you will need. This will depend very much on the particular strategy you will be using. For example, if you are planning a social action campaign, you may need access to typing and photocopying facilities, telephones and stationery. You may also need a hall for large meetings and smaller rooms for committee meetings, easily accessible to members of the community. Or, if you are planning a formal health education program, you may need teaching aids, an appropriate venue and perhaps child care facilities.

Once you have assessed which resources you require, you may need to find out which resources are available elsewhere. For example, if you decide that your plans cannot be implemented without outside assistance, you will need to find out which outside resources are available. Once again, people are probably the most valuable resources. Health promotion specialists, perhaps working in other areas of the health department, may be able to contribute a great deal of expertise. People from volunteer or self-help groups may also contribute much about the issues they face.

Another form of outside resources is money. External funding sources may be available to fund some of the activity you want to carry out. Most funding of this kind is available only at certain times of the year rather than on a continual basis, but it is well worth checking whether any funds are available at the time you need them. Keep an eye on the major newspapers in your area for details.

Plan how you will evaluate your action

Planning an evaluation is vital to the development of any health promotion program and will be an integral part of it. Evaluating what you are doing will enable you to improve what you are doing as you are doing it, thus maximising the chances that your activity will be successful. It will also enable you to report any successes and lessons learned to other people working for health promotion and to the community, funding bodies and administrators to whom you are accountable.

You will need to plan how you are going to evaluate so that you can ask the appropriate questions throughout the implementation of your activity. It will not be possible to evaluate effectively if you leave consideration of evaluation until after your activity has finished. We examined evaluation in some depth in Chapter 4, to which you are referred for more detail.

Implement your plans

When the time comes to put your plans into action, you should have a fairly strong sense of what you are doing and how you are doing it. You will need to remain flexible, however, being sensitive to the possibility that needs, circumstances and available resources may change and your responses may thus need to change. Continued communication and critique will therefore be an important component of your action.

Conclusion

In this book we have reviewed the importance of health workers promoting health, the values that should drive health promotion practice and some of the key strategies of use in working with members of the community to promote their health. In drawing those elements together to help create effective health promotion action, this chapter has provided an overview of several important issues. The challenge for each health worker lies in drawing the same elements together for the purpose of effective action based on the principles of social justice and on the right of ordinary people to make effective decisions about their lives.

References and further reading

Australian Community Health Association 1990, *Healthy Environments in the 90's: the Community Health Approach,* papers from the 3rd National Conference of the Australian Community Health Association, Australian Community Health Association, Sydney.

Bear-Wingfield, R. 1996, *Sharing Good Tucker Stories: a Guide for Aboriginal and Torres Strait Island Communities,* Commonwealth Department of Health and Family Services, Canberra.

Central Sydney Area Health Service 1994, *Program Management Guidelines for Health Promotion,* New South Wales Health Department, Sydney.

Checkley, G. 1990, 'Talking to Teenagers', *Healthright,* 9 (4), 25, 196–8.

Clark, M. A. 1984, *Facts, Myths and Stigma: a Report on Teenage Pregnancy and Parenting,* NSW Department of Health, Sydney.

Clarke, B. and MacDougall, C. (eds) 1993, *The 1993 Community Health Conference, Vol. 1, Papers and Workshops,* proceedings of the Fourth National Australian Community Health Association Conference, Australian Community Health Association, Sydney.

Cox, M. 1994, *Good Practices in Women's Mental Health: Training and Resource Kit,* Healthsharing Women's Health Resource Service, Melbourne.

Egger, G., Spark, R. and Lawson, J. 1990, *Health Promotion Strategies and Methods,* McGraw-Hill, Sydney.

Ewles, L. and Simnett, I. 1999, *Promoting Health: a Practical Guide,* Bailliere Tindall in association with the Royal College of Nursing, Edinburgh.

Hawe, P., Noort, M., King, L. and Jordens, C. 1997, 'Multiplying Health Gains: the Critical Role of Capacity-Building Within Health Promotion Programs', *Health Policy,* 39, 29–42.

Johnson, S. 1992, 'Aboriginal Health Through Primary Health Care', in Gray, G. and Pratt, R. (eds), *Issues in Australian Nursing 3,* Churchill Livingstone, Melbourne.

Lorig, K. 1991, *Common Sense Patient Education,* Fraser Publications, Ivanhoe, Vic.

May, A., Herriot, M., Sinclair, A., Boyce, M. and Anear, E. 1994, *Developing Policies Around Primary Health Care: a Guide For Your Health Unit,* South Australian Health Commission and CHASP (SA), Adelaide.

McKenzie, J. F. and Jurs, J. L. 1993, *Planning, Implementing, and Evaluating Health Promotion Programs: a Primer,* Macmillan, New York.

Phillips-Rees, S., Sanderson, C., Herriot, M. and May, A. 1992, *The Changing Face of Health: a Primary Health Care Casebook,* South Australian Health Commission and South Australian Community Health Association, Adelaide.

Renhard, R. 1996, 'Best Practice in Health Care: Confusion and Contribution?', *Australian Journal of Primary Health – Interchange,* 2, (1), 3–8.

Ryan, P. 1992, *Cases for Change: CHASP in Practice,* Australian Community Health Association, Sydney.

Shaw, L. and Tilden, J. 1990, *Creating Health for Women: a Community Health Promotion Handbook,* Women's Health Development Program, Brisbane Women's Community Health Centre, Brisbane.

Stoker, L. 1988, *Healthy Women: an Introduction to Health for Women from Non-English-Speaking Backgrounds,* New South Wales Department of Health, Sydney.

Wadsworth, Y. 1997, *Everyday Evaluation on the Run,* Allen and Unwin, Sydney.

Conclusion

Where to from here?

Having read through this book and used the information in it to further develop your skills, where do you go from here? As has become progressively clearer throughout the preceding 10 chapters, this book can only provide an introduction to the particular skills you can use in promoting health and the approaches you can take. It is now up to you to build on this information. Some things you can do from this point on to keep developing your skills and expertise in the area of health promotion are:

- *Use the information here to develop your skills.* Put the ideas into practice and see which ones work for you and your community.
- *Keep reading about the areas covered in this book.* Each of them has a wealth of theoretical basis, and as you develop your background in the areas, you'll be more effective in developing your own theory and practice. The references and further readings at the end of each chapter is a valuable place to start.
- *Talk with your colleagues.* Discuss your ideas, your successes and your failures, with anyone who is interested to learn with you.
- *Ask questions.* Get help when you need it, and don't be afraid to ask for help. Successful people use their expertise, and the expertise of others, to its best advantage. And don't forget to include those people you are employed to serve among the people you ask questions of. The partnership with community members needs to include learning from each other as you develop.
- *Share your learning professionally, by joining professional associations, attending conferences and presenting papers on your work.* So many people who do great work fail to recognise how many people would like to hear about their work and learn from it. Don't judge your work too harshly.
- *Work together, supporting and encouraging each other and promoting the health of the team.* A great many of the strategies described in this book cannot be implemented fully if health workers themselves have not experienced the strategies themselves. This is particularly so with the empowerment strategies. Traditionally the health care system has encouraged compliance and discouraged lateral thinking and creativity. It has worked to stifle, rather than empower, people working within the health system. If you, as a health worker, do not feel able to impact on the world around you, it is going to be very difficult for you to help develop these skills in others. If you are one of these people, or you are working in a team with people with these experiences, then a vital step to working to promote the health of your community is to use these strategies within the team, to develop the team and the self-efficacy of everyone in the team. Too often health workers write each other off, ignoring the strong socialisation processes that have impacted on each other. It is not possible to ignore these health promotion issues within your own team yet achieve your potential in promoting the health of the community. Work together, supporting and encouraging each other and promoting the health of the team. The ripples of this work will be felt far beyond the confines of the staff room and you will

be able to establish a team environment that will achieve so much more than that which individuals alone may achieve.

- *Continue working to keep the development of a Primary Health Care system on the agenda, and to ensure that the system develops towards a greater emphasis on the promotion of health.* There is some important work to be done in lobbying to break up the current trend toward medicalisation of community health, which is threatening the establishment of a comprehensive Primary Health Care approach. An important component of this will be working for the continuing reorientation of undergraduate and postgraduate education of health workers and others whose actions impact on health towards a Primary Health Care approach.

Effective reorientation of the health care system to a focus on the promotion of health and the needs of the community will only come from a concerted effort by health workers and community members. Don't underestimate the importance of your role in this process. You *can* make a difference, and I wish you all the best in your health promotion work!

The Declaration of Alma-Ata

On 12 September 1978, at Alma-Ata in Soviet Kazakhstan, representatives of 134 nations agreed to the terms of a solemn Declaration pledging urgent action by all governments, all health and development workers, and the world community to protect and promote the health of all the people of the world. The climax of a major International Conference on Primary Health Care, jointly sponsored by WHO and UNICEF, this Declaration stated:

1. The conference strongly reaffirms that health, which is a state of complete physical, mental and social well-being, and not merely the absence of disease or infirmity, is a fundamental human right and that the attainment of the highest possible level of health is a most important world-wide social goal whose realisation requires the action of many other social and economic sectors in addition to the health sector.

2. The existing gross inequality in the health status of the people, particularly between developed and developing countries as well as within countries, is politically, socially and economically unacceptable and is, therefore, of common concern to all countries.

3. Economic and social development, based on a New International Economic Order, is of basic importance to the fullest attainment of health for all and to the reduction of the gap between the health status of the developing and developed countries. The promotion and protection of the health of the people is essential to sustained economic and social development and contributes to a better quality of life and to world peace.

4. The people have the right and duty to participate individually and collectively in the planning and implementation of their health care.

5. Governments have a responsibility for the health of their people which can be fulfilled only by the provision of adequate health and social measures. A main social target of governments, international organizations and the whole world community in the coming decades should be the attainment by all peoples of the world by the year 2000 of a level of health that will permit them to lead a socially and economically productive life. Primary health care is the key to attaining this target as part of development in the spirit of social justice.

6. Primary health care is essential health care based on practical, scientifically sound and socially acceptable methods and technology made universally accessible to individuals and families in the community through their full participation and at a cost that the community and country can afford to maintain at every stage of their development in the spirit of self-reliance and self-determination. It forms an integral part both of the country's health system, of which it is the central function and main focus, and of the overall social and economic development of the community. It is the first level of contact of individuals, the family and community with the national health system, bringing

health care as close as possible to where people live and work, and constitutes the first element of a continuing health care process.

7. Primary health care:

    i.   reflects and evolves from the economic conditions and socio-cultural and political characteristics of the country and its communities, and is based on the application of the relevant results of social, biomedical and health services research and public health experience;

    ii. addresses the main health problems in the community, providing promotive, preventive, curative, and rehabilitative services accordingly;

    iii. includes at least: education concerning prevailing health problems and the methods of preventing and controlling them; promotion of food supply and proper nutrition; an adequate supply of safe water and basic sanitation; maternal and child health care, including family planning; immunization against the major infectious diseases; prevention and control of locally endemic diseases; appropriate treatment of common diseases and injuries; and provision of essential drugs;

    iv. involves, in addition to the health sector, all related sectors and aspects of national and community development, in particular agriculture, animal husbandry, food, industry, education, housing, public works, communication and other sectors; and demands the coordinated efforts of all those sectors;

    v. requires and promotes maximum community and individual self-reliance and participation in the planning, organization, operation and control of primary health care, making fullest use of local, national and other available resources, and to this end develops through appropriate education the ability of communities to participate;

    vi. should be sustained by integrated, functional and mutually supportive referral systems, leading to the progressive improvement of comprehensive health care for all, and giving priority to those most in need;

    vii. relies, at local and referral levels, on health workers, including physicians, nurses, midwives, auxiliaries and community workers as applicable, as well as traditional practitioners as needed, suitably trained socially and technically to work as a health team and to respond to the expressed health needs of the community.

8. All governments should formulate national policies, strategies and plans of action to launch and sustain primary health care as part of a comprehensive national health system and in coordination with other sectors. To this end, it will be necessary to exercise political will, to mobilize the country's resources and to use available external resources rationally.

9. All countries should cooperate in a spirit of partnership and service to ensure primary health care for all people since the attainment of health by people in any one country directly concerns and benefits every other country. In this context the joint WHO/UNICEF report on primary health care constitutes a solid basis for the further development and operation of primary health care throughout the world.

10. An acceptable level of health for all the people of the world by the year 2000 can be attained through a fuller and better use of the world's resources, a

considerable part of which is now spent on armaments and military conflicts. A genuine policy of independence, peace, détente and disarmament could and should release additional resources that could well be devoted to peaceful aims and in particular to the acceleration of social and economic development of which primary health care, as an essential part, should be allotted its proper share.

The International Conference on Primary Health Care calls for urgent and effective national and international action to develop and implement primary health care throughout the world and particularly in developing countries in a spirit of technical cooperation and in keeping with a New International Economic Order. It urges governments, WHO and UNICEF, and other international organizations, as well as multilateral and bilateral agencies, non-governmental organizations, funding agencies, all health workers and the whole world community to support national and international commitment to primary health care and to channel increased technical and financial support to it, particularly in developing countries. The Conference calls on all the aforementioned to collaborate in introducing, developing and maintaining primary health care in accordance with the spirit and content of this Declaration.

World Health Organization 1978, The Declaration of Alma-Ata, *World Health*, August/September 1988, 16–17.

The Ottawa Charter for Health Promotion

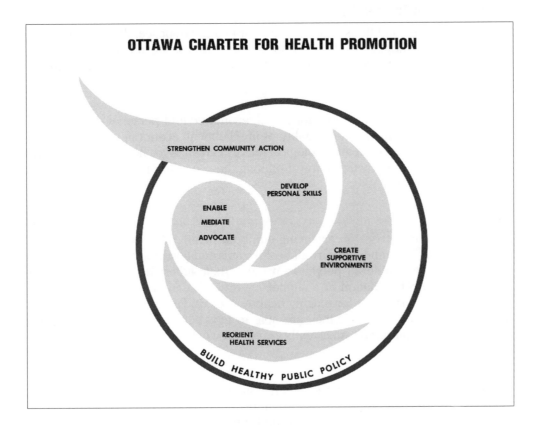

The first International Conference on Health Promotion, meeting in Ottawa this 21st day of November 1986, hereby presents this CHARTER for action to achieve Health for All by the year 2000 and beyond.

This conference was primarily a response to growing expectations for a new public health movement around the world. Discussions focused on the needs in industrialized countries, but took into account similar concerns in all other regions. It built on the progress made through the Declaration on Primary Health Care at Alma Ata, the World Health Organization's Targets for Health for All document, and the recent debate at the World Health Assembly on intersectoral action for health.

Health promotion

Health promotion is the process of enabling people to increase control over, and to improve, their health. To reach a state of complete physical, mental and social well-being, an individual or group must be able to identify and to realize aspirations, to satisfy needs, and to change or cope with the environment. Health is, therefore, seen as a resource for everyday life, not the objective of living. Health is a positive concept emphasizing social and personal resources, as well as physical capacities. Therefore, health promotion is not just the responsibility of the health sector, but goes beyond healthy lifestyles to well-being.

Prerequisites for health

The fundamental conditions and resources for health are peace, shelter, education, food, income, a stable ecosystem, sustainable resources, social justice and equity. Improvement in health requires a secure foundation in these basic prerequisites.

Advocate

Good health is a major resource for social, economic and personal development and an important dimension of quality of life. Political, economic, social, cultural, environmental, behavioral and biological factors can all favor health or be harmful to it. Health promotion action aims at making these conditions favorable through advocacy for health.

Enable

Health promotion focuses on achieving equity in health. Health promotion action aims at reducing differences in current health status and ensuring equal opportunities and resources to enable all people to achieve their fullest health potential. This includes a secure foundation in a supportive environment, access to information, life skills and opportunities for making healthy choices. People cannot achieve their fullest health potential unless they are able to take control of those things which determine their health. This must apply equally to women and men.

Mediate

The prerequisites and prospects for health cannot be ensured by the health sector alone. More importantly, health promotion demands coordinated action by all concerned: by governments, by health and other social and economic sectors, by non-governmental and voluntary organizations, by local authorities, by industry and by the media. People in all walks of life are involved as individuals, families and communities. Professional and social groups and health personnel have a major responsibility to mediate between differing interests in society for the pursuit of health.

Health promotion strategies and programmes should be adapted to the local needs and possibilities of individual countries and regions to take into account differing social, cultural and economic systems.

Health promotion action means:

Build healthy public policy

Health promotion goes beyond health care. It puts health on the agenda of policy makers in all sectors and at all levels, directing them to be aware of the health consequences of their decisions and to accept their responsibilities for health.

Health promotion policy combines diverse but complementary approaches including legislation, fiscal measures, taxation and organizational change. It is coordinated action that leads to health, income and social policies that foster greater equity. Joint action contributes to ensuring safer and healthier goods and services, healthier public services, and cleaner, more enjoyable environments.

Health promotion policy requires the identification of obstacles to the adoption of healthy public policies in non-health sectors, and ways of removing them. The aim must be to make the healthier choice the easier choice for policy makers as well.

Create supportive environments

Our societies are complex and interrelated. Health cannot be separated from other goals. The inextricable links between people and their environment constitutes the basis for a socio-ecological approach to health. The overall guiding principle for the world, nations, regions and communities alike, is the need to encourage reciprocal maintenance — to take care of each other, our communities and our natural environment. The conservation of natural resources throughout the world should be emphasized as a global responsibility.

Changing patterns of life, work and leisure have a significant impact on health. Work and leisure should be a source of health for people. The way society organizes work should help create a healthy society. Health promotion generates living and working conditions that are safe, stimulating, satisfying and enjoyable.

Systematic assessment of the health impact of a rapidly changing environment — particularly in areas of technology, work, energy production and urbanization — is essential and must be followed by action to ensure positive benefit to the health of the public. The protection of the natural and built environments and the conservation of natural resources must be addressed in any health promotion strategy.

Strengthen community action

Health promotion works through concrete and effective community action in setting priorities, making decisions, planning strategies and implementing them to achieve better health. At the heart of this process is the empowerment of communities, their ownership and control of their own endeavors and destinies.

Community development draws on existing human and material resources in the community to enhance self-help and social support, and to develop flexible systems for strengthening public participation and direction of health matters. This requires full and continuous access to information, learning opportunities for health, as well as funding support.

Develop personal skills

Health promotion supports personal and social development through providing information, education for health and enhancing life skills. By so doing, it increases the options available to people to exercise more control over their own health and over their environments, and to make choices conducive to health.

Enabling people to learn throughout life, to prepare themselves for all of its stages and to cope with chronic illness and injuries is essential. This has to be facilitated in school, home, work and community settings. Action is required through educational, professional, commercial and voluntary bodies, and within the institutions themselves.

Reorient health services

The responsibility for health promotion in health services is shared among individuals, community groups, health professionals, health service institutions and governments. They must work together towards a health care system which contributes to the pursuit of health.

The role of the health sector must move increasingly in a health promotion direction, beyond its responsibility for providing clinical and curative services. Health services need to embrace an expanded mandate which is sensitive and respects cultural needs. This mandate should support the needs of individuals and communities for a healthier life, and open channels between the health sector and broader social, political, economic and physical environmental components.

Reorienting health services also requires stronger attention to health research as well as changes in professional education and training. This must lead to a change of attitude and organization of health services, which refocuses on the total needs of the individual as a whole person.

Moving into the future

Health is created and lived by people within the settings of their everyday life; where they learn, work, play and love. Health is created by caring for oneself and others, by being able to take decisions and have control over one's life circumstances, and by ensuring that the society one lives in creates conditions that allow the attainment of health by all its members.

Caring, holism and ecology are essential issues in developing strategies for health promotion. Therefore, those involved should take as a guiding principle that, in each phase of planning, implementation and evaluation of health promotion activities, women and men should become equal partners.

Commitment to health promotion

The participants in this conference pledge:
* to move into the arena of healthy public policy, and to advocate a clear political commitment to health and equity in all sectors;
* to counteract the pressures towards harmful products, resource depletion, unhealthy living conditions and environments, and bad nutrition; and to focus attention on public health issues such as pollution, occupational hazards, housing and settlements;
* to respond to the health gap within and between societies, and to tackle the inequities in health produced by the rules and practices of these societies;
* to acknowledge people as the main health resource; to support and enable them to keep themselves, their families and friends healthy through financial and other means, and to accept the community as the essential voice in matters of its health, living conditions and well-being;
* to reorient health services and their resources towards the promotion of health; and to share power with other sectors, other disciplines and most importantly with people themselves;
* to recognize health and its maintenance as a major social investment and challenge; and to address the overall ecological issue of our ways of living.

The conference urges all concerned to join them in their commitment to a strong public health alliance.

Call for international action

The Conference calls on the World Health Organization and other international organizations to advocate the promotion of health in all appropriate forums and to support countries in setting up strategies and programmes for health promotion.

The Conference is firmly convinced that if people in all walks of life, non-governmental and voluntary organizations, governments, the World Health Organization and all other bodies concerned join forces in introducing strategies for health promotion, in line with the moral and social values that form the basis of this CHARTER, Health For All by the year 2000 will become a reality.

This CHARTER for action was developed and adopted by an international conference, jointly organized by the World Health Organization, Health and Welfare Canada and the Canadian Public Health Association. Two hundred and twelve participants from 38 countries met from November 17 to 21, 1986, in Ottawa, Canada to exchange experiences and share knowledge of health promotion.

The Conference stimulated an open dialog among lay, health and other professional workers, among representatives of governmental, voluntary and community organizations, and among politicians, administrators, academics and practitioners. Participants coordinated their efforts and came to a clearer definition of the major challenges ahead. They strengthened their individual and collective commitment to the common goal of Health for All by the year 2000.

This CHARTER for action reflects the spirit of earlier public charters through which the needs of people were recognized and acted upon. The CHARTER presents fundamental strategies and approaches for health promotion which the participants considered vital for major progress. The Conference report develops the issues raised, gives concrete examples and practical suggestions regarding how real advances can be achieved, and outlines the action required of countries and relevant groups.

The move towards a new public health is now evident worldwide. This was reaffirmed not only by the experiences but by the pledges of Conference participants who were invited as individuals on the basis of their expertise. The following countries were represented: Antigua, Australia, Austria, Belgium, Bulgaria, Canada, Czechoslovakia, Denmark, Eire, England, Finland, France, German Democratic Republic, Federal Republic of Germany, Ghana, Hungary, Iceland, Israel, Italy, Japan, Malta, Netherlands, New Zealand, Northern Ireland, Norway, Poland, Portugal, Romania, St. Kitts-Nevis, Scotland, Spain, Sudan, Sweden, Switzerland, Union of Soviet Socialist Republics, United States of America, Wales and Yugoslavia.

APPENDIX 3

The Jakarta Declaration on Leading Health Promotion into the 21st Century

Preamble

The 4th International Conference on Health Promotion—*New Players for a New Era: Leading Health Promotion into the 21st Century*, meeting in Jakarta from 21 to 25 July 1997 has come at a critical moment in the development of international strategies for health. It is almost 20 years since the World Health Organization's member states made an ambitious commitment to a global strategy for *Health for All*, and the principles of primary health care through the *Declaration of Alma-Ata*. It is 11 years since the First International Conference on Health Promotion was held in Ottawa, Canada. That conference resulted in proclamation of the *Ottawa Charter for Health Promotion*, which has been a source of guidance and inspiration for health promotion since that time. Subsequent international conferences and meetings have further clarified the relevance and meaning of key strategies in health promotion, including healthy public policy (Adelaide, Australia, 1988), and supportive environments for health (Sundsvall, Sweden, 1991).

The Fourth International Conference on Health Promotion is the first to be held in a developing country, and the first to involve the private sector in supporting health promotion. It has provided an opportunity to reflect on what has been learned about effective health promotion, to re-examine the determinants of health, and to identify the directions and strategies that must be adopted to address the challenges of promoting health in the 21st century.

The participants in the Jakarta Conference hereby present this declaration on action for health promotion into the next century.

Health promotion is a key investment

Health is a basic human right and is essential for social and economic development.

Increasingly, health promotion is being recognised as an essential element of health development. It is a process of enabling people to increase control over, and to improve, their health. Health promotion, through investment and action, has a marked impact on the determinants of health so as to create the greatest health gain for people, to contribute significantly to the reduction of inequities in health, to further human rights, and to build social capital. The ultimate goal is to increase health expectancy, and to narrow the gap in health expectancy between countries and groups.

The Jakarta Declaration on Health Promotion offers a vision and focus for health promotion into the next century. It reflects the firm commitment of participants in the Fourth International Conference on Health Promotion to draw upon the widest possible range of resources to tackle health determinants in the 21st century.

Determinants of health: new challenges

The prerequisites for health are peace, shelter, education, social security, social relations, food, income, empowerment of women, a stable ecosystem, sustainable resource use, social justice, respect for human rights and equity. Above all, poverty is the greatest threat to health.

Demographic trends such as urbanisation, an increase in the number of older people and the high prevalence of chronic diseases pose new problems in all countries. Other social, behavioural and biological changes such as increased sedentary behaviour, resistance to antibiotics and other commonly available drugs, increased drug abuse, and civil and domestic violence, threaten the health and well-being of hundreds of millions of people.

New and re-emerging infectious diseases, and the greater recognition of mental health problems, require an urgent response. It is vital that approaches to health promotion evolve to meet changes in the determinants of health.

Transnational factors also have a significant impact on health. These include the integration of the global economy, financial markets and trade, wide access to media and communications technology, and environmental degradation as a result of the irresponsible use of resources.

These changes shape people's values, their lifestyles throughout the lifespan, and living conditions across the world. Some have great potential for health, such as the development of communications technology, while others, such as international trade in tobacco, have a major negative impact.

Health promotion makes a difference

Research and case studies from around the world provide convincing evidence that health promotion is effective. Health promotion strategies can develop and change lifestyles, and have an impact on the social, economic and environmental conditions that determine health. Health promotion is a practical approach to achieving greater equity in health.

The five strategies set out in the Ottawa Charter for Health Promotion are essential for success:
• build healthy public policy;
• create supportive environments;
• strengthen community action;
• develop personal skills;
• re-orient health services.

There is now clear evidence that:
• **comprehensive approaches to health development are the most effective —** those which use combinations of the five strategies are more effective than single track approaches;

- **particular settings offer practical opportunities for the implementation of comprehensive strategies** — these include mega-cities, islands, cities, municipalities, local communities, markets, schools, the workplace, and health care facilities;
- **participation is essential to sustain efforts** — people have to be at the centre of health promotion action and decision-making processes for it to be effective;
- **health learning fosters participation** — access to education and information is essential to achieving effective participation and the empowerment of people and communities.

These strategies are core elements of health promotion and are relevant for all countries.

New responses are needed

To address emerging threats to health, new forms of action are needed. The challenge for the coming years will be to unlock the potential for health promotion inherent in many sectors of society, among local communities and within families.

There is a clear need to break through traditional boundaries within government sectors, between government and non-government organisations, and between the public and private sectors. Co-operation is essential; this requires the creation of new partnerships for health, on an equal footing between the different sectors at all levels of governance in societies.

Priorities for health promotion in the 21st century

1. Promote social responsibility for health

Decision-makers must be firmly committed to social responsibility. Both the public and private sectors should promote health by pursuing policies and practices that:
- avoid harming the health of individuals;
- protect the environment and ensure sustainable use of resources;
- restrict production of and trade in inherently harmful goods and substances such as tobacco and armaments, as well as unhealthy marketing practices;
- safeguard both the citizen in the marketplace and the individual in the workplace;
- include equity-focused health impact assessments as an integral part of policy development.

2. Increase investments for health development

In many countries, current investment in health is inadequate and often ineffective. Increasing investment for health development requires a truly multi-sectoral approach, including, for example, additional resources for education and housing as well as for the health sector. Greater investment for health and re-orientation of existing investments, both within and among countries, has the potential to achieve significant advances in human development, health and quality of life.

Investments for health should reflect the needs of particular groups such as women, children, older people, indigenous, poor and marginalised populations.

3. Consolidate and expand partnerships for health

Health promotion requires partnerships for health and social development between the different sectors at all levels of governance and society. Existing partnerships need to be strengthened and the potential for new partnerships must be explored.

Partnerships offer mutual benefit for health through the sharing of expertise, skills and resources. Each partnership must be transparent and accountable and be based on agreed ethical principles, mutual understanding and respect. WHO guidelines should be adhered to.

4. Increase community capacity and empower the individual

Health promotion is carried out *by* and *with* people, not *on* or *to* people. It improves both the ability of individuals to take action, and the capacity of groups, organisations or communities to influence the determinants of health.

Improving the capacity of communities for health promotion requires practical education, leadership training and access to resources. Empowering individuals demands more consistent, reliable access to the decision-making process and the skills and knowledge essential to effect change.

Both traditional communication and the new information media support this process. Social, cultural and spiritual resources need to be harnessed in innovative ways.

5. Secure an infrastructure for health promotion

To secure an infrastructure for health promotion, new mechanisms of funding it locally, nationally and globally must be found. Incentives should be developed to influence the actions of governments, non-governmental organisations, educational institutions and the private sector to make sure that resource mobilisation for health promotion is maximised.

'Settings for health' represent the organisational base of the infrastructure required for health promotion. New health challenges mean that new and diverse networks need to be created to achieve intersectoral collaboration. Such networks should provide mutual assistance within and among countries and facilitate exchange of information on which strategies have proved effective in which settings.

Training in and practice of local leadership skills should be encouraged in order to support health promotion activities. Documentation of experiences in health promotion through research and project reporting should be enhanced to improve planning, implementation and evaluation.

All countries should develop the appropriate political, legal, educational, social and economic environments required to support health promotion.

Call for action

The participants in this conference are committed to sharing the key messages of the Jakarta Declaration with their governments, institutions and communities, putting the actions proposed into practice, and reporting back to the Fifth International Conference on Health Promotion.

In order to speed progress towards global health promotion, the participants endorse the formation of a global health promotion alliance. The goal of this alliance is to advance the priorities for action in health promotion set out in this declaration.

Priorities for the alliance include:

* raising awareness of the changing determinants of health;
* supporting the development of collaboration and networks for health development;
* mobilising resources for health promotion;
* accumulating knowledge on best practice;
* enabling shared learning;
* promoting solidarity in action;
* fostering transparency and public accountability in health promotion.

National governments are called upon to take initiative in fostering and sponsoring networks for health promotion both within and among their countries.

The participants call on WHO to take the lead in building such a global health promotion alliance and enabling its member states to implement the outcomes of the conference. A key part of this role is for WHO to engage governments, non-governmental organisations, development banks, organisations of the United Nations system, inter-regional bodies, bilateral agencies, the labour movement and cooperatives, as well as the private sector in advancing the priorities for action in health promotion.

World Health Organization, *Health Promotion International,* 12 (4), pp. 261–4.

APPENDIX 4

Annotated bibliography — practice examples from around Australia

Books

Baum, F. (ed.) 1995, *Health For All: the South Australian Experience,* Wakefield Press, Kent Town, SA.

This edited book sets out to document South Australia's progress in its 20-year commitment to the Primary Health Care approach. After examining the policy context in South Australia, 23 chapters then each examine a different aspect of the work in South Australia, ranging from exploration of how certain principles of Primary Health Care were implemented, such as community participation, through the responses to the needs of population groups, such as Aboriginal people, to the approaches taken to address particular health problems, such as injury.

Its presentation of the bigger picture, through examining the effects of practice over a longer time frame and in a supportive policy environment, gives the reader a strong sense of what can be achieved using the Primary Health Care approach over a longer time frame.

Bear-Wingfield, R. 1996, *Sharing Good Tucker Stories: a Guide for Aboriginal and Torres Strait Island Communities,* Commonwealth Department of Health and Family Services, Canberra.

This book presents an overview of Aboriginal health and the issues affecting it and explains the processes of developing a nutrition program. It then presents the stories of 11 Aboriginal communities from around Australia in planning, implementing and evaluating community food and nutrition programs. The stories are written by the indigenous health workers involved in the programs and reflect positive community approaches to health and nutrition. The book concludes with a section on funding submissions and a useful reference list.

Butler, P., Legge, D., Wilson, G. and Wright, M. 1995, *Towards Best Practice in Primary Health Care,* Centre for Development and Innovation in Health, Northcote, Vic.

This working paper includes an annotated bibliography of 185 case studies of Primary Health Care, chosen for their contribution to our understanding of what constitutes best practice in primary health care. The document itself is one of a series produced by CDIH as part of their Best Practice in Primary Health Care project. The case studies are listed under a variety of subject headings and cross-referenced to other subjects in the index.

Butler, P. (ed.) 1994, *Innovation and Excellence in Community Health,* Centre for Development and Innovation in Health, Northcote, Vic.

This booklet presents the stories of 13 Victorian Primary Health Care and health promotion projects, winners of the first Awards for Excellence and Innovation in Community Health, an initiative of the Victorian Community Health Association and the Centre for Development and Innovation in Community Health. Each example is a story of innovative practice, conducted within the context of a community health centre or other community based organisation. Each story represents a winning project in one of a number of categories and, as they have been judged by peers as award winning work, it is little wonder that they are exciting community health practice examples.

Butler, P. and Cass, S. (eds) 1993, *Case Studies of Community Development in Health,* Centre for Development and Innovation in Health, Northcote, Vic.

After briefly exploring the principles of community development, this book presents 16 case studies of community development in Victoria, New South Wales, South Australia and Queensland, written by people actively involved in the process, either as workers or as local residents. While all of the case studies represent good Primary Health Care practice, they each reflect the principles of community development to varying degrees. As a result, the book provides an opportunity for readers to analyse community development principles in practice.

Ellis, R. (ed.) 1996, *Indigenous Health Promotion Resources: a National Information Guide for Aboriginal and Torres Strait Islander Health Workers,* Aboriginal and Islander Health Worker Journal, Sydney.

This booklet lists over 500 resources designed specifically for Aboriginal and Torres Strait Islander people and of use in indigenous health promotion, from pamphlets and posters to cross-cultural education packages. The resources are categorised under 72 different headings. Each resource listed is briefly described and contact details to obtain copies of the resources are provided.

Gill, M. and Cobb, J. 1994, *The Power to Change: Interviews with Projects Funded by the NSW National Women's Health Program, 1989-1993,* NSW Department of Health, Sydney.

This booklet presents 18 case studies of women's health practice from around New South Wales. As examples of good women's health practice, they are also good examples of Primary Health Care at work.

Hanrick, P. (ed.) 1996, *Better All Round: Best Practice in Queensland Primary Health Care,* Community Health Association Queensland, Brisbane.

This booklet presents 24 brief summaries of Primary Health Care practice in Queensland, linking them to various aspects of the Community Health Accreditation and Standards program.

Health Advancement Standing Committee, National Health and Medical Research Council 1996, *Promoting the Health of Australians: Case Studies of Achievements in Improving the Health of the Population,* **Australian Government Publishing Service, Canberra.**

This monograph, produced as part of the 1996 review of infrastructure support for health promotion in Australia, examines six case studies of Australia's achievements in improving population health, in the areas of smoking and tobacco control, road injury and trauma, cervical cancer, cardiovascular disease, HIV/ AIDS and asthma. The monograph identifies that these areas were chosen because they have been identified as being preventable, they have been the targets of 20 years of concerted activity across a range of levels, there is evidence that health outcomes in these areas have improved over the last 20 years and information on the Australian experience with these problems is available. Thus, while there is a focus on these specific areas, each case study presents a review of both the process and outcome of public health activity in these areas over a 20-year period, emphasising the importance of a range of different strategies to address the cause of the problem, the active contribution of the health sector and the importance of work with and by other sectors. As a review of 20 years of activity on specific illnesses, these case studies represent a perspective quite different to those presented in most of the other publications listed here.

Health Advancement Standing Committee, National Health and Medical Research Council 1996, *Promoting the Health of Aboriginal and Torres Strait Island Communities: Case Studies and Principles of Good Practice,* **Australian Government Publishing Service, Canberra.**

This booklet, prepared as part of the 1996 review of infrastructure support for Indigenous health promotion in Australia, presents nine case studies of good practice among Aboriginal and Torres Strait Island communities in Queensland, Western Australia and New South Wales. It then presents and briefly explores six principles of good practice in indigenous health promotion — needs identified by communities; partnerships between indigenous health workers; communities and non-indigenous health workers; adequate resources and organisational support; implementation in the control of communities and Indigenous health workers; identified outcomes and sustainability.

James, C. 1996, *Asking Women: Case Studies in Women's Health,* **Queensland Women's Health Network, Brisbane.**

This booklet briefly examines the framework for women's health then presents 10 case studies of women's health practice from around Queensland. It then briefly explores some of the important issues in implementing good women's health practice.

Phillips-Rees, S., Sanderson, C., Herriott, M. and May, A. 1992, *The Changing Face of Health: a Primary Health Care Casebook,* **South Australian Health Commission, Adelaide.**

This South Australian publication begins with a critical examination of the Australian health system and presents the case for a greater reorientation to Primary Health Care. It then outlines 26 examples of good Primary Health Care practice from throughout South Australia. They reflect some of the diversity of Primary Health Care practice across a range of situations and contexts.

Ryan, P. 1992, *Cases for Change: CHASP in Practice,* **Australian Community Health Association, Sydney.**

This book provides a brief overview of the Community Health Accreditation and Standards Program, then presents 33 case studies of community health practice from New South Wales, Victoria, South Australia, Queensland and the Australian Capital Territory, each written to demonstrate one of the 10 principles around which the Community Health Accreditation and Standards Project (CHASP) is organised. Because the case studies are written to demonstrate a particular principle in the context of practice, many reflect other aspects of good practice in addition to that which they have been chosen to highlight.

Shaw, L. and Tilden, J. 1990, *Creating Health for Women: a Community Health Promotion Handbook,* **Brisbane Women's Community Health Centre, Brisbane.**

This book examines the principles of the women's health movement and the Australian context for women's health promotion, before exploring practical issues in planning, implementing and evaluating women's health promotion. It includes 17 short case studies of innovative women's health promotion practice from around Australia.

Webster, K. 1993, *Australian Case Studies in Community Development 1972–1992: an Annotated Bibliography,* **CDIH, Melbourne.**

This annotated bibliography lists and summarises over 220 published Australian examples of community development, particularly those relating to health. Examples are categorised under a number of subject headings, and cross-referenced where relevant.

Webster, K. and Wilson, G. 1993, *Mapping the Models,* **Centre for Development and Innovation in Health, Northcote, Vic.**

This book reviews the development of the Victorian Women's Health Services Program, then presents a set of 12 case studies of good women's health practice from across Victoria. These examples demonstrate the value of working *with* women in a respectful way, to together address health issues meaningfully and appropriately.

Yangulla Centre 1995, *Making It Happen: a Casebook of Primary Health Care.* **Queensland Health Central Region, Rockhampton.**

This booklet of examples was put together as a result of a Rural Health and Support, Education and Training (RHSET) grant. After briefly explaining Primary Health Care, the booklet presents 26 practice examples from rural Queensland, under four categories that make up Queensland's Primary Health Care Implementation Plan (1992). It then presents a number of suggestions for greater implementation of Primary Health Care, such as support and education for rural health workers and use of databases such as HealthWIZ. The examples presented are only very brief, so it is not possible to explore them in any depth. However, contact numbers are available for those wishing to obtain further information about the examples.

Journals

The following multidisciplinary journals are of particular value for Primary Health Care and health promotion because they focus on discussing and critically analysing practice and the theory that informs practice.

Aboriginal and Islander Health Worker Journal

This Australian journal includes a wide range of articles on indigenous health promotion and Primary Health Care practice, and interviews with people involved in contemporary indigenous issues. It also includes information about conferences and workshops of direct relevance to those working in Aboriginal and Torres Strait Islander health. From 1995–1997 the journal ran a series of articles on models of excellence in Indigenous community health.

Australian and New Zealand Journal of Public Health

This refereed journal, the official journal of the Public Health Association of Australia, contains predominantly research articles on public health and health promotion from Australia and New Zealand, as well as some comparative articles examining other countries. It also contains editorial comment on contemporary public health issues by Australian experts.

Australian Journal of Primary Health – Interchange

This Australian refereed journal, the official journal of the Victorian Community Health Association, includes a wide range of material of value to practitioners. In addition to key academic papers on issues relevant to Primary Health Care, the journal regularly documents practice examples in a 'Community Health Live' section. The Journal regularly lists upcoming conferences and reviews books of interest to Primary Health Care practitioners. The Journal also publishes papers from Awards for Innovation and Excellence in Primary Health Care (see, e.g. Vol. 3, nos 2 and 3, 1997).

The Community Development Journal

This international refereed journal, with its focus on theory and practice in community development, has much to offer the reader looking to understand the challenges in community development and other community participation approaches.

Community Quarterly

This Australian journal focuses on community development practice, with short, readable examples from practitioners of their experiences of community development.

Health Education Research and Health Education Quarterly

These two international refereed journals, while focusing on health education, include some articles that address the broader range of issues that arise in health promotion.

Health Promotion International

This international refereed journal publishes articles describing and critically examining health promotion practice and the theory that underpins practice, predominantly from industrialised countries around the world. In addition to the regular smattering of Australian articles published here, many of the papers from other countries examine issues of direct relevance to Australia.

Health Promotion Journal of Australia

This Australian refereed journal, the official journal of the Australian Association of Health Promotion Professionals, contains research and practice articles from Australian health promotion, as well as conference notices, book reviews and other material of interest to health promotion practitioners.

Social Science and Medicine

This international refereed journal contains papers that critically analyse key issues in health systems and health practice, including many of direct relevance to Primary Health Care. Its strengths include the fact that it presents a broad range of papers from both industrialised and developing countries.

Some useful internet sites

There is a wide range of valuable information of relevance for health promotion on the worldwide web. Below are some web site addresses that may be useful to people working in Primary Health Care and health promotion. This list is by no means meant to be definitive. Rather, it is intended as a starting point, to encourage you to explore the web and to get a taste of the information that can be of use to you in working to promote health. Many of the sites also have links to other useful sites, so this really is designed as a beginning only.

Health Communications Network — Australian Health

http://www.hcn.net.au/info

This site has links to over 180 Australian health-related sites, including the sites of professional associations, community groups and government bodies. With links to so many useful sites, it is a great place to start if you want to explore the range of health-related information available on the web. Many of the sites listed below are linked to this one.

National Aboriginal and Torres Strait Islander Health Clearinghouse

http://www.cowan.edu.au/clearinghouse

Australian Institute of Health and Welfare

http://www.aihw.gov.au

Australian Institute of Health and Welfare

http://www.aihw.gov.au

The Australian Institute of Health and Welfare site provides a wide range of information on the AIHW, its publications, major health-and-welfare-related conferences and workshops. In addition, it contains an 'Infobytes' section, which provides commonly requested health and welfare statistics, and links to a number of related organisations.

National Aboriginal and Torres Strait Islander Health Clearinghouse

http://www.cowan.edu.au/clearinghouse

The National Aboriginal and Torres Strait Islander Health Clearinghouse brings together a wide range of information on indigenous health issues. It contains a bibliographical database, with information on Aboriginal and Torres Strait Islander health publications and unpublished material from 1988, a discussion group for those wishing to debate issues related to indigenous health, and an online publication, the *Aboriginal and Torres Strait Islander Health Bulletin*. Links are provided to related internet sites, as well as to relevant documents and journals.

Public Health Association of Australia

http://www.pha.org.au

The site of this professional association includes information about Public Health Association conferences and campaigns, and information about the Association's journal *(Australian and New Zealand Journal of Public Health)* and newsletter. It also contains specific information for members only.

Consumers Health Forum of Australia

http://www.chf.org.au

The Consumers Health Forum site provides all the necessary information about the Consumers Health Forum, its publications, deatils of membership etc. In addition, it includes links to a range of health-related and health consumer-related sites.

Commonwealth Department of Health and Aged Care

http://www.health.gov.au

The Commonwealth health site provides a range of information about the Department, including current campaigns and provides a search engine with which to explore the material here. Linked in to this page are other strategy sites (for example, the National Mental Health Strategy home page at www.health.gov.au/hsdd/mentalhe). Of note also is a link to Health Insite (www.healthinsite.gov.au), a new site which will provide a wide range of health information about Australia.

Queensland Department of Health

http://www.health.qld.gov.au/

Health Department of Western Australia

http://www.health.wa.gov.au

Victorian Department of Human Services

http://www.vichealth.vic.gov.au/

Department of Health and Human Services Tasmania

http://www.dchs.tas.gov.au

South Australian Department of Human Services

http://www.health.sa.gov.au

New South Wales Department of Health

http://www.health.nsw.gov.au

Australian Capital Territory

http://www.health.act.gov.au

Territory Health Services (NT)

http://www.nt.gov.au/nths

These web sites of the various State and Territory health departments around Australia contain a wide range of information of direct relevance to each state and territory, including local priorities, policies and other publications. Many of them also have links to other useful sites.

Prometheus Information

http://www.prometheus.com.au

This site provides access to HealthWIZ, the computer-based database containing a wide range of health information (see pp. 93–4 of this book), HEAPS (a health promotion database; see pages 247–8) and the Social Health Atlas. The site has a range of links to other useful health-related sites.

World Health Organization

http://www.who.ch

This site provides all the latest information about aspects of the World Health Organization's work, including its policies, the work of the various Collaborating Centres (some of which focus on health promotion, injury prevention and Primary Health Care, for example) and health topics of current interest.

Amnesty International Australia

http://www.amnesty.org.au

The Amnesty International site provides access to much material of relevance to those wishing to learn more about Amnesty's work or become more actively involved. It contains the latest information on current and urgent human rights issues.

Community Aid Abroad

http://www.caa.org.au

The site of Community Aid Abroad includes news of current issues and details of ongoing campaigns. It also includes material on ethical business, and provides a range of suggestions on how individuals may become involved in Community Aid Abroad activites.

INDEX

TO THE OWNER OF THIS BOOK

We are interested in your reaction to *Promoting Health*, 2nd edition by Andrea Wass.

1. What was your reason for using this book?

    _____ university course

    _____ college course

    _____ TAFE course

    _____ continuing education course

    _____ personal interest

    _____ other (please specify)

2. In which school are you enrolled? _____

3. Approximately how much of the book did you use?

    _____ ¼   _____ ½   _____ ¾   _____ all

4. What is the best aspect of the book?

5. Have you any suggestions for improvement?

6. Would more diagrams/ illustrations help?

7. Is there any topic that should be added?

Fold here
- -

(Tape shut)

Reply Paid 5
The Marketing Coordinator, College Division
Harcourt Australia Pty Limited
Locked Bag 16
ST PETERS 2044